Echocardiographic Evaluation of Patients with Implanted Devices

Despina-Manuela Toader

Echocardiographic Evaluation of Patients with Implanted Devices

Springer

Despina-Manuela Toader
EuroEchoLab Craiova Cardiology Center
Emergency Hospital Craiova Romania
Craiova, Romania

ISBN 978-3-031-64078-0 ISBN 978-3-031-64079-7 (eBook)
https://doi.org/10.1007/978-3-031-64079-7

This Springer imprint is published by the registered company Springer Nature Switzerland AG
The registered company address is: Gewerbestrasse 11, 6330 Cham, Switzerland

Contents

General Description of Types and Modes of Pacing

1

Abstract

There are currently many categories of cardiac device carriers: patients with pacemakers, cardiac resynchronization therapy, and implanted cardio defibrillators. In the last years, His bundle pacing has been widely used because it provides a physiological simultaneous electrical activation of both ventricles. Echocardiographic evaluation of these patients has some particularities linked to the presence of intracardiac leads.

1. **Endocardial Pacing**

An endocardial pacemaker is a pulse generator placed in the pectoral region and transvenous leads implanted into the myocardium that senses cardiac activity and produces cardiac stimulation.

There are two categories of pacing: two-chamber stimulation, with a lead in the right atrium (RA), and another in the right ventricle (RV) (Fig. 1.1, supplementary material 1), and single-chamber stimulation, with a single lead in the RV (Burri et al. 2021) (Fig. 1.2, supplementary material 2).

2. **Cardiac Resynchronization Therapy (CRT)**

CRT or biventricular pacing consists of transvenous positioning of the RA and RV pacing leads, and a left ventricle (LV) epicardial lead in a branch of the coronary sinus, to correct mechanical dyssynchrony (Glikson et al. 2021) (Fig. 1.3, supplementary material 3). CRT is followed by coordinated myocardial contraction and relaxation, increasing cardiac performance, determined by the pattern of electrical activation correction (Kydd et al. 2012). CRT has shown a significant decrease in morbidity and mortality in patients with reduced left ventricular ejection fraction (LVEF) (Tang et al. 2010; Ponikowski et al. 2016).

3. Patients with **Implanted Cardiac Defibrillator (ICD)** for sudden cardiac death prevention (Fig. 1.4, supplementary material 4)

4. **Conduction System Pacing**

His bundle pacing (HBP) provides a physiological simultaneous electrical activation of the ventricles via the His Purkinje system. HBP may restore conduction in patients with high-degree AVB and shorten QRS duration in patients with left bundle branch block (LBBB) or right bundle branch block (RBBB) (Verma and Knight 2019; Ali et al. 2018). Studies evaluating the advantage of HBP over CRT or RV pacing are

Supplementary Information The online version contains supplementary material available at https://doi.org/10.1007/978-3-031-64079-7_1.

D.-M. Toader, *Echocardiographic Evaluation of Patients with Implanted Devices*,
https://doi.org/10.1007/978-3-031-64079-7_1

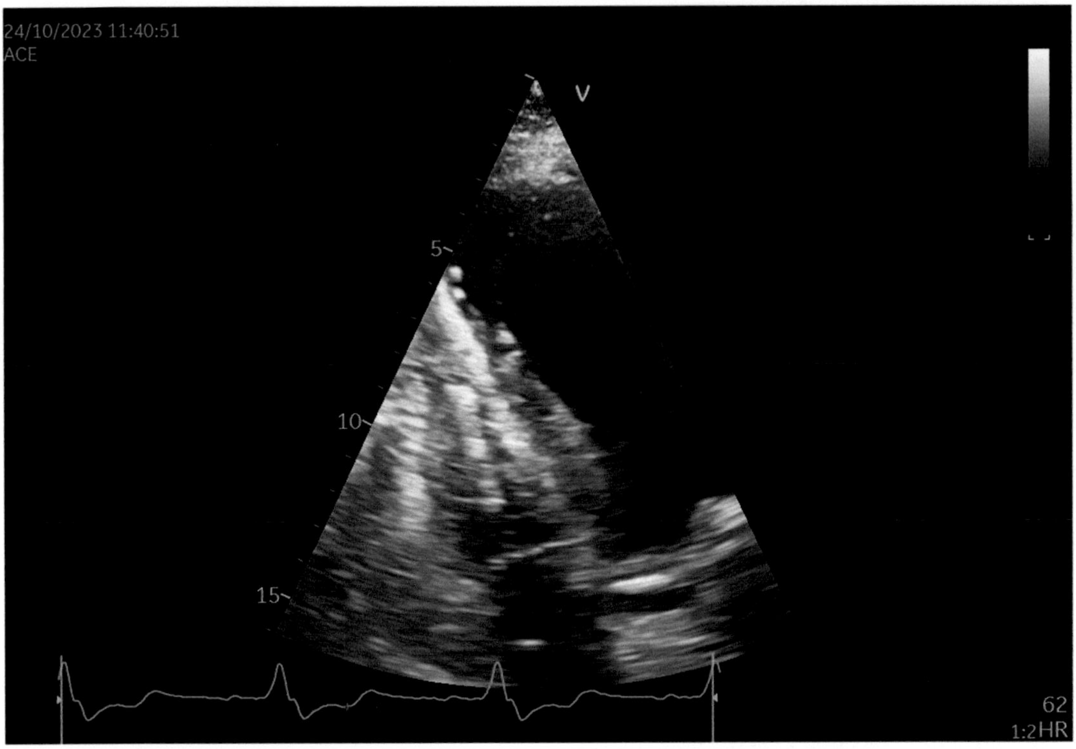

Fig. 1.1 Two chamber stimulation, with two leads, one in the RA and one in the RV

ongoing (Tang et al. 2010) (Fig. 1.5, supplementary material 5).

The patients with intracardiac devices have echocardiographic particularities linked to the lead presence.

Evaluation of the patients with **pacemakers** is linked to the RV position at the RV apex or RV septum (Liu et al. 2008; Hussain et al. 2015; Shimony et al. 2012; Merchant et al. 2017; Kaye et al. 2018). In this case, mid-term, and long-term follow-up consist in

– Lead position evaluation
– LV systolic function and LV volume measurement
– LV diastolic function evaluation
– RV morphology and function measurement
– Mitral regurgitation (MR), tricuspid regurgitation (TR), and pulmonary artery systolic pressure (PASP) reevaluation and comparison with the aspect before implantation
– The presence of dyssynchrony signs, linked to the RV electrode or is a de novo LVBB (Kiehl et al. 2016; Dreger et al. 2012; Kaye et al. 2018).
– Criteria for upgrading to CRT according to the last guidelines
– Complications identification, due to the lead presence: pericardial effusion, endocarditis pacemaker-induced cardiomyopathy (PICM) or linked to baseline cardiac disease.

Evaluation of the patients with **CRT**.

Clinical trials and guidelines recommend CRT in symptomatic heart failure patients with reduced ejection fraction (HFrEF) and wide QRS. CRT acutely decreases LV dyssynchrony, and increases LV contractility and LV stroke volume. In the long term, LV volumes decrease and LVEF increases, a phenomenon known as LV reverse remodeling (Yancy et al. 2017). CRT also produces left atrial (LA) reverse

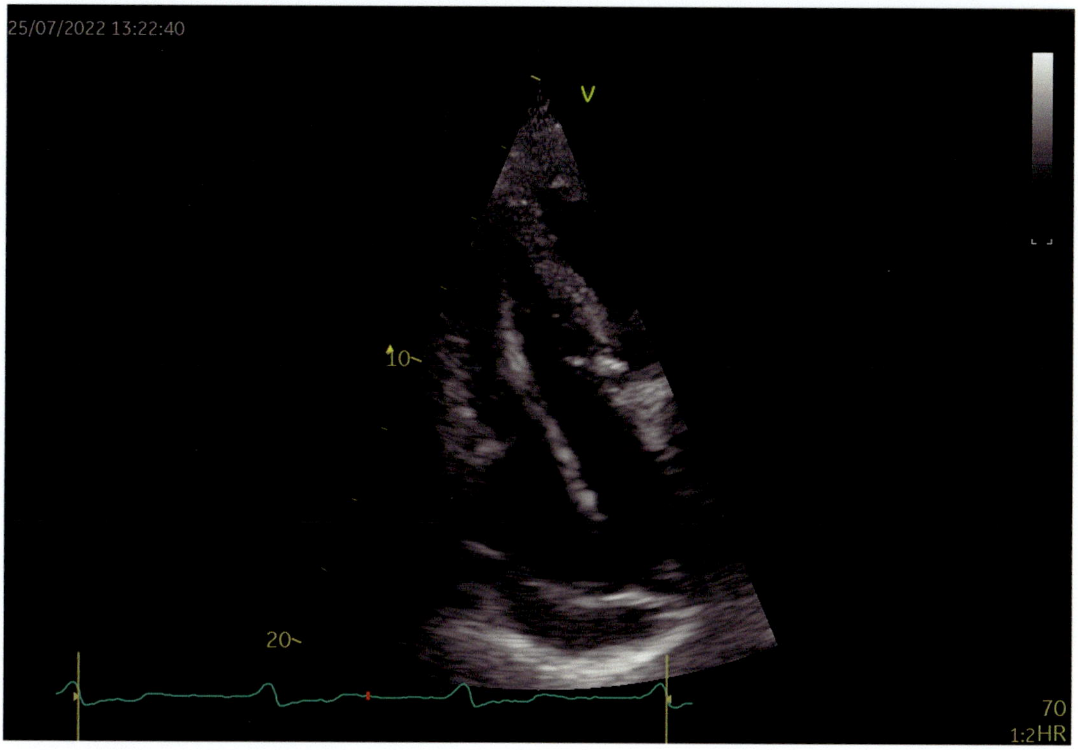

Fig. 1.2 A single chamber stimulation with a single lead in the RV

remodeling, LV diastolic function improvement, decreasing LV diastolic pressures and LA pressure, and a decrease in the severity of MR. All these anatomical and functional improvements are linked to the RV systolic function amelioration (Yancy et al. 2017).

Echocardiographic and Doppler imaging techniques have an essential role in the care of the patient with CRT (Gorcsan et al. 2008). Echocardiography evaluates the LVEF, but it also provides several additional parameters that may be used to predict the CRT response, assess prognosis, and guide the implant by identifying the optimal pacing site, optimizing the device, following up the implanted patients, and diagnose the complications (Mele et al. 2017).

Besides the fact that only ECG criteria are accepted by the guidelines as CRT implantation, the research identified some characteristics that must be provided by echocardiography before and after the implantation.

1. Before CRT: baseline mechanical dyssynchrony—area with the last activation and areas of scar identification. The lead implantation accordingly with this feature is one of the strongly linked to CRT response determination in some studies (Ypenburg et al. 2008; Bleeker et al. 2006; Becker et al. 2011).
2. After the implant: optimization of the device—the RV pacing site and optimization of the intervals—atrioventricular activation (AV) delay, and the interventricular (VV) delay. Optimization of the AV and intraventricular delays have been shown in some studies to provide additional benefits, improving mechanical dyssynchrony and LV performance (Glikson et al. 2021)—CRT response evaluation according to the parameters used in clinical trials: LVEF, end-systolic volume (ESV), and dyssynchrony—follow up in the short-term (3 months), mid-term (6 months), and long-term (after one year). LV

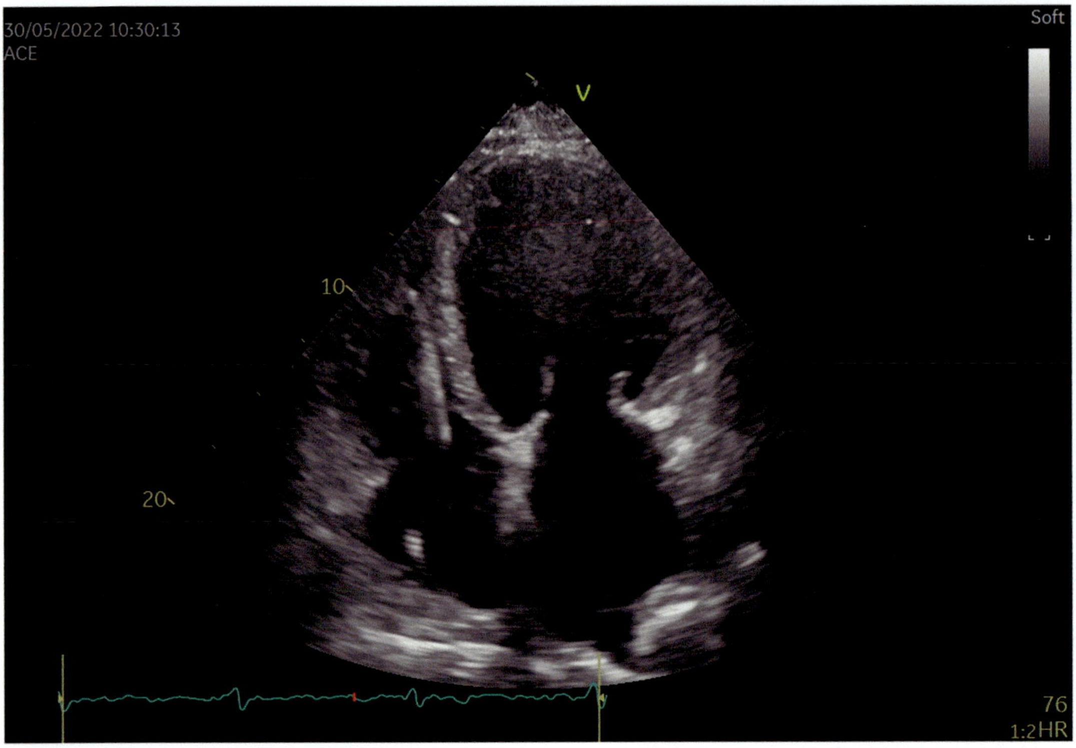

Fig. 1.3 CRT 3 leads: one in the right atrium, one in the right ventricular, and an LV epicardial lead in a branch of the coronary sinus

systolic and diastolic function evaluation, MR and TR reevaluation, RV morphology and function, PASP measurement (Ypenburg et al. 2009; Ichibori et al. 2017).

- Complications linked to the leads presence or baseline cardiac disease.
- Echocardiographic evaluation of the patients with implanted **ICD:**
- If the patient has an ICD with pacemaker function, evaluation must be performed as in patients with pacemakers.
- It is important to underlie the importance of TR and right heart evaluation, taking into consideration of the higher dimension of the ICD lead.

This book aims to indicate how to use appropriate echocardiography in patients with implanted devices.

Conclusions

Echocardiographic and Doppler imaging techniques are essential in patient care with intracardiac devices. These patients have echocardiographic particularities linked to the number and position of intracardiac leads. Consequently, the evaluation must provide data regarding the cardiac chamber's dimensions and function and about complications.

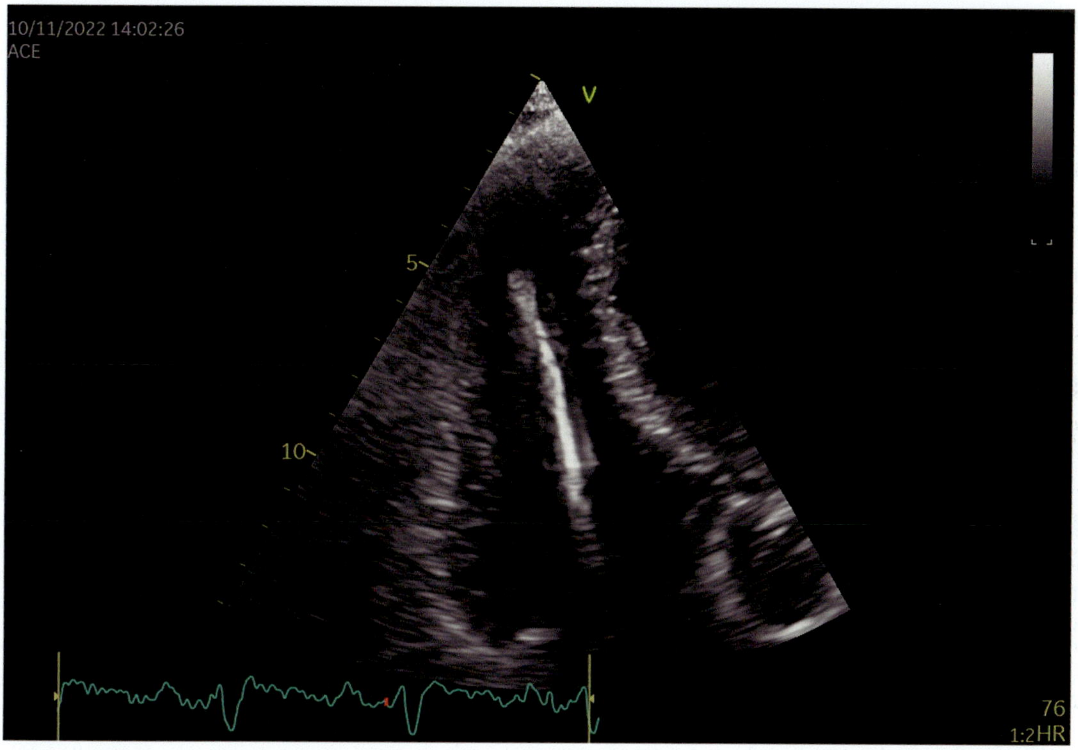

Fig. 1.4 ICD

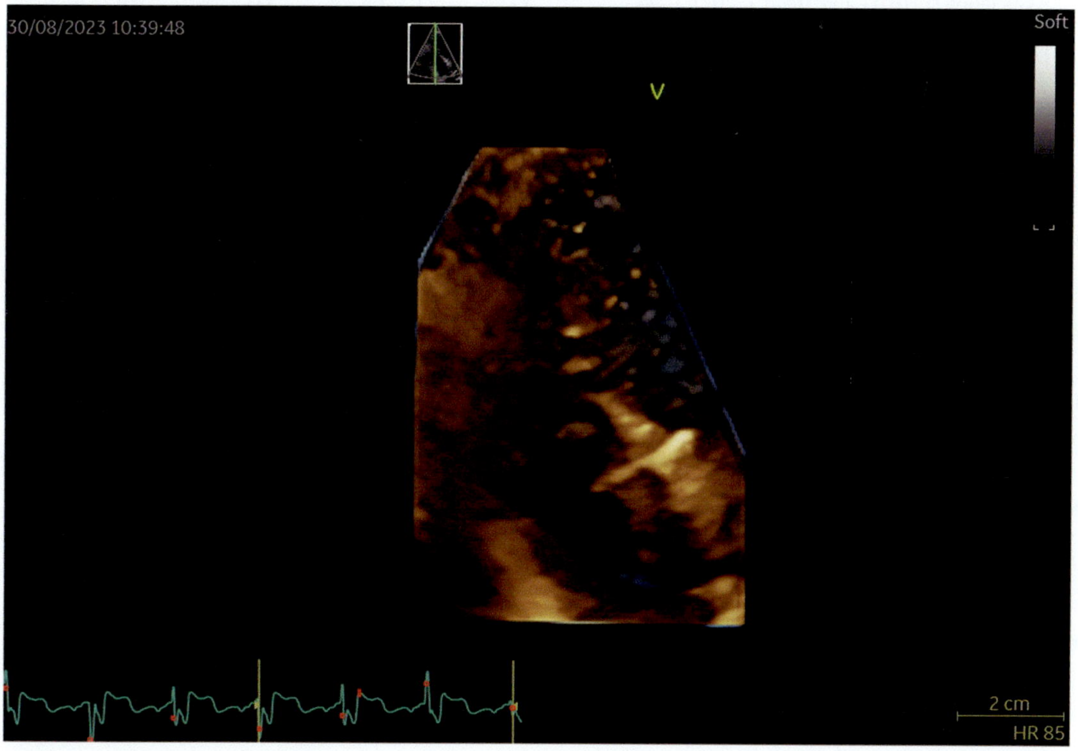

Fig. 1.5 Conduction system pacing

References

Ali N, Keene D, Arnold A, et al. His bundle pacing: a new frontier in the treatment of Heart failure. Arrhythm Electrophysiol Rev. 2018;7:103–10.

Becker M, Zwicker C, Kaminski M, et al. Dependency of cardiac resynchronization therapy on myocardial viability at the LV lead position. JACC Cardiovasc Imaging. 2011;4:366–74.

Bleeker GB, Kaandorp TA, Lamb HJ, et al. Effect of posterolateral scar tissue on clinical and echocardiographic improvement after cardiac resynchronization therapy. Circulation. 2006;113:969–76.

Burri H, Starck C, Auricchio A, et al. EHRA expert consensus statement and practical guide on optimal implantation technique for conventional pacemakers and implantable cardioverter-defibrillators: endorsed by the Heart Rhythm Society (HRS), the Asia Pacific Heart Rhythm Society (APHRS), and the Latin-American Heart Rhythm Society (LAHRS). Europace. 2021;23:983–1008.

Dreger H, Maethner K, Bondke H, Baumann G, Melzer C. Pacing induced cardiomyopathy in patients with right ventricular stimulation for >15 years. Europace. 2012;14(2):238–42.

Glikson M, Nielsen JC, Kronborg MB, et al. 2021 ESC Guidelines on cardiac pacing and cardiac resynchronization therapy developed by the task force on cardiac pacing and cardiac resynchronization therapy of the European Society of Cardiology (ESC) with the special contribution of the European Heart Rhythm Association (EHRA). Eur Heart J. 2021;1–94.

Gorcsan J III, Abraham T, Agler DA, Bax JJ, Derumeaux G, et al. ASE expert consensus statement echocardiography for cardiac resynchronization therapy: recommendations for performance and reporting—a report from the American Society of Echocardiography Dyssynchrony Writing Group Endorsed by the Heart Rhythm Society. J Am Soc Echocardiogr. 2008;21(3):191–213.

Hussain MA, Furuya-Kanamori L, Kaye G, Clark J, Doi SA. The effect of right ventricular apical and non-apical pacing on the shortand long-term changes in left ventricular ejection fraction: a systematic review and meta-analysis of randomized-controlled trials. Pacing Clin Electrophysiol. 2015;38(9):1121–1136.

Ichibori H, Fukuzawa K, Kiuchi FHRS. Predictors and clinical outcomes of transient responders to cardiac resynchronization therapy. Paced Clin Electrophysiol. 2017;40(3):301–309.

Kaye GC, Linker NJ, Marwick TH, et al. Effect of right ventricular pacing lead site on left ventricular function in patients with highgrade atrioventricular block: results of the Protect-Pace study. Eur Heart J. 2015;3614):856–862.

Kaye G, Ng JY, Ahmed S, Valencia D, Harrop D, Ng ACT. The Prevalence of Pacing-Induced Cardiomyopathy (PICM) in patients with long-term right ventricular pacing—is it a matter of definition? Heart Lung Circ. 2018;27pii: S1443–9506(18)30726-1.

Kiehl EL, Makki T, Kumar R, et al. Incidence and predictors of right ventricular pacing-induced cardiomyopathy in patients with complete atrioventricular block and preserved left ventricular systolic function. Heart Rhythm. 2016;13(12):2272–8.

Kydd AC, McCormick LM, Dutka DP. Optimizing benefit from CRT: role of speckle tracking echocardiography, the importance of LV lead position and scar. Expert Rev Med Devices. 2012;9(5):521–36.

Liu WH, Chen MC, Chen YL, et al. Right ventricular apical pacing acutely impairs left ventricular function and induces mechanical dyssynchrony in patients with sick sinus syndrome: a real-time three-dimensional echocardiographic study. J Am Soc Echocardiogr. 2008;21(3):224–9.

Mele D, Bertini M, Malagù M. Current role of echocardiography in cardiac resynchronization therapy. Heart Fail Rev. 2017;22:699–722.

Merchant FM, Hoskins MH, Musat DL, et al. Incidence and time course for developing heart failure with high-burden right ventricular pacing. Circ Cardiovasc Qual Outcomes. 2017;10(6):pii: e003564

Ponikowski P, Voors AA, Anker SD, et al. 2016 ESC Guidelines for the diagnosis and treatment of acute and chronic heart failure: the task force for the diagnosis and treatment of acute and chronic heart failure of the European Society of Cardiology (ESC) developed with the special contribution of the Heart Failure Association (HFA) of the ESC. Eur Heart J. 2016;37:2129–200.

Shimony A, Eisenberg MJ, Filion KB, Amit G. Beneficial effects of right ventricular non-apical vs. apical pacing: a systematic review and meta-analysis of randomized-controlled trials. Europace. 2012;14:81–91.

Tang AS, Wells GA, Talajic M, et al. Cardiac-resynchronization therapy for mild-to-moderate heart failure. N Engl J Med. 2010;363:2385–95.

Verma N, Knight BP. Update in cardiac pacing. Arrhythm Electrophysiol Rev. 2019;8:228–33.

Yancy CW, Jessup M, Bozkurt B, et al. 2017 ACC/AHA/HFSA focused update of the 2013 ACCF/AHA guideline for the management of heart failure: a report of the American College of Cardiology/American Heart Association task force on clinical practice guidelines and the Heart Failure Society of America. Circulation. 2017;136:e137–61.

Ypenburg C, van Bommel RJ, Delgado V, et al. Optimal left ventricular lead position predicts reverse remodeling and survival after cardiac resynchronization therapy. J Am Coll Cardiol. 2008;52(17):1402–9.

Ypenburg C, van Bommel RJ, Borleffs CJ, et al. Long-term prognosis after cardiac resynchronization therapy is related to the extent of left ventricular reverse remodeling at midterm follow-up. J Am Coll Cardiol. 2009;53:483–90.

Left Ventricle Systolic Function Evaluation in Patients with Implanted Devices

2

Abstract

Echocardiography is the most common method of examination of cardiac patients. Left ventricle dimension and function evaluation is a cornerstone in patients with implanted devices. The measurement includes classical parameters and variables from advanced techniques such as three-dimensional echocardiography and two and three-speckle tracking echocardiography. Wall motion abnormalities also need special attention, according to implanted devices.

2.1 Evaluation of Classical Parameters of Systolic Function in Patients with Implanted Devices

Quantitative assessment of left ventricle (LV) size and function is essential for the diagnosis, treatment, and prognosis of heart diseases in any patient (Lang et al. 2015).

Two-dimensional (2D) echocardiography has an established role in LV function assessment. The limitations are foreshortening, malrotation, and angulation; therefore, the measurements may be inaccurate (Lang et al. 2012).

The most used parameters to describe LV cavity size are linear internal dimensions and volumes. Measurements are commonly reported for end-diastole and end-systole and should be reported indexed to body surface area (BSA). Linear measurements are representative only in normally shaped ventricles and should be avoided in heart failure (HF) patients with dilated cardiomyopathy (DCM) and cardiac resynchronization therapy (CRT) (Lang et al. 2015).

2.2 LV Volumes Measurement

According to the guideline's recommendations for chamber quantification, LV size should be assessed by calculating volumes using the biplane method of disks summation technique (modified Simpson's rule) (Lang et al. 2015). Acquisition will be obtained from the apical 4- and 2-chamber views, focused on the LV (Fig. 2.1). Contrast agents for endocardial delineation improvement will be used when two or more contiguous LV segments are poorly visualized in apical views (Mulvagh et al. 2008). Volumes provided by contrast-enhanced images are closer to those obtained with cardiac magnetic resonance (CMR) (Hoffmann et al. 2006). Left ventricle end-diastolic volume (LVEDV)

Supplementary Information The online version contains supplementary material available at https://doi.org/10.1007/978-3-031-64079-7_2.

D.-M. Toader, *Echocardiographic Evaluation of Patients with Implanted Devices*, https://doi.org/10.1007/978-3-031-64079-7_2

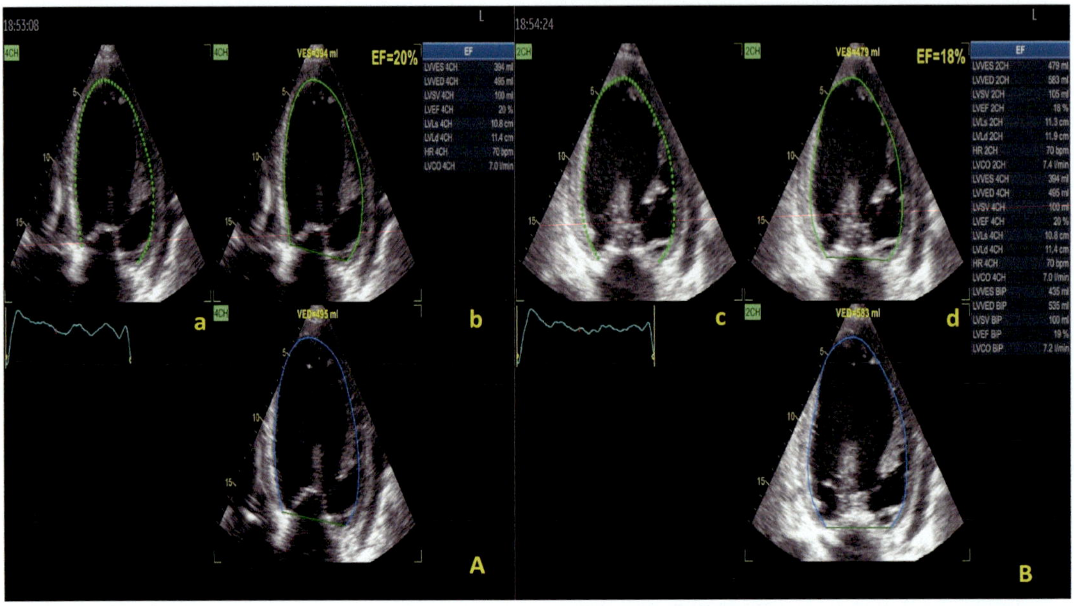

Fig. 2.1 Left ventricle volume measurement by Simpson method. Left ventricle end-diastolic volume evaluation at end-diastole—the first frame after mitral valve closure or the frame where the LV volume is largest: **Aa** in four-chamber view, **Bc** in two-chamber view. Left ventricle end-systolic volume will be evaluated at end-systole—the first frame after aortic valve closure or the frame where the LV volume is smallest. **Ab** in four-chamber view, **Bd** in two-chamber view

will be evaluated at end-diastole—the first frame after mitral valve closure or the frame where the largest LV volume is the largest (Fig. 2.1Aa, Bc). Left ventricle end-systolic volume (LVESV) will be evaluated at end-systole—the first frame after aortic valve closure or the frame where the LV volume is smallest (Lang et al. 2015) (Fig. 2.1Aa, Bd).

The guidelines also recommend:

- tracing the endocardial border at the blood pool interface, between the compacted myocardium and the cavity, using the images with clear endocardial border definition
- excluding papillary muscles from the LV cavity tracing
- maximizing LV area
- avoiding foreshortening.

At the mitral valve level, the contour is closed by connecting the two opposite sections of the mitral ring with a straight line. LV length is the distance between the middle of this line and the most and the apical point of the LV contour (Lang et al. 2015).

LV EDVs of 74 mL/m^2 for men and 61 mL/m^2 for women and LVESVs of 31 mL/m^2 for men and 24 mL/m^2 for women are the upper limits of the normal range (Lang et al. 2015).

2.3 LVEF

Ejection Fraction (EF) is the primary method for the global systolic function measurement and uses LVEDV and LVESV.

LVEF by Biplane Method of Disks (modified Simpson's rule)

$$LVEF = LVEDV - LVESV/LVEDV$$

The average value of ejection fraction is 53–73% (52–72% for men, 54–74% for women) (Lang et al. 2015; Potter 2018).

Another LV systolic function assessment parameter is **Global Longitudinal Strain (GLS**), derived from 2D speckle tracking echocardiography (2D STE). GLS represents the change in the length of cardiac fiber within a certain direction: longitudinal, circumferential, and radial planes, relative to its baseline length (Tops et al. 2017; Negishi and Negishi 2015).

Strain (%) = (Lt – Lo) / Lo o Lt is the length at time t, Lo is the length at time 0 (Potter 2018). PW of the LVOT should be used to time the aortic valve opening and closure (Fig. 2.2a). Longitudinal and circumferential shortening have a negative value (Fig. 2.2b), while radial thickening has a positive value (Fig. 2.2c, d) (Potter 2018; Negishi and Negishi 2015).

Peak global LV strain measurement involves averaging 3 standard apical views GLS values. The three, four, and two apical LV-focused views should be acquired by optimizing endocardial borders. The acquisition should be performed at a frame rate of 60–90 Hz. Heart rate variation should not vary more than five bpm. (Potter 2018).

Strain is a frame-by-frame automatic tracking of acoustic markers throughout the cardiac cycle. The operator can manually adjust the segments that failed to track correctly. After tracing the endocardial border, the time–longitudinal strain curves for the apical four-chamber (A4ch), two-chamber (A2ch), and three-chamber (A3ch) views will be obtained. The left ventricle is divided into six segments in each apical view. The final bull's eye plot will display the regional longitudinal strain value for every 17 segments, and the LV averaged GLS (Tops et al. 2017) (Fig. 2.3). Peak GLS is a negative number, and average values range from 15.9% to 22.1% (Potter and Marwick 2018). Normal values usually differ depending on the vendor or the software version, but generally, the cut-off is – 20%. A smaller absolute number represents a pathological value (Negishi and Negishi 2015) (Fig. 2.4).

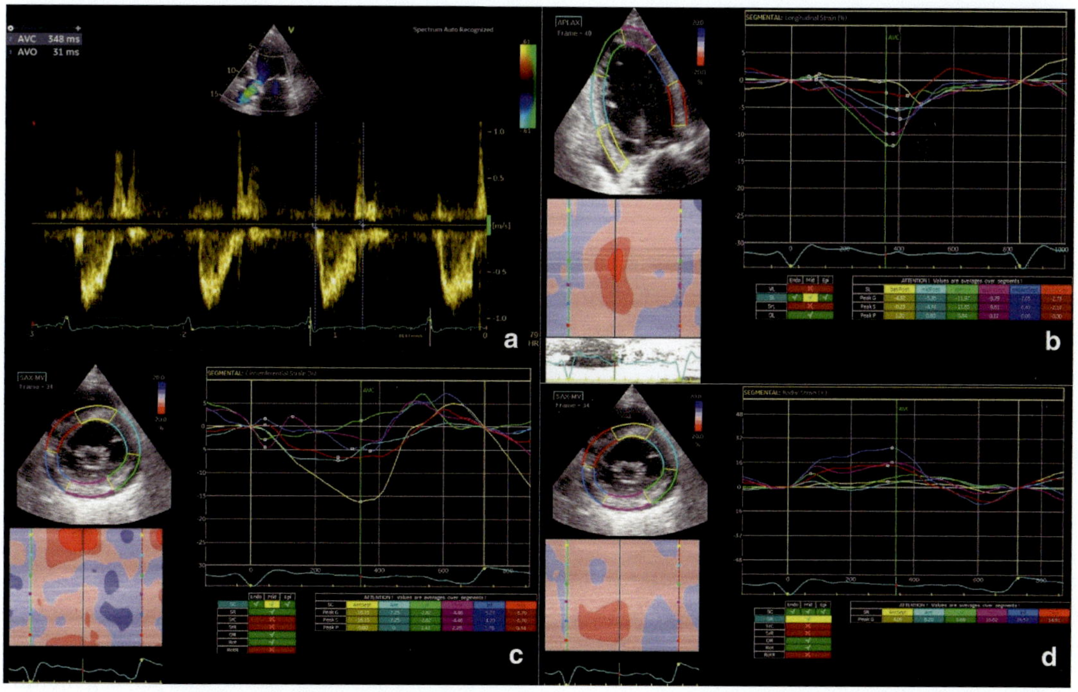

Fig. 2.2 Speckle tracking strain curves in a patient with CRT: **a** Aortic valve timing, **b** longitudinal strain curve in apical three-chamber view, **c** circumferential strain curve at the mitral valve level, **d** radial strain curve at the mitral valve level

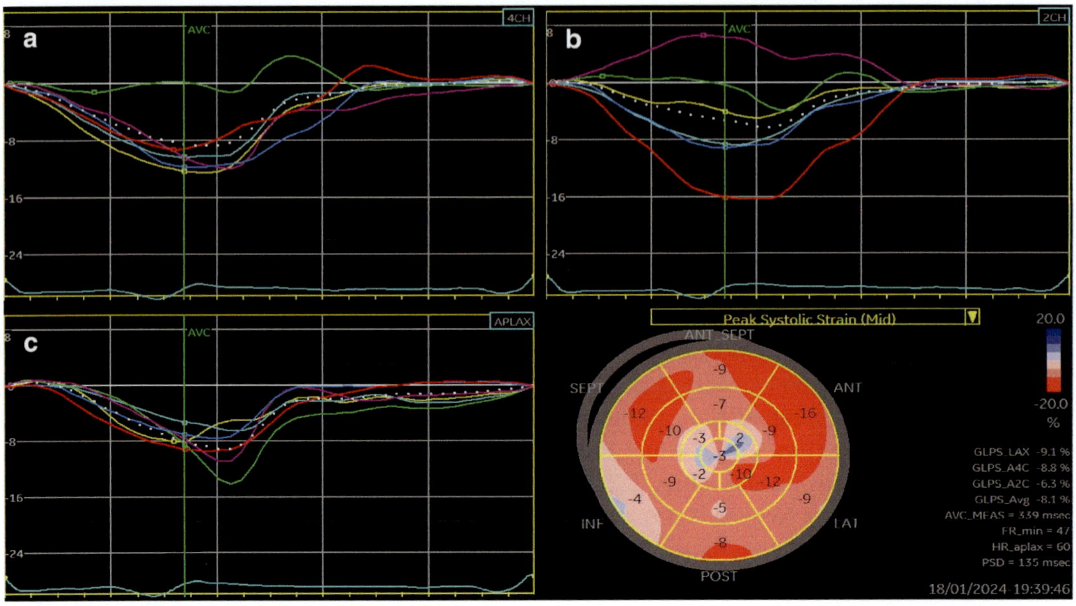

Fig. 2.3 BE display obtained after tracing the endocardial border in apical three-, four-, and two-chamber view

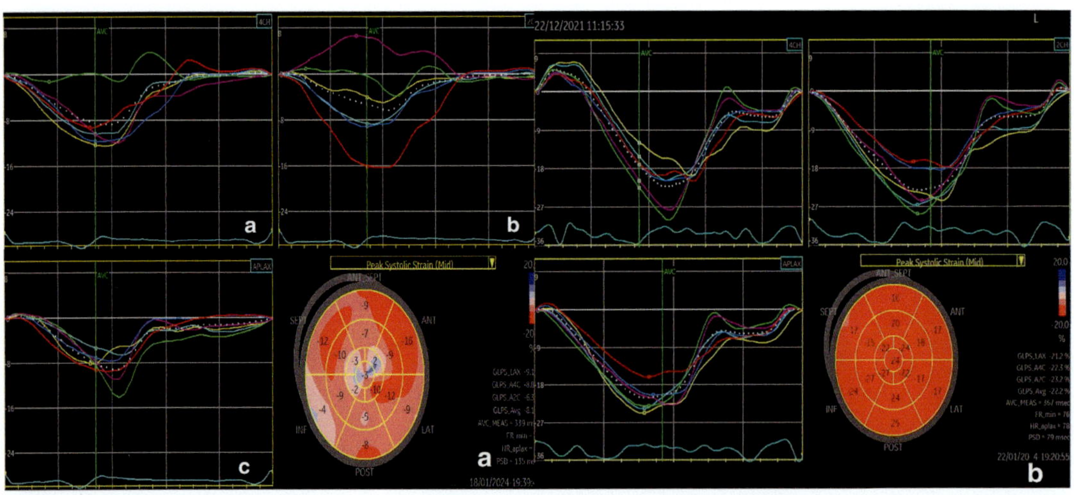

Fig. 2.4 BE in a patient with CRT vs BE in a healthy individual

The *peak strain* can be measured as peak systolic strain, peak strain at end-systole (in the moment of aortic valve closure), or peak strain during the cardiac cycle regardless of timing (Negishi and Negishi 2015).

The strain has three main components: longitudinal (LS) (motion from base to apex) (Fig. 2.5), circumferential (CS) (change in radius of the short axis, perpendicular to the radial and long axis) (Fig. 2.6) and radial (RS) (wall thickening and thinning) (Fig. 2.7). Analysis can be performed either for individual segments or the entire LV. The radial strain data have generally shown an increased variability compared with longitudinal and circumferential strain (Chan et al. 2006a; Oxborough et al. 2012) because the

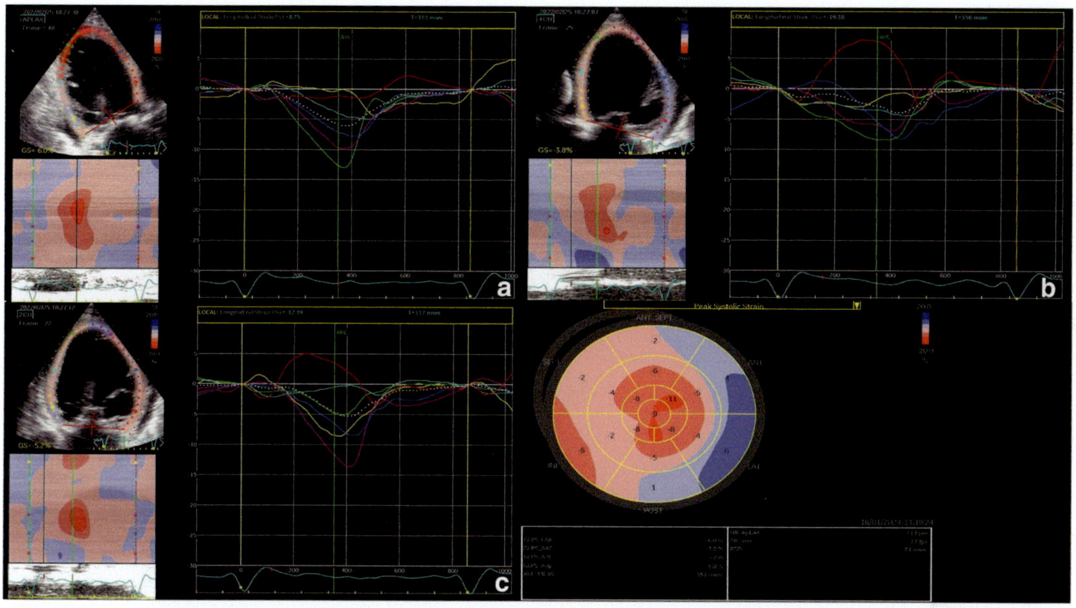

Fig. 2.5 Global longitudinal strain in **a,** apical tree-chamber view, **b** apical four-chamber view, **c** apical two-chamber view, and **d** BE display in a patient with DCM and CRT

lower lateral resolution produces lateral drop-out and out-of-plane motion of the LV basal segments (Geyer et al. 2010). Nonuniform segmental thickness of the scar area could produce variability of the region of interest during stain analysis, with variability in strain parameters (Biaggi et al. 2011). Myocardial shear strain in the circumferential longitudinal plane provides the *twist and torsion* (Geyer et al. 2010) (Fig. 2.8). LV wall strain will impair according to the involved myofiber.

The damage to the subendocardium, the most sensitive layer with longitudinally oriented fibers, will decrease the longitudinal strain (Fig. 2.9). Involvement of the mid myocardium with circumferential fiber or subepicardial layer with oblique fiber alignment results in impairment of CS (Fig. 2.10) and RS (Fig. 2.11) and twist mechanics (Fig. 2.12). Acute transmural damage or a disease affecting all three layers will damage all vectors of mechanics (Mor-Avi et al. 2011).

The *strain rate* represents the change of strain over time (Potter and Marwick 2018) (Fig. 2.13).

Systolic dyssynchrony index (SDI) is calculated by STE averaging values from A-3ch, A4ch, and A-2ch view. For each view, SDI is quantified by calculating the standard deviation of time to peak systolic strain of six segments (Fig. 2.14) (Kusumoto et al. 2018).

Myocardial work evaluates LV performance, incorporating afterload into strain measurement. The method uses cuff systolic blood pressure, providing a more load-independent measurement than GLS. Measured parameters are: myocardial work efficiency, global work index (GWI), global constructive work (GCW), global wasted work (GWW), global work efficiency (GWE).

Myocardial work efficiency = GCW/[GCW + GWW]) (Fig. 2.15) (Kusumoto et al. 2018).

Three-dimensional transthoracic echocardiographic (3DE TTE) LV assessment is more accurate than 2D echocardiography (Yoshitani et al. 2009) and includes volumes, ejection fraction, shape, and regional and global strain (Lang et al. 2012). Depending on image quality and availability, 3D LV evaluation is recommended when feasible (Lang et al. 2015). The most important contribution of 3D echocardiography is the LV quantification (Monaghan 2006). The advantage of 3D echocardiographic

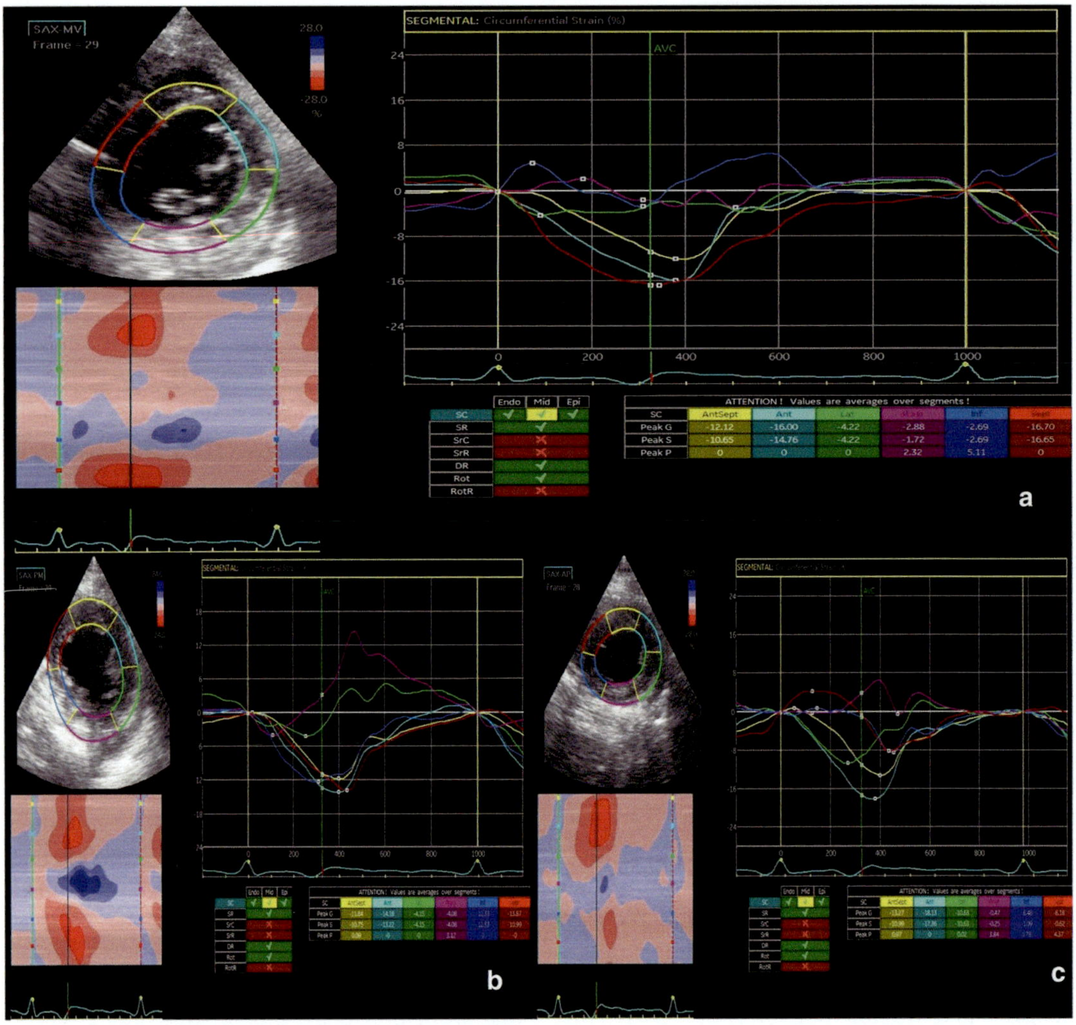

Fig. 2.6 Circumferential strain: **a** the mitral valve level, **b** papillary muscles level, **c** apical level in a patient with dilated cardiomyopathy and CRT

volume measurements is that they do not rely on geometric assumptions (Monaghan 2006). This is the method of choice in patients with good image quality (Dorosz et al. 2012).

Acquisition modes for 3D LV analyses are:

1. *"Full volume" LV-focused acquisition will allow LV volume measurement.* Multiple-beat 3D echocardiography image acquisition should include the entire left ventricle within the pyramidal data set, maximizing the temporal resolution without compromising spatial resolution. This approach will increase the accuracy of end-systole identification (Lang et al. 2012). Acquisitions of multiple narrow volumes of data over up to seven cardiac cycles, stitched together, ECG gated, will create a single volumetric data set. The breath hold will minimize the risk of stitch artifacts (Nucifora et al. 2009; Jenkins et al. 2009). The pyramidal data set should include LV, and the settings should reveal a good endocardial border. The volume/frame rate should be 15 Hz or higher (Nucifora et al. 2009; Jenkins et al. 2009).

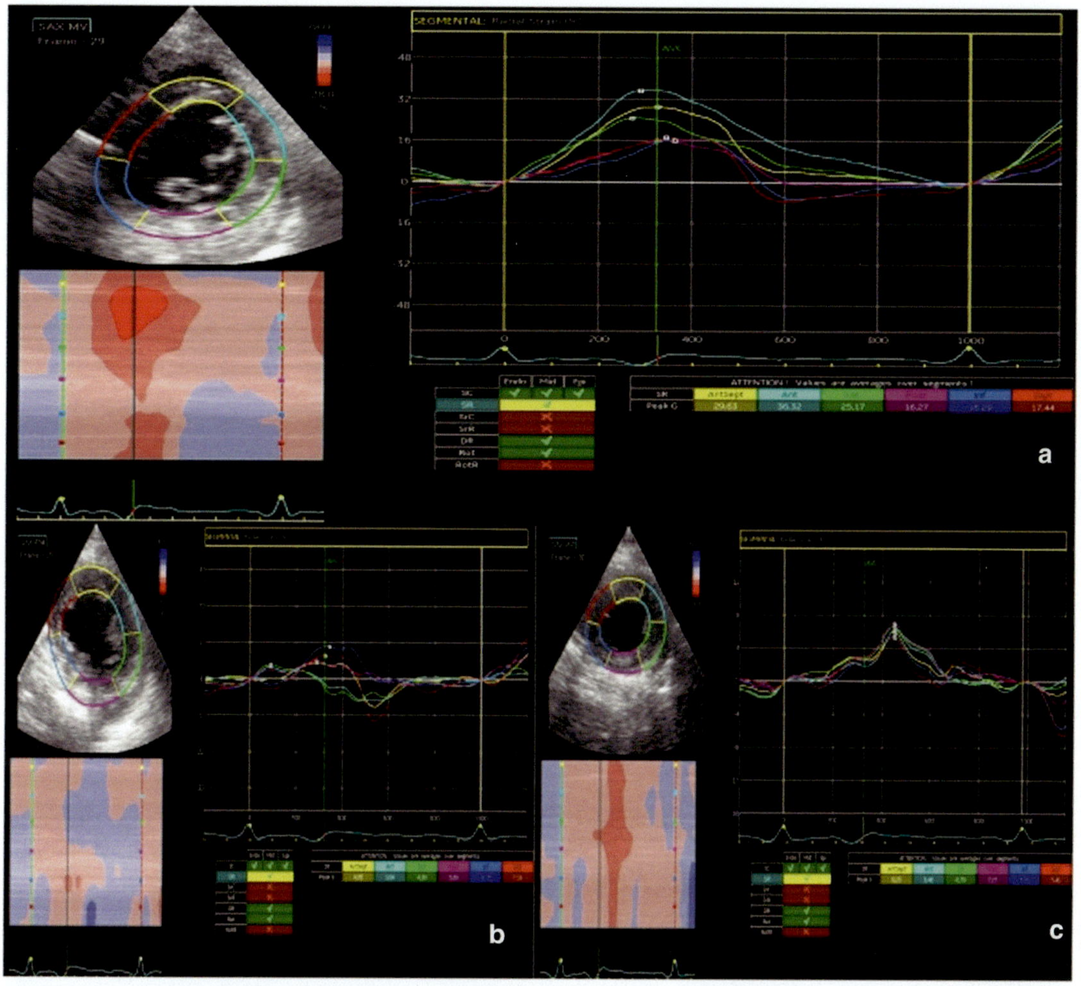

Fig. 2.7 Radial strain: **a** the mitral valve level, **b** papillary muscles level, **c** apical level in a patient with dilated cardiomyopathy and CRT

2. Simultaneous multi-plane imaging.

Display modes are:

– *Simultaneous orthogonal* two or three *orthogonal planes display:* coronal, sagittal, and transverse. This mode provides multiple visualizations of the same segment within a single cardiac cycle, useful for ventricular function analysis (Yoshitani et al. 2009) (Fig. 2.16).
– *Surface rendering* technique allows visualization of the surface of structures (Fenster et al. 2001) and the LV functional measurements: volumes, ejection fraction, and mass (Lang et al. 2012).

3D LVQ is a semiautomated quantification software used for edge detection and tracing. This algorithm allows:

– The calculation of cavity contours and evaluation of changes during the cardiac cycle, resulting in a volume-versus-time curve.
– Surface-rendered cavity cast display with volume computation.

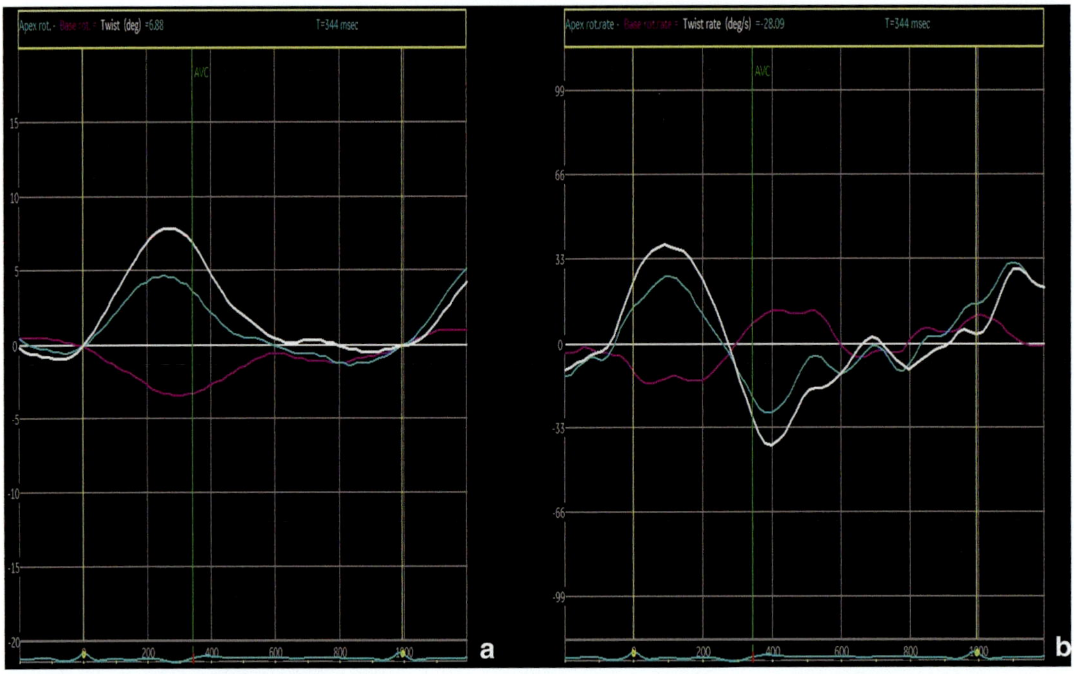

Fig. 2.8 Twist, twist rate in a patient with dilated cardiomyopathy and CRT

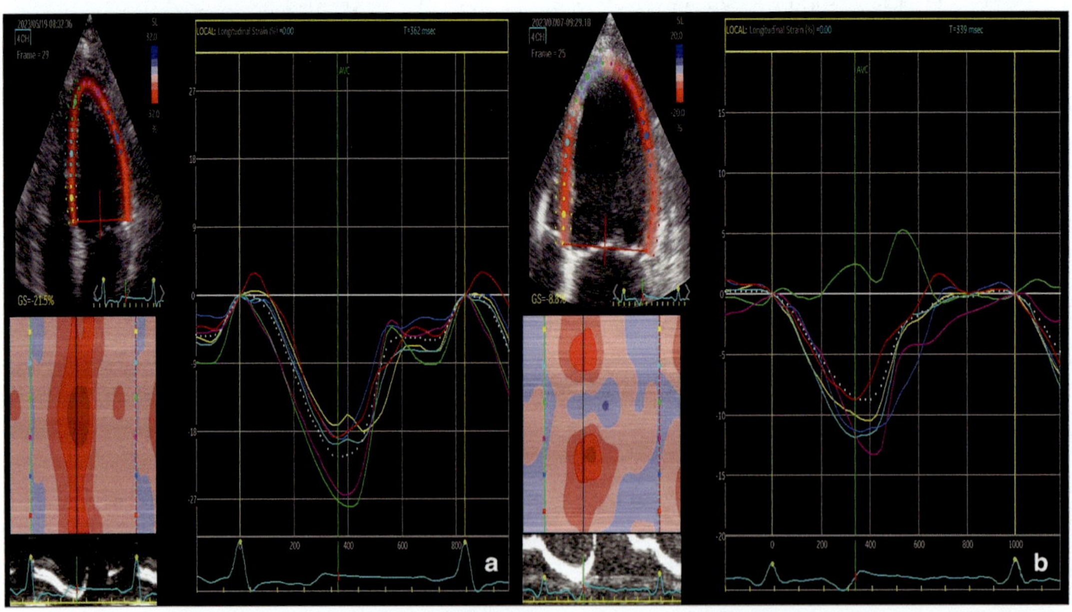

Fig. 2.9 Decrease global longitudinal strain in patient with CRT: **a** healthy volunteer, **b** a patient with dilated cardiomyopathy and CRT

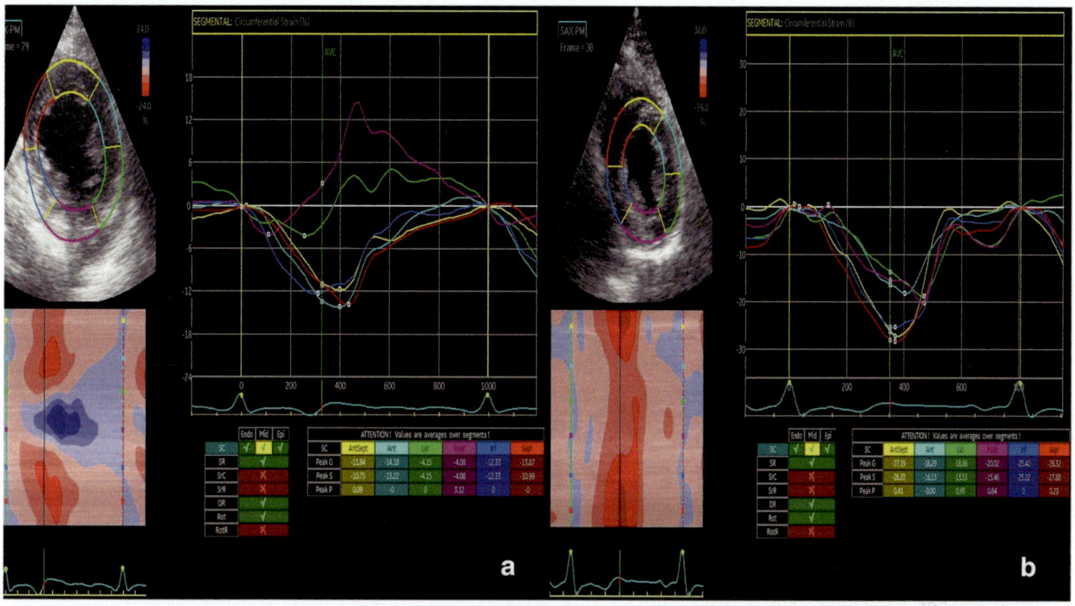

Fig. 2.10 Circumferential strain in a patient with CRT: **a** healthy volunteer, **b** a patient with dilated cardiomyopathy and CRT measured in short axis view at the level of papillary muscles by speckle tracking echocardiography

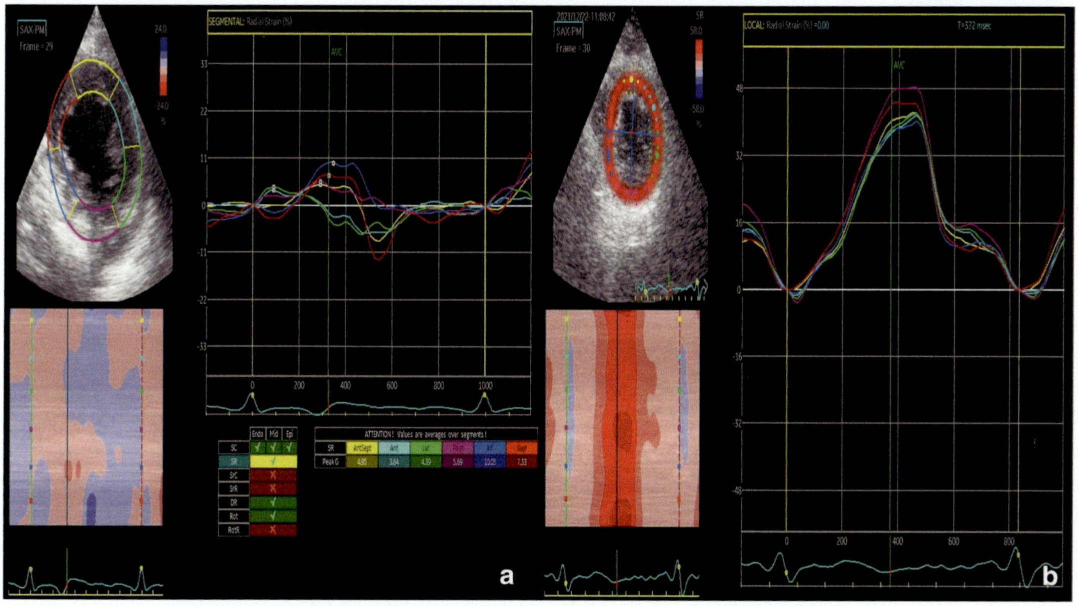

Fig. 2.11 Radial strain in a patient with CRT: **a** healthy volunteer, **b** a patient with dilated cardiomyopathy and CRT measured in short axis view at the level of papillary muscles by speckle tracking echocardiography

Wireframe models allow the definition of sections of the left ventricle in position and time, and they are used to assess LV synchrony, regional strain, curvature, and wall stress. The analysis of regional function uses a polar map display incorporating wall motion scoring or a contraction front mapping, the spatial distribution of contraction, and relaxation (Lang

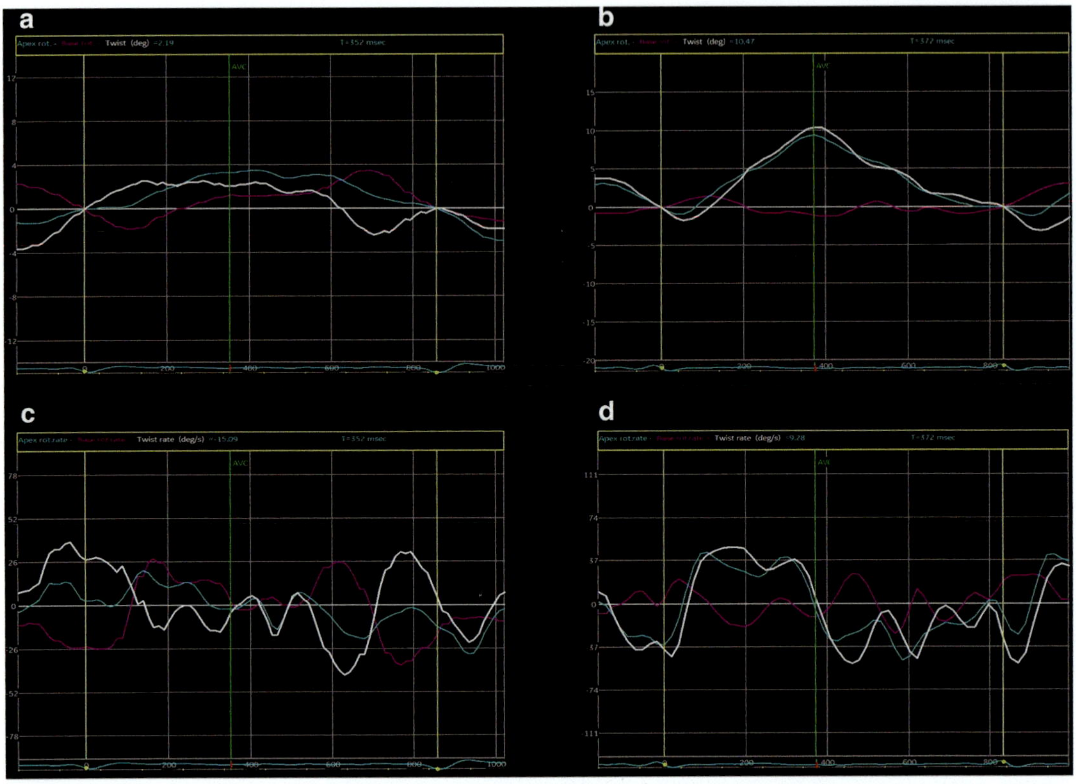

Fig. 2.12 Rotation in a patient with CRT: **a** twist, **c** torsion in a patient with CRT, **b** twist, **d** torsion in a healthy volunteer

et al. 2012). The method uses manual tracing or semiautomatic border detection algorithms to trace the endocardium in three orthogonal imaging planes generated from the 3D data set segmentation. The anatomic landmarks are the mitral annulus and apex (Muraru et al. 2010). The borders are checked in ED and ES, with manual corrections to the endocardial borders, if necessary, and approved. Finally, the volume is computed. 3DE can measure LV volume and EF without geometric assumptions (Monaghan 2006) (Fig. 2.17). Obtained contours will be combined to generate a 3D shape, visualized as a solid or a wireframe object, to create a 3D perspective (Pandian et al. 1994). Wireframe reconstruction generates 3D images of subsets of the entire data set in a cage-like picture. Combining the solid and wireframe surface-rendering techniques, we can appreciate the extent of cardiac structure motion or cardiac chamber volume changes during the cardiac cycle (Lang et al. 2012). Semiautomated contour detection by 3DE underestimates LV volumes and EF (Chan et al. 2006a, 2006b; Caiani et al. 2005; Jenkins et al. 2004; Jacobs et al. 2006; Lee et al. 2001) because echocardiography cannot accurately differentiate between the myocardium and the trabeculae (Mor-Avi et al. 2008). To minimize these differences, the guidelines recommend excluding trabeculae in the LV cavity when tracing the endocardium. LV opacification with contrast agents improve this structure identification (Nucifora et al. 2009; Jenkins et al. 2009; Muraru et al. 2010; Caiani et al. 2005; Krenning et al. 2007). 3D LV volume and EF are similar to magnetic resonance imaging (Mor-Avi et al. 2008). LV volumes and EF by 3D echocardiography have closer agreement with cardiac magnetic resonance measurements than 2D echocardiography (Muraru et al. 2010; Jenkins

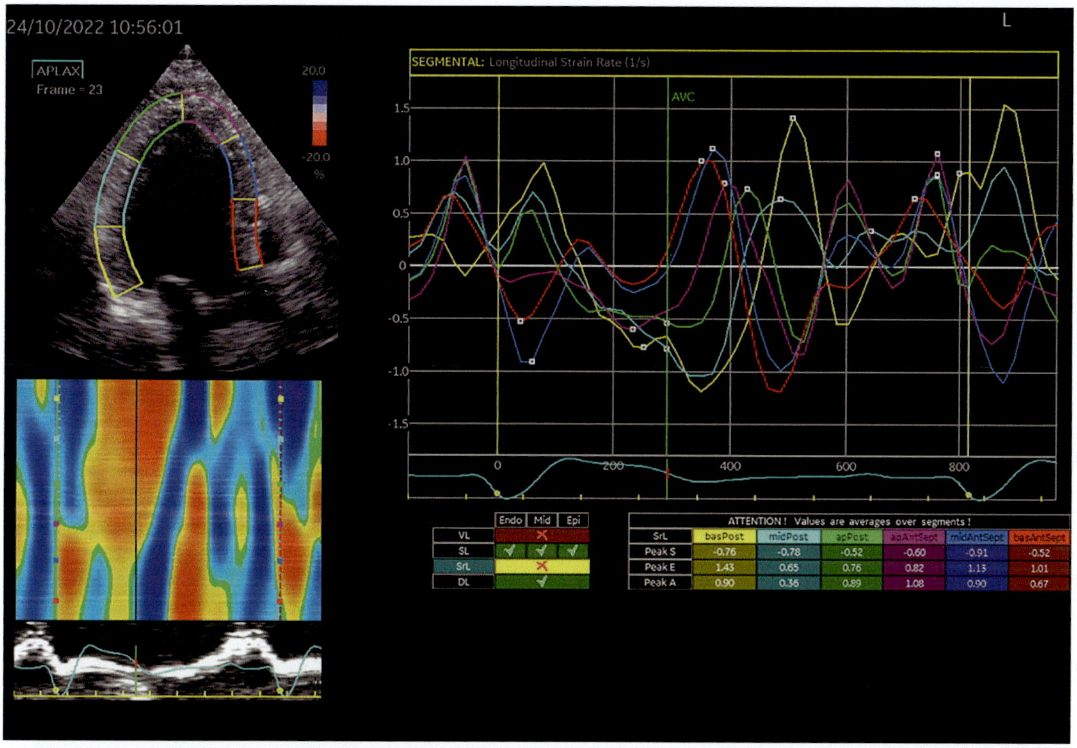

Fig. 2.13 Strain rate in a patient with dilated cardiomyopathy and CRT

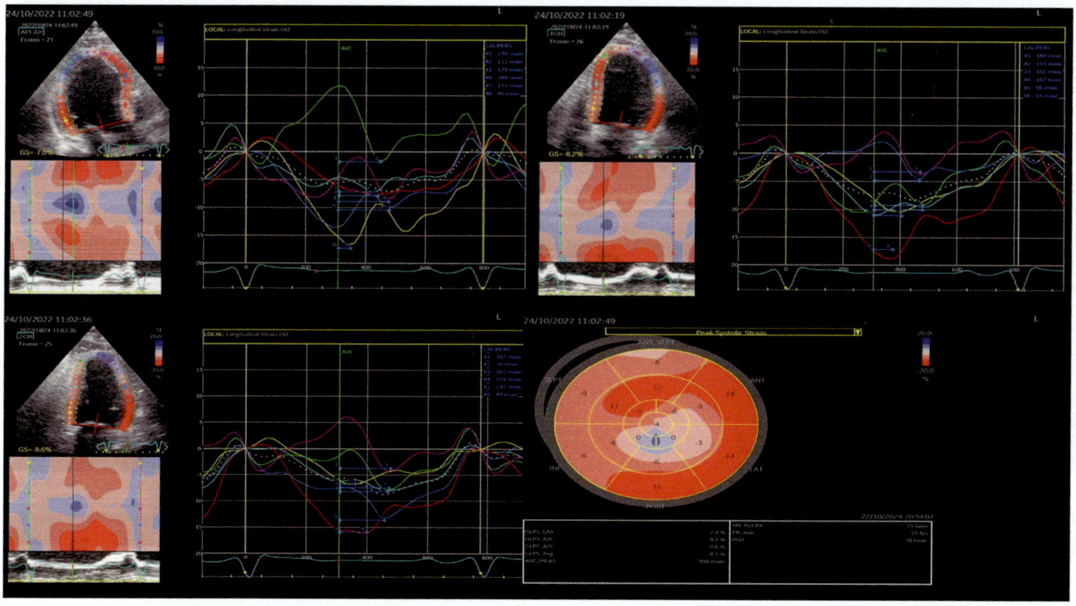

Fig. 2.14 Two-dimensional systolic dyssynchrony index calculation in a patient with dilated cardiomyopathy and CRT

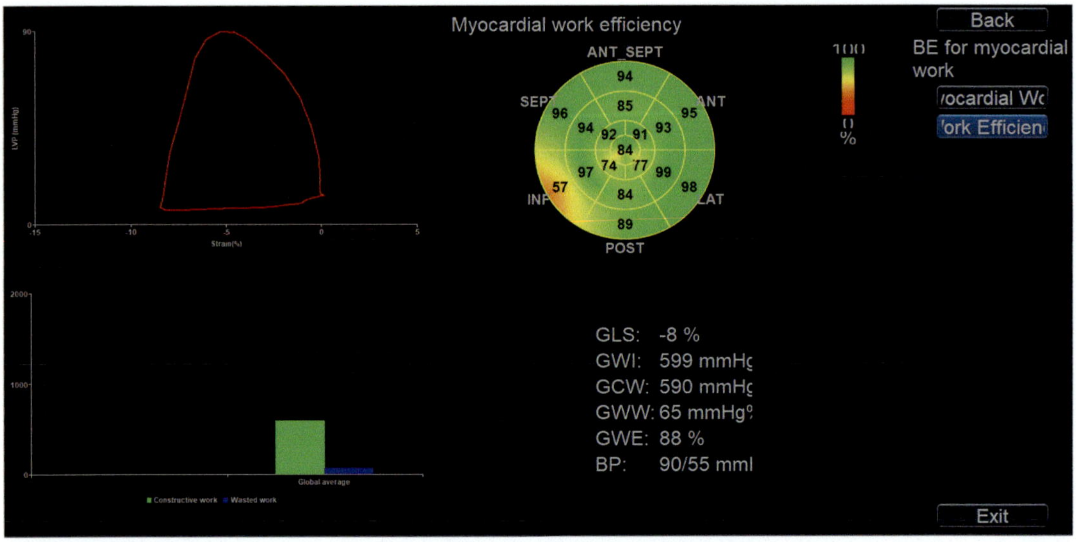

Fig. 2.15 Myocardial work efficiency calculation in a patient with dilated cardiomyopathy and CRT

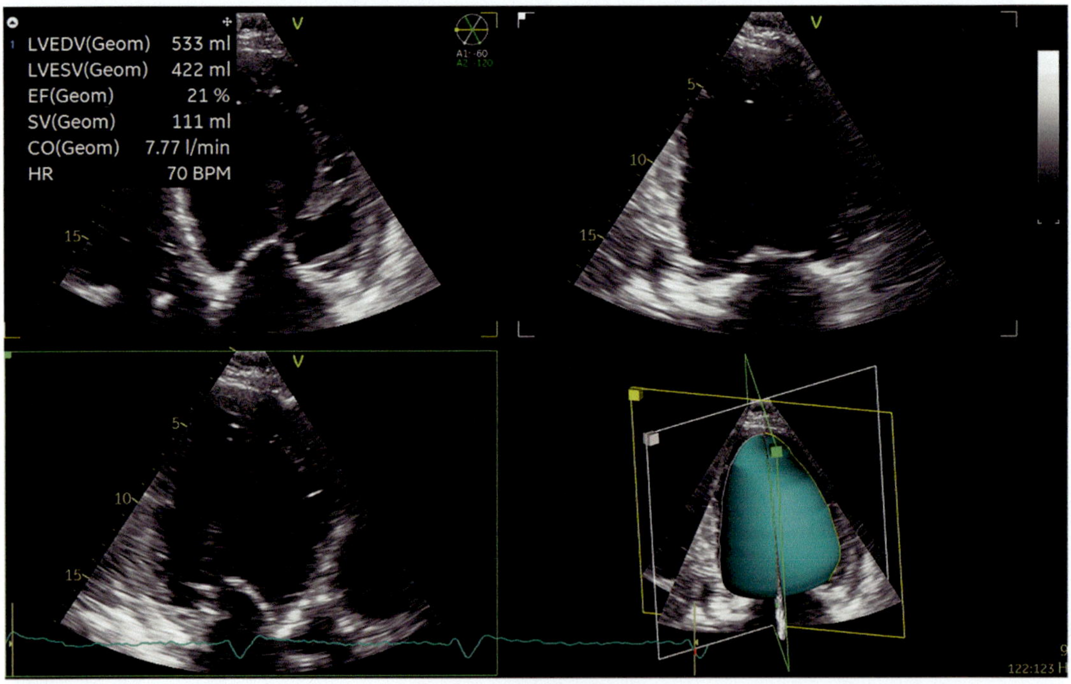

Fig. 2.16 Left ventricle ejection fraction and volumes calculation from triplane echocardiography acquisition in a patient with dilated cardiomyopathy and CRT

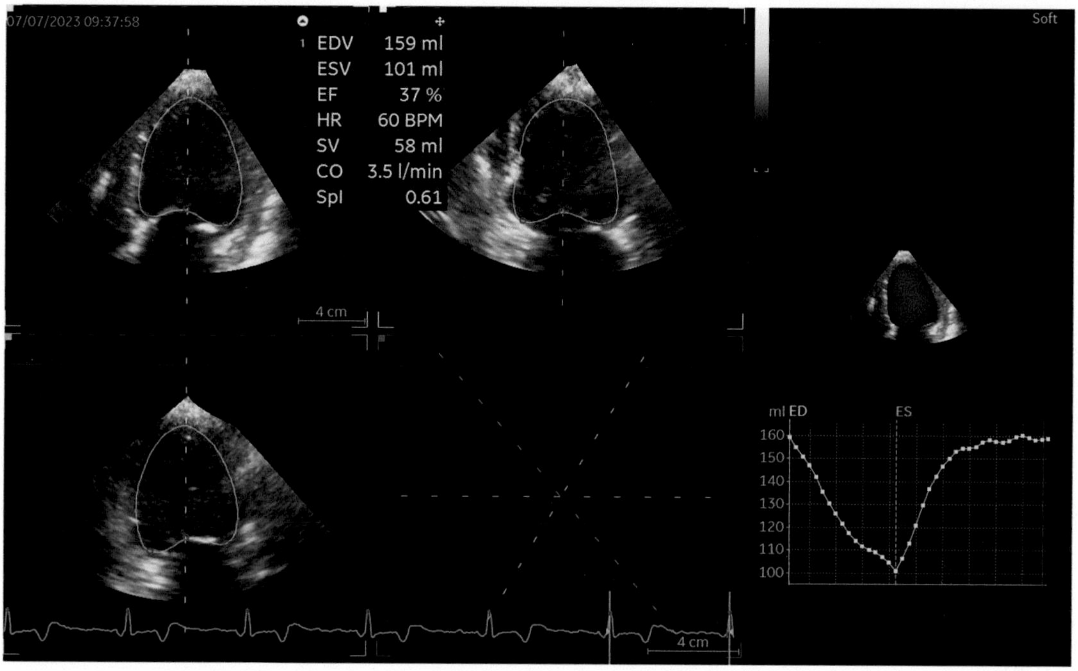

Fig. 2.17 Left ventricle ejection fraction and calculation by 3DE using left ventricle quantification software in a patient with cardiomyopathy and CRT

et al. 2004, 2006; Mor-Avi and Lang 2009; Soliman et al. 2008).

The *3D sphericity index* is a quantitative parameter extracted from cavity shape in patients with LV dysfunction (Mannaerts et al. 2004).

LV dyssynchrony 3D analysis provides the LV segmental individual volumes plotted versus time throughout the cardiac cycle, allowing the measurement of temporal differences in segmental time to minimum volume. Regional minimal volume corresponding to maximal contraction must be concordant during the ventricular systole for all segments (Lang et al. 2012). LV dyssynchrony translates into a discrepancy in minimal volume achievement for each segment. This anomaly is responsible for dispersion in the timing of regional segments reaching minimal volume. The systolic dyssynchrony index (SDI) represents the standard deviation of regional ejection times or time to reach the regional minimal volume. Different color schemes representing timing differences in segmental contraction can be displayed in a "bull's-eye" format, allowing the areas of dyssynchrony localization (Lang et al. 2012).

In *3D STE,* the deformation or strain can be performed in multiple planes, and all the s egments can be assessed simultaneously with a single beat acquisition, without beat-to-beat variability or out-of-plane motion, with a sequential assessment of basal, mid, and apical regions. Multiple strain parameters are provided by the left ventricular quantification (LVQ) software imaging technique (Nesser et al. 2009) (Fig. 2.18).

2.4 LV Mass

The methods for LV mass calculation use M-mode echocardiography, 2DE, and 3DE. The measurements should be performed at the end of diastole (the frame before mitral valve closure or the frame during the cardiac cycle in which the ventricular dimension is largest). As already underlined, M-Mode echocardiography is not an appropriate method for LV mass

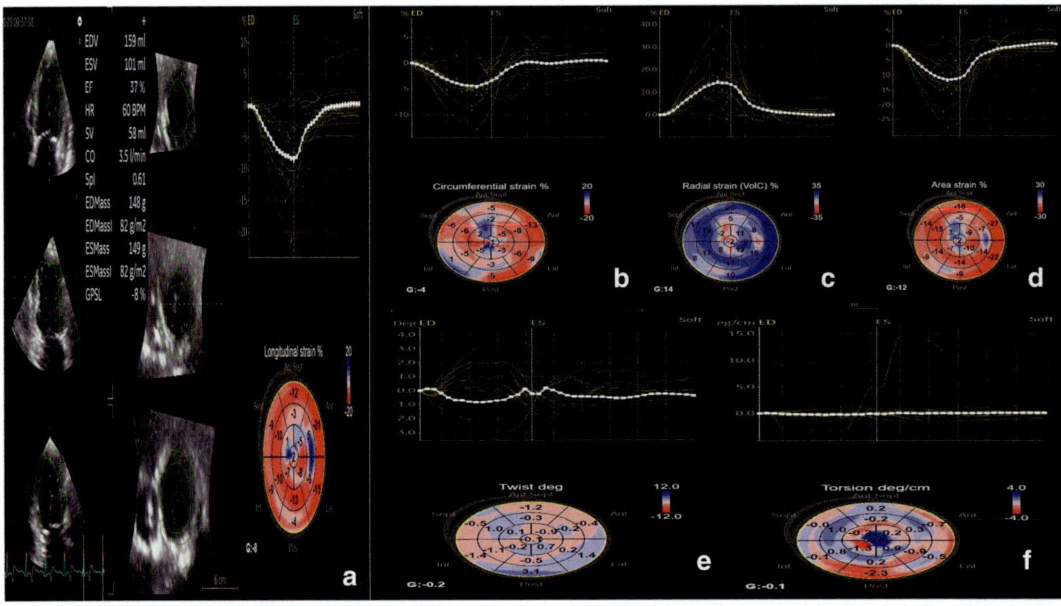

Fig. 2.18 Strain 3D calculation by 3DE using left ventricle quantification software in a patient with cardiomyopathy and CRT

calculation in CRT patients (Lang et al. 2015). 2D echocardiographic methods have advantages compared with the linear dimension technique in patients with LV shape abnormalities (Lang et al. 2015). 2DE uses the area-length or truncated ellipsoid technique for LV mass calculation. Both methods convert the LV volume to mass by multiplying the measured volume of the myocardium by the myocardial density (1.05 g/mL) (Lang et al. 2005). LV mass must be indexed to BSA. Reference upper limits of normal LV mass by 2D measurements are 88 g/m^2 in women and 102 g/m^2 in men with 2D methods) (Lang et al. 2005).

3DE can measure LV mass directly and is the most appropriate approach to calculate the LV mass (Mor-Avi et al. 2004). This is the only echocardiographic technique that measures myocardial volume directly, without geometric assumptions regarding LV shape and distribution of wall thickening (Lang et al. 2005). The accuracy of 3D echocardiography in LV mass measurement is similar to that of magnetic resonance imaging, with a slight overestimation (Bicudo et al. 2008; Caiani et al. 2006; Qin et al. 2005; Oe et al. 2005; Bosch et al. 2006) (Fig. 2.19).

2.5 LV Regional Function Segmentation of the LV

Myocardial segments are attributed to the three major coronary arteries. The 17-segment model allows wall motion evaluation by identifying six segments (inferoseptal, anteroseptal, anterior, lateral, inferolateral, inferior) in the base and mid left ventricle, four segments (septal, anterior, lateral, inferior) in the apex, and the apical cap (Lang et al. 2005). In the longitudinal dimension, the landmarks are the mitral annulus, papillary muscles, and LV apical segment. In the transverse dimension, the segments are distributed in 60-degree arcs from the midpoint of the septum. The septum's anterior and posterior RV insertion points define the interventricular septum (Lang et al. 2005) (Fig. 2.20).

2.6 Visual Assessment

According to its visual assessment contraction, every segment receives a score from 1 to 4. The final value will be divided by the number of evaluated segments, resulting in the LV wall

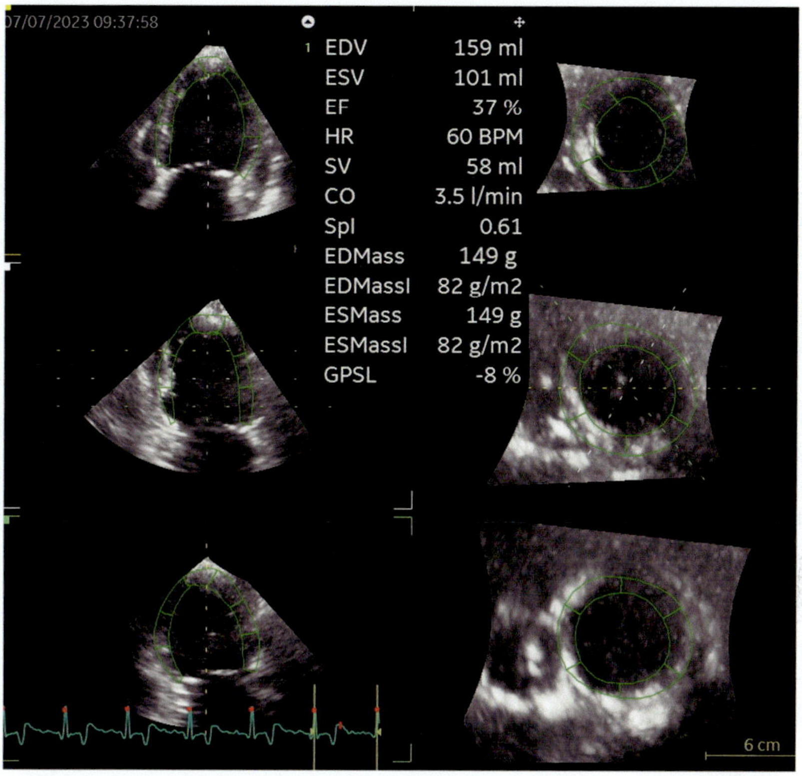

Fig. 2.19 Left ventricle mass calculation by 3DE using left ventricle quantification software in a patient with cardiomyopathy and CRT

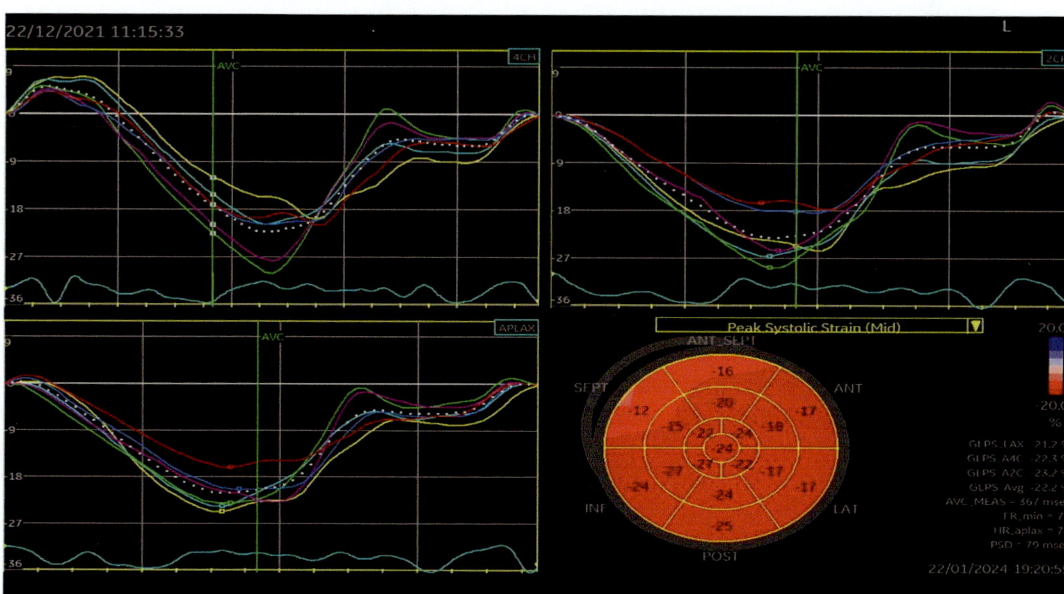

Fig. 2.20 Left ventricle segmentation

motion score index (sum score of all segments assessed /number of segments assessed)

Visual assessment of the contraction:

1. Normal or hyperkinetic
2. Hypokinetic (reduced thickening)
3. Akinetic (absent contraction or negligible -scar)
4. Dyskinetic systolic thinning or stretching (aneurysm).

Echocardiography may over- or underestimate the amount of ischemic or scared myocardium, depending on the adjacent regions' contraction, regional loading conditions, and stunning areas (Lang et al. 2015).

2.7 Abnormal Wall Motion Abnormalities in Patients with Implanted Devices

The patients with RV pacing or CRT present an abnormal motion of the interventricular septum named *septal bounce (septal beaking or septal flash (SF)*, and abnormal motion of the V apex, called *apical rocking*. SF is a hallmark of intraventricular dyssynchrony and can be visualized by 2D echocardiographic views (slowed-down loops and manual frame-by-frame advance) and confirmed by M-mode echocardiography. Mechanical dyssynchrony represents a non-homogeneous regional myocardial motion, assessed mainly through echocardiography (Smiseth et al. 2012).

It is essential to identify this motion in patients with implanted devices. This pattern will attenuate after the implant in CRT responders and predict CRT response in patients with right ventricular pacing needing an upgrade to CRT (Stankovic et al. 2017).

Septal flash

RVA pacing induces dyssynchronous left ventricular (LV) electric activation and contraction, with detrimental effects on LV structure and function, which is associated with an increased risk of cardiac morbidity and mortality (Kusumoto et al. 2018; Upadhyay et al. 2019; Zhang et al. 2019). Pacing from the RV apex causes early activation of the interventricular septum and late activation of the lateral wall of the LV (Sarvari et al. 2017). The main reason for LV dysfunction in patients with RVA pacing is the reduced contribution of the septum in global myocardial deformation (Sarvari et al. 2017).

Intraventricular dyssynchrony is identified by the presence of an SF in patients with conventional RV pacing, and its magnitude is related to LV dysfunction and remodeling. SF severity predicts the development of LV dysfunction and adverse remodelling in patients with conventional RV pacing. SF is characterized by pre-ejection shortening, followed abruptly by septal stretch during ejection (Leenders et al. 2012; Lumens et al. 2015; Remme et al. 2016; Gorcsan and Lumens 2019).

SF is usually assessed by echocardiography using M-mode (Fig. 2.21a). SF excursion is quantified by the highest amplitude of the early inward motion (measured from QRS onset to maximal inward motion) in M-mode at basal, mid-, and apical segments of the septum (Sarvari et al. 2017). The SF can also be easily detected by tissue Doppler imaging in short (Fig. 2.21b) or long axis view (Parsai et al. 2009; Oosterhout et al. 1998) (Fig. 2.21c) and by speckle tracking imaging (Calle et al. 2020) (Fig. 2.21d).

The presence and extent of SF correlate with *post systolic shortening (PSS)* (Fig. 2.21b, c,d). The development of PSS results from regional variations in the magnitude and duration of the contraction forces within the LV at the beginning of systole (Claus et al. 2007). PSS is assessed and quantified by the amplitude of the late inward motion after aortic valve closure in the same M-mode image where SF and systolic septal excursion were assessed (Sarvari et al. 2017). SF is associated with decreased LV function and adverse remodelling in patients with RV apical pacing (Curtis et al. 2013; Wilkoff 2003).

SF correlates with EF decreasing and increased in end-systolic volumes as an

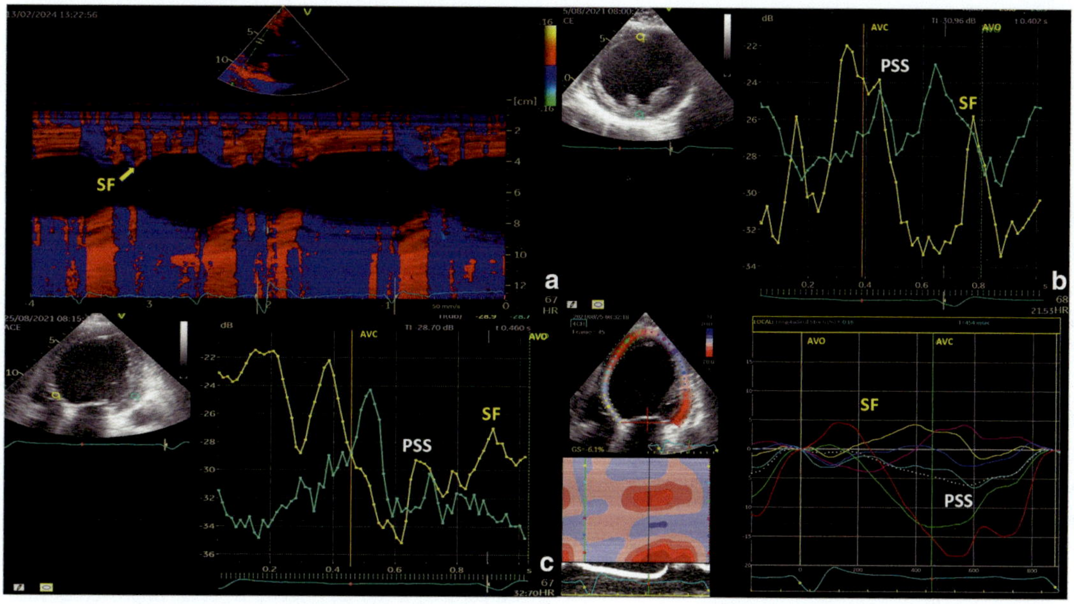

Fig. 2.21 Septal flush A Mmode, B tissue Doppler apical short axis view at the level of papillary muscles, C Tissue Doppler apical four-chamber view, D Speckle tracking echocardiography Apical four-chamber view

expression of adverse LV remodelling, and also with the presence and magnitude of PSS evaluated by STE (Sarvari et al. 2017). 45–50% of patients with RV pacing and normal EF present intra-ventricular dyssynchrony, and the prevalence increases parallel with decreasing LV function (Pastore et al. 2008; Fang et al. 2010). EF, GLS, and apical strain decrease over two years of permanent RV apical and septal pacing in patients with normal baseline LV function (Saito et al. 2015). Studies have shown decreased apical strain and reversed apicobasal strain gradient in patients with an SF. Basal function was similar in patients with or without SF (Saito et al. 2015). Mechanical dyssynchrony revealed by SF is associated with the percentage of RV pacing (Sarvari et al. 2017; Pastore et al. 2008). The SF's magnitude depends on the lead's exact place in the septal wall. The evaluation during implantation is the best approach for the appropriate lead position, minimizing future LV deterioration (Sarvari et al. 2017).

SF does not occur with ischemia or scar at the level of the posterior lateral wall. In this situation, the septum stretch is absent.

Requirements for SF are as follows:

- Delayed posterolateral electrical activation;
- Viable and functioning septal and posterolateral myocardium;
- Preserved RV conduction and function (Leenders et al. 2012; Lumens et al. 2015; Remme et al. 2016).

Factors that may influence SF:

- During the pre-ejection: septum shortening occurs only in the presence of electrical delay of the posterior lateral wall.
- The septal scar attenuates septal contraction as well as posterior wall pre-stretch.
- During ejection: severe posterolateral dysfunction or scar attenuates septal stretch and SF will be absent.
- The SF will not occur if the scar involves both the septum and posterior walls because of the diminishing of posterolateral pre-stretch and septal rebound stretch.
- RV conduction delay and function may influence SF (Walmsley et al. 2016).

Apical rocking (AR) is a consequence of SF (Beela et al. 2019; Gorcsan and Lumens 2017). AR from apical views consists of pre-ejection septal shortening stretches the lateral wall, shifting the LV apex, followed by lateral wall contraction, which stretches the septum, pulling the LV apex in the opposite direction (Gorcsan and Lumens 2017) AR can be qualitatively visually evaluated best using 2DE (Gorcsan and Lumens 2017) (Supplementary material 1), (Supplementary material 2).

The early activation and contraction of the septum pull the apex towards the RV. The delayed activation and contraction of the lateral wall pulls the apex back to the left and stretches the relaxed septum (Szulik et al. 2010).

Following CRT implant, synchrony is restored (with the disappearance of SF), and septal wall thickness and contractility should improve (Sze and Daubert 2018). This achievement might be explained by the electrical activation of the septal wall restoration, irrespective of the modality of ventricle pacing biventricular or LV pacing only (Sharma et al. 2018).

2.8 Conclusion

In patients with implanted devices, LV systolic evaluation follows the same approach as in patients without intracardiac leads, with some peculiarities linked to the specific device. Wall motion abnormalities should be carefully evaluated. Apical rocking and septal flush persistence in CRT patients should pay attention to the absence of synchrony restoration. Patients with pacemakers should conclude about the moment of CRT updating after LV dimension and function evaluation. In both cases, three echocardiography is the best imaging evaluation technique for LV volumes and function. Evaluating the strain by speckle tracking echocardiography adds essential information.

References

Beela AS, Ünlü S, Duchenne J, et al. Assessment of mechanical dyssynchrony can improve the prognostic value of guideline-based patient selection for cardiac resynchronization therapy. Eur Heart J Cardiovasc Imaging. 2019;20:66–74.

Biaggi P, Carasso S, Garceau P, et al. Comparison of two different speckle tracking software systems: does the method matter? Echocardiography. 2011;28(5):539–47.

Bicudo LS, Tsutsui JM, Shiozaki A, et al. Value of real-time three-dimensional echocardiography in patients with hypertrophic cardiomyopathy: comparison with two-dimensional echocardiography and magnetic resonance imaging. Echocardiography. 2008;25:717–26.

Caiani EG, Corsi C, Zamorano J, et al. Improved semi-automated quantification of left ventricular volumes and ejection fraction using 3-dimensional echocardiography with a full matrix-array transducer: comparison with magnetic resonance imaging. J Am Soc Echocardiography. 2005;18:779–88.

Caiani EG, Corsi C, Sugeng L, et al. Improved quantification of left ventricular mass based on endocardial and epicardial surface detection with real-time three-dimensional echocardiography. Heart. 2006;92:213–9.

Calle S, Delens C, Kamoen V, De Pooter J, Timmermans F. Septal flash: At the heart of cardiac dyssynchrony. Trends Cardiovasc Med. 2020;30:115–22.

Chan J, Hanekom L, Wong C, et al. Differentiation of subendocardial and transmural infarction using two-dimensional strain rate imaging to assess short-axis and long-axis myocardial function. J Am Coll Cardiol. 2006a;48(10):2026–33.

Chan J, Jenkins C, Khafagi F, Du L, Marwick T. What is the optimal clinical technique for measurement of left ventricular volume after myocardial infarction? A comparative study of 3-dimensional echocardiography, single photon emission computed tomography, and cardiac magnetic resonance imaging. J Am Soc Echocardiogr. 2006b;19:192–201.

Claus P, Weidemann F, Dommke C, Bito V, Heinzel FR, D'Hooge J, et al. Mechanisms of postsystolic thickening in ischemic myocardium: mathematical modelling and comparison with experimental ischemic substrates. Ultrasound Med Biol. 2007;33:1963–70.

Curtis AB, Worley SJ, Adamson PB, et al. Biventricular pacing for atrioventricular block and systolic dysfunction. N Engl J Med. 2013;368:1585–93.

Dorosz JL, Lezotte DC, Weitzenkamp DA, Allen LA, Salcedo EE. Performance of 3-dimensional echocardiography in measuring left ventricular volumes and ejection fraction: a systematic review and meta-analysis. J Am Coll Cardiol. 2012;59:1799–808.

Fang F, Chan JY, Yip GW, Xie JM, Zhang Q, Fung JW, et al. Prevalence and determinants of left ventricular systolic dyssynchrony in patients with normal ejection fraction received right ventricular apical pacing: a real-time three-dimensional echocardiographic study. Eur J Echocardiogr. 2010;11:109–18.

Fenster A, Downey DB, Cardinal HN. Three-dimensional ultrasound imaging. Phys Med Biol. 2001;46:R67-99.

Geyer H, Caracciolo G, Abe H, et al. Assessment of myocardial mechanics using speckle tracking echocardiography: fundamentals and clinical applications. J Am Soc Echocardiogr. 2010;23(4):351–63.

Geyer H, Caracciolo G, Abe H, et al. Assessment of myocardial mechanics using speckle tracking echocardiography: fundamentals and clinical applications. J Am Soc Echocardiogr. 2010;23(4):351–369.

Gorcsan J III, Lumens J. Opposing wall pushing and stretching response to cardiac resynchronization therapy requires electrical delay and viability. JACC: Cardiovasc Imaging. 2019;(12)12:2414–2416.

Gorcsan J III, Lumens J. Rocking and flashing with RV pacing: implications for resynchronization therapy. J Am Coll Cardiol Img. 2017;10:1100–2.

Hoffmann R, von Bardeleben S, Kasprzak JD, et al. Analysis of regional left ventricular function by cineventriculography, cardiac magnetic resonance imaging, and unenhanced and contrast-enhanced echocardiography: a multicenter comparison of methods. J Am Coll Cardiol. 2006;47:121–8.

Jacobs LD, Salgo IS, Goonewardena S, et al. Rapid online quantification of left ventricular volume from real-time three-dimensional echocardiographic data. Eur Heart J. 2006;27:460–8.

Jenkins C, Bricknell K, Hanekom L, Marwick TH. Reproducibility and accuracy of echocardiographic measurements of left ventricular parameters using real-time three-dimensional echocardiography. J Am Coll Cardiol. 2004;44:878–86.

Jenkins C, Chan J, Hanekom L, Marwick TH. Accuracy and feasibility of online 3-dimensional echocardiography for measurement of left ventricular parameters. J Am Soc Echocardiogr. 2006;19:1119–28.

Jenkins C, Moir S, Chan J, Rakhit D, Haluska B, Marwick TH. Left ventricular volume measurement with echocardiography: a comparison of left ventricular opacification, three-dimensional echocardiography, or both with magnetic resonance imaging. Eur Heart J. 2009;30:98–106.

Krenning BJ, Kirschbaum SW, Soliman OI, et al. Comparison of contrast agent-enhanced versus non-contrast agent-enhanced real-time three-dimensional echocardiography for analysis of left ventricular systolic function. Am J Cardiol. 2007;100:1485–9.

Kusumoto FM, Schoenfeld MH, Barrett C, et al. ACC/AHA/HRS guideline on the evaluation and management of patients with bradycardia and cardiac conduction delay: a report of the American College of Cardiology/American Heart Association Task Force on clinical practice guidelines and the heart rhythm society. Circulation. 2018;2019:140.e382-e482.

Lang RM, Bierig M, Devereux RB, et al. Recommendations for chamber quantification: a report from the American Society of Echocardiography's Guidelines and Standards Committee and the Chamber Quantification Writing Group, developed in conjunction with the European Associate of Echocardiography, a branch of the European Society of Cardiology. J Am Soc Echocardiogr. 2005;18:1440–63.

Lang RM, Badano LP, Tsang W, et al. EAE/ASE recommendations for image acquisition and display using three-dimensional echocardiography. J Am Soc Echocardiogr. 2012;25:3–46.

Lang RM, Badano LP, Mor-Avi V, et al. Recommendations for cardiac chamber quantification by echocardiography in adults: an update from the American society of echocardiography and the European association of cardiovascular imaging. Eur Heart J Cardiovasc Imaging. 2015;16:233–71.

Lee D, Fuisz AR, Fan PH, Hsu TL, Liu CP, Chiang HT. Real-time 3-dimensional echocardiographic evaluation of left ventricular volume: correlation with magnetic resonance imaging-a validation study. J Am Soc Echocardiogr. 2001;14:1001–9.

Leenders GE, Lumens J, Cramer MJ, et al. Septal deformation patterns delineate mechanical dys-synchrony and regional differences in contractility: analysis of patient data using a computer model. Circ Heart Fail. 2012;5:87–96.

Lumens J, Tayal B, Walmsley J, et al. Differentiating electromechanical from non-electrical substrates of mechanical discoordination to identify responders to cardiac resynchronization therapy. Circ Cardiovasc Imaging. 2015;8:e003744.

Mannaerts HF, van der Heide JA, Kamp O, Stoel MG, Twisk J, Visser CA. Early identification of left ventricular remodelling after myocardial infarction, assessed by transthoracic 3D echocardiography. Eur Heart J. 2004;25:680–7.

Monaghan MJ. Role of real-time 3D echocardiography in evaluating the left ventricle. Heart. 2006;92:131–6.

Monaghan MJ. Role of real-time 3D echocardiography in evaluating the left ventricle. Heart. 2006;92:131–136.

Mor-Avi V, Lang RM. The use of real-time three-dimensional echocardiography for the quantification of left ventricular volumes and function. Curr Opin Cardiol. 2009;24:402–9.

Mor-Avi V, Sugeng L, Weinert L, MacEneaney P, Caiani EG, Koch R, et al. Fast measurement of left ventricular mass with real-time three-dimensional echocardiography: comparison with magnetic resonance imaging. Circulation. 2004;110:1814–8.

Mor-Avi V, Jenkins C, Kuhl HP, Nesser HJ, Marwick TH, Franke A, et al. Real-time 3-dimensional echocardiographic quantification of left ventricular volumes: multicenter study for validation with magnetic resonance imaging and investigation of sources of error. JACC Cardiovasc Imaging. 2008;1:413–23.

Mor-Avi V, Lang RM, Badano LP, et al. Current and evolving echocardiographic techniques for the quantitative evaluation of cardiac mechanics: ASE/EAE consensus statement on methodology and indications endorsed by the Japanese Society of Echocardiography. J Am Soc Echocardiogr. 2011;24(3):277–313.

Mulvagh SL, Rakowski H, Vannan MA, et al. American society of echocardiography consensus statement on the clinical applications of ultrasonic contrast agents in echocardiography. J Am Soc Echocardiogr. 2008;21:1179–201.

Muraru D, Badano LP, Piccoli G, et al. Validation of a novel automated border-detection algorithm for rapid and accurate quantitation of left ventricular volumes based on three-dimensional echocardiography. Eur J Echocardiogr. 2010;11:359–68.

Negishi K, Negishi T, Kurosawa K, et al. Practical guidance in echocardiographic assessment of global longitudinal strain. JACC: Cardiovasc Imaging. 2015;8(4):489–492.

Nesser HJ, Mor-Avi V, Gorissen W, et al. Quantification of left ventricular volumes using three-dimensional echocardiographic speckle tracking: comparison with MRI. Eur Heart J. 2009;30(13):1565–73.

Nucifora G, Marsan NA, Holman ER, et al. Real-time 3-dimensional echocardiography early after acute myocardial infarction: incremental value of echo-contrast for assessment of left ventricular function. Am Heart J. 2009;157:882–8.

Oe H, Hozumi T, Arai K, Matsumura Y, et al. Comparison of accurate measurement of left ventricular mass in patients with hypertrophied hearts by real-time three-dimensional echocardiography versus magnetic resonance imaging. Am J Cardiol. 2005;95:1263–7.

Oxborough D, George K, Birch KM. Intraobserver reliability of two-dimensional ultrasound derived strain imaging in the assessment of the left ventricle, right ventricle, and left atrium of healthy human hearts. Echocardiography. 2012;29(7):793–802.

Pandian NG, Roelandt J, Nanda NC, et al. Dynamic three-dimensional echocardiography: methods and clinical potential. Echocardiography. 1994;11:237–59.

Parsai C, Bijnens B, Sutherland GR, Baltabaeva A, Claus P, Marciniak M, et al. Toward understanding response to cardiac resynchronization therapy: left ventricular dyssynchrony is only one of multiple mechanisms. Eur Heart J. 2009;30(8):940–9.

Pastore G, Noventa F, Piovesana P, et al. Left ventricular dyssynchrony resulting from right ventricular apical pacing: relevance of baseline assessment. Pacing Clin Electrophysiol. 2008;31:1456–62.

Potter E, Marwick TH. Assessment of left ventricular function by echocardiography the case for routinely adding global longitudinal strain to ejection fraction. JACC: Cardiovasc Imaging. 2018;11(2):260–274.

Qin JX, Jones M, Travaglini A, et al. The accuracy of left ventricular mass determined by real-time three-dimensional echocardiography in chronic animal and clinical studies: a comparison with postmortem examination and magnetic resonance imaging. J Am Soc Echocardiogr. 2005;18:1037–43.

Remme EW, Niederer S, Gjesdal O, et al. Factors determining the magnitude of the pre-ejection leftward septal motion in left bundle branch block. Europace. 2016;18:1905–13.

Saito M, Kaye G, Negishi K, et al. Dyssynchrony, contraction efficiency and regional function with apical and non-apical RV pacing. Heart. 2015;101:600–8.

Sarvari SI, Sitges M, Sanz M, et al. Left ventricular dysfunction is related to the presence and extent of a septal flash in patients with right ventricular pacing. Europace. 2017;19:289–96.

Sharma PS, Dandamudi G, Herweg B, et al. Permanent His-bundle pacing as an alternative to biventricular pacing for cardiac resynchronization therapy: A multicenter experience. Heart Rhythm. 2018;15(3):413–20.

Smiseth OA, Russell K, Skulstad H. The role of echocardiography in quantification of left ventricular dyssynchrony: state of the art and future directions. Eur Heart J Cardiovasc Imaging. 2012;13(1):61–68.

Soliman OI, Kirschbaum SW, van Dalen BM, et al. Accuracy and reproducibility of quantitation of left ventricular function by real-time three-dimensional echocardiography versus cardiac magnetic resonance. Am J Cardiol. 2008;102:778–83.

Stankovic I, Prinz C, Ciarka A, Daraban AM, Mo Y, Aarones M, et al. Long-term outcome after CRT in the presence of mechanical dyssynchrony seen with chronic RV pacing or intrinsic LBBB. JACC Cardiovasc Imaging. 2017;10(10 Pt A):1091–1099.

Sze E, Daubert EJ. Left bundle branch block-induced left ventricular remodeling and its potential for reverse remodeling. J Interv Card Electrophysiol. 2018;52:343–52.

Szulik M, Tillekaerts M, Vangeel V, et al. Assessment of apical rocking: a new, integrative approach for selection of candidates for cardiac resynchronization therapy. Eur J Echocardiogr. 2010;11:863–9.

Tops LF, Delgado V, Marsan NA, Bax JJ. Myocardial strain to detect subtle left ventricular systolic dysfunction. Eur J Heart Fail. 2017;19:307–13.

Upadhyay GA, Vijayaraman P, Nayak HM, et al. His corrective pacing or biventricular pacing for cardiac resynchronization in heart failure. J Am Coll Cardiol. 2019;74:157–9.

van den Bosch AE, Robbers-Visser D, Krenning BJ, McGhie JS, Helbing WA, Meijboom FJ, et al. Comparison of real-time three-dimensional echocardiography to magnetic resonance imaging for assessment of left ventricular mass. Am J Cardiol. 2006;97:113–7.

van Oosterhout MF, Prinzen FW, Arts T, Schreuder JJ, Vanagt WY, Cleutjens JP, et al. Asynchronous electrical activation induces asymmetrical hypertrophy of the left ventricular wall. Circulation. 1998;98(6):588–95.

Walmsley J, Huntjens PR, Prinzen PW, et al. Septal flash and septal rebound stretch have different underlying mechanisms. Am J Physiol Heart Circ Physiol. 2016;310:H394-403.

Wilkoff BL. The dual chamber and VVI implantable defibrillator (DAVID) trial: rationale, design, results, clinical implications and lessons for future trials. Card Electrophysiol Rev. 2003;7:468–72.

Yoshitani H, Takeuchi M, Mor-Avi V, Otsuji Y, Hozumi T, Yoshiyama M. Comparative diagnostic accuracy of multiplane and multislice three-dimensional dobutamine stress echocardiography in the diagnosis of coronary artery disease. J Am Soc Echocardiogr. 2009;22:437–42.

Zhang S, Zhou X, Gold MR. Left bundle branch pacing. J Am Coll Cardiol. 2019;74:3039–49.

3 Left Ventricle Diastolic Function Evaluation in Patients with Implanted Devices

Abstract

Compared with patients without intracardiac devices, patients with implanted devices will present some inconvenience in diastolic dysfunction evaluation linked to dyssynchrony due to the right ventricle lead presence and atrioventricular interval optimization. Small studies provide some information about diastolic dysfunction parameters in these patients. The probability of normal diastolic function in patients with cardiac resynchronization therapy or right ventricular pacing is low because they usually present structural heart disease. The more advanced diastolic dysfunction, the more increased left ventricle filling pressure. There are no specific indications for diastolic dysfunction evaluation in patients with implanted devices. The last guidelines may be used mainly for grading diastolic dysfunction, considering the accuracy of presented parameters in this situation.

The diastolic function represents heart filling during diastole. Diastole comprises four phases: relaxation, rapid filling, slow filling (diastasis), and active filling (Kossaify and Nasr 2019) (Fig. 3.1). During *isovolumic relaxation*, all four heart valves are closed (Nagueh et al. 2009; Schirmer et al. 2000), and the gradient between the left atrium (LA) and the left ventricle (LV) increases. This phase depends on load conditions, contraction inactivation, and asynchrony (Fukuta and Little 2008). When LV pressure falls below LA pressure, the atrioventricular valves will open, and rapid filling will start (passive filling) (Kossaify and Nasr 2019). It stops when the gradient ends. Isovolumic relaxation represents the interactions between LV suction (active relaxation) and viscoelastic proprieties of the myocardium (compliance) (Fukuta and Little 2008). The process is represented by spectral Doppler echocardiography by the E wave (Kossaify and Nasr 2019) (Fig. 3.2).

During diastasis, the LV filling decreases or is absent because of increased intraventricular pressure (Kossaify and Nasr 2019). During this phase, the blood enters the LV from pulmonary veins, depending on LV pressure and compliance. LA has a passive conduit phase during diastasis (Fukuta and Little 2008).

Atrial contraction determines the active LV filling and is represented on spectral Doppler echocardiography by the A wave (Kossaify and Nasr 2019; Nagueh et al. 2009; Schirmer et al. 2000) (Fig. 3.2). This period is mainly influenced by LV compliance but also depends on the pericardial resistance, the atrial force, and the atrioventricular synchrony (Fukuta and Little 2008).

Diastolic function correlates to heart rate, atrial systolic function, ventricular compliance, preload, heart rhythm, and atrioventricular valve function (Fukuta and Little 2008).

D.-M. Toader, *Echocardiographic Evaluation of Patients with Implanted Devices*,
https://doi.org/10.1007/978-3-031-64079-7_3

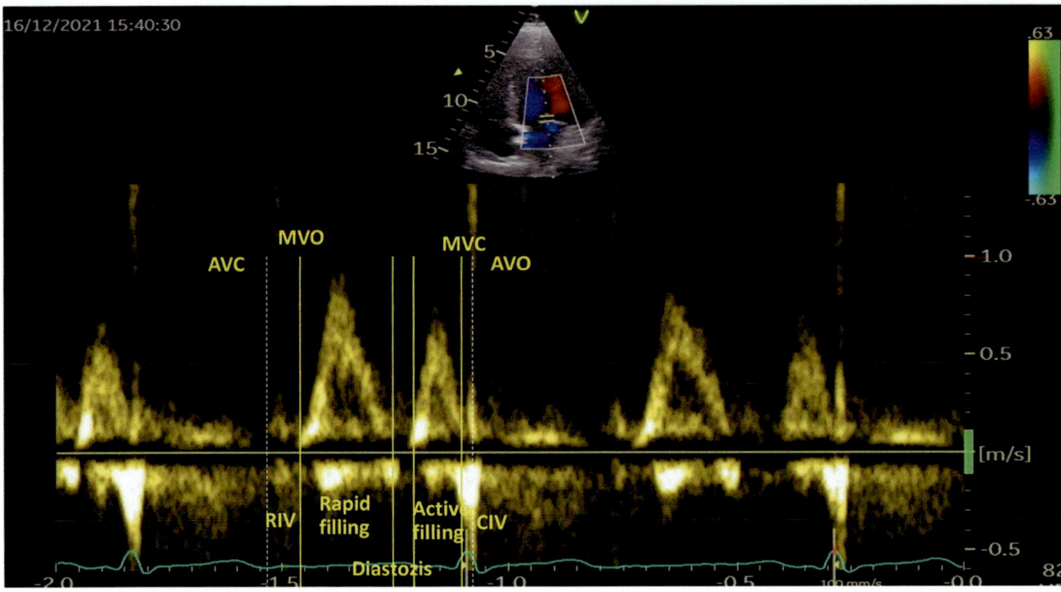

Fig. 3.1 Diastole phases

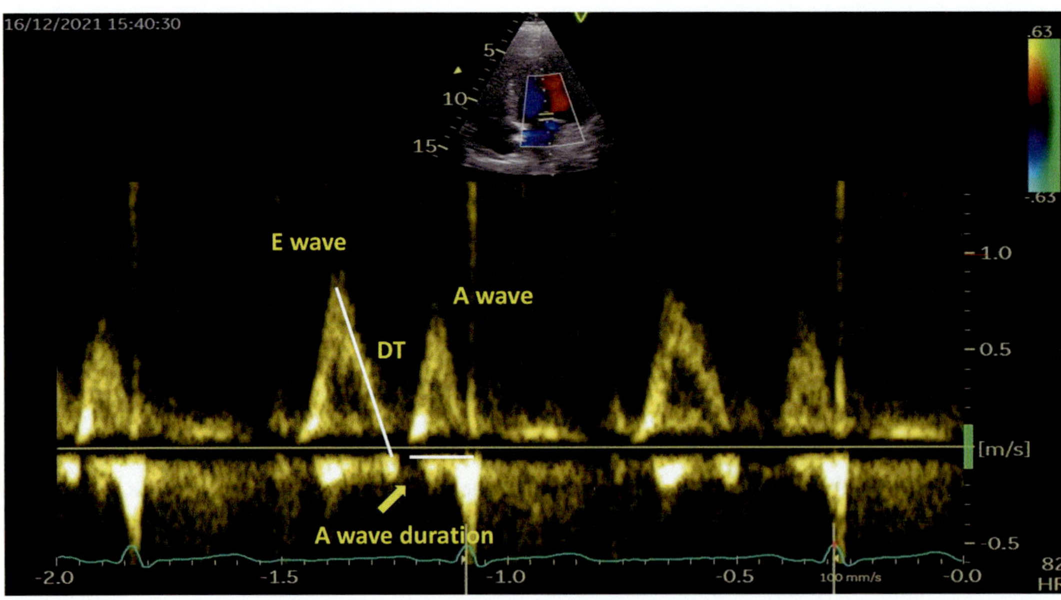

Fig. 3.2 Mitral valve diastolic inflow components evaluated by pulsed wave Doppler echocardiography

Filling pressures represent the left atrial pressure (LAP) and the LV end-diastolic pressure (LVEDP) (Kossaify and Nasr 2019). A mean pulmonary capillary wedge pressure (PCWP) > 12 mm Hg or an LV end-diastolic pressure (left ventricular filling pressure (LVFP)) > 16 mm Hg (hemodynamic measured) describes an increased LV pressure (Brutsaert et al. 1993).

Increased LV filling pressure is the main pathophysiological consequence of diastolicdysfunction (Fukuta and Little 2008). LVFP and

LAP are often used interchangeably to describe increased filling pressure (Paulus et al. 2007; Brutsaert et al. 1993).

Echocardiographic techniques used for DD evaluation are pulsed wave Doppler (PW) echocardiographic evaluation of mitral valve diastolic inflow and the pulmonary veins flow, tissue Doppler (TD) evaluation of mitral annulus velocities, color-M mode evaluation of flow velocity propagation (vp) in LV during diastole, strain, and strain rate during diastole by speckle tracking echocardiography (STE) (Nagueh et al. 2016).

The 2016 ASE/EACVI guideline DD recommendations for the LV diastolic function assessment identifies six *classical* parameter measurements. Special conditions need other additional parameters (Nagueh et al. 2016).

The classical parameters are E wave velocity from the PW mitral inflow, E/A ratio, e′ velocity at the level of septal and mitral annulus measured by TDI, average E/e′ ratio, left atrial volume indexed (LAVi), and peak tricuspid regurgitation (TR) velocity (Nagueh et al. 2016).

Indications for mitral inflow velocities recording are:

- pulse wave (PW) Doppler imaging guided by color flow imaging for an adequate alignment with color flow
- apical four-chamber (A4c) view
- 1–3 mm sample volume placed at the level of mitral leaflets tips
- recording at end-expiration
- sweep speed of 50–100 mm/s
- averaging three consecutive cardiac cycles in sinus rhythm patients and five cardiac cycles in atrial fibrillations (Fukuta and Little 2008) (Fig. 3.2).

Mitral inflow measurements include:

- Peak of early filling (E velocity) (Fig. 3.2) - depends on LVEDP and LV relaxation and is also very sensitive to loading conditions, heart rate, the presence of mitral valve (MV) diseases like mitral valve stenosis (Popović et al. 2018; Thomas et al. 1991) or mitral regurgitation (MR) (Thomas et al. 1997).
- Deceleration time (DT) of E velocity (Fig. 3.2)—is the time interval from peak E-wave along the slope of LV filling extrapolated to the zero-velocity baseline (Nagueh et al. 2016). This variable depends on LV diastolic pressure after MV opening, LV relaxation, LV compliance E wave peak velocity and DT represent LA—LV gradient during early diastole, affected by LV preload, relaxation, elastic recoil (suction), compliance, and MV orifice area. The E wave amplitude decreases with age, and the DT increases with relaxation abnormalities (Kossaify and comNasr 2019) (Fig. 3.3).
- Peak E velocity—cutoff value is > 50 cm/s
- Peak of late atrial filling (A velocity) - represents LA—LV pressure gradient during late diastole, mainly influenced by LV compliance and LA contractile function.
- The E/A ratio
- Mitral A velocity duration (Fig. 3.2, arrow)

Velocities will be expressed in m/s and time intervals in ms (Fukuta and Little 2008; Nagueh et al. 2016).

Indications for wave tissue Doppler annular diastolic velocities recording are:

- a 3-mm PW Doppler sample volume
- placed at 1 cm within the septal or lateral MV insertion of MV leaflets
- A4c view
- gain and velocity scale adequately setted
- minimal angulation between the ultrasound beam and the plane of cardiac motion (< 20 degrees)
- recording at the end-expiration
- sweep speed of 50–100 mm/s
- averaging three consecutive cardiac cycles in sinus rhythm patients and five cardiac cycles in atrial fibrillations (Fukuta and Little 2008; Nagueh et al. 2016).

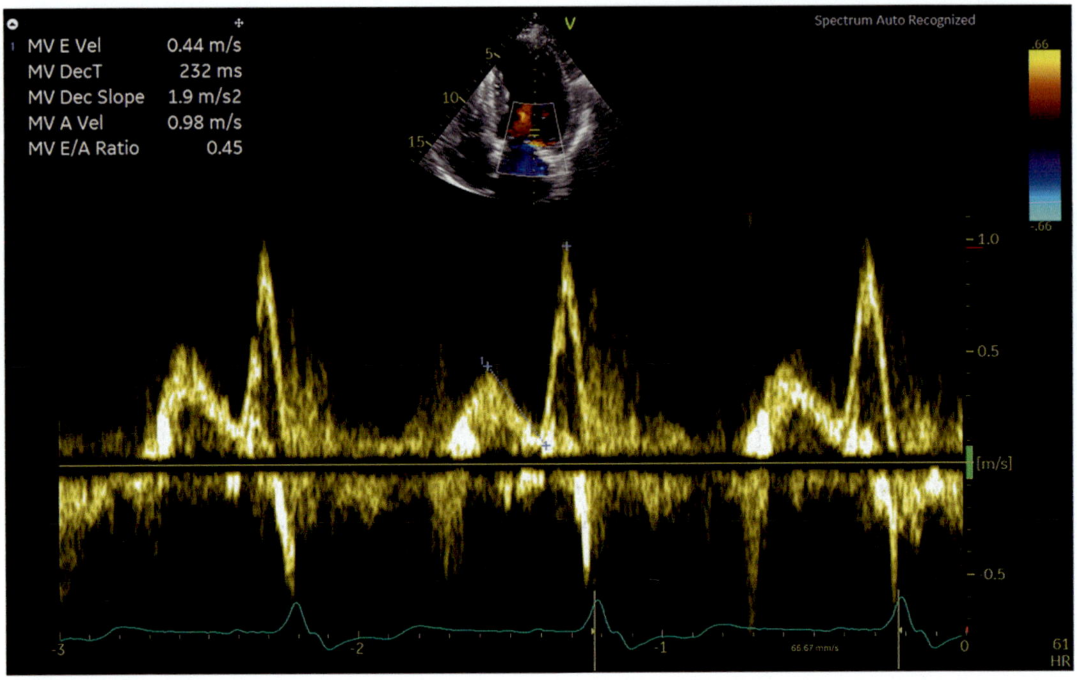

Fig. 3.3 Abnormal relaxation pattern of mitral valve diastolic inflow

PW TD diastolic measurements include:

- Early diastolic velocity (e′)—represents the peak modal velocity in early diastole at the leading edge of the spectral waveform influenced by LV relaxation The cutoff values are septal e′ < 7 cm/s and lateral e′ < 10 cm/s.
- Late atrial velocity (a′)—represents the peak modal velocity in late diastole at the leading edge of the spectral waveform influenced by LA function and LVEDP
- The e′/a′ ratio (Fig. 3.4) Annular velocities are expressed in cm/s. A reduced and delayed e′ velocity value reflects LV relaxation abnormalities (Nagueh et al. 2009; Waggoner and Bierig 2001) E/e′ ratio calculation estimates LV filling pressure. Cutoff values are: septal > 15, lateral > 13, average > 14 TD velocities are also influenced by age (Fukuta and Little 2008).

Indications for pulmonary venous flow recording are:

- pulse wave (PW) Doppler imaging guided by color flow imaging for an adequate alignment with color flow
- A4c view
- A 2–3 mm PW sample volume placed 1–2 cm into the right upper pulmonary vein (PV)
- the wall filter setting is low enough (100–200 MHz) to distinguish the onset and the end of atrial reversal activity
- low signal gain
- the spectral waveforms should not display signal spikes or feathering.

Measurements include:

- peak systolic v (S) velocity (fusion of systolic waves S1 and S2)—represents the peak modal velocity in early systole at the leading edge of the spectral waveform (Nagueh et al. 2016). This parameter corresponds to the reservoir function.
- peak diastolic (D) velocity—the peak modal velocity in early diastole after MV opening at the leading edge of the spectral waveform (Nagueh et al. 2016) represents the conduit function and corresponds temporarily to the mitral inflow E velocity (cm/s).

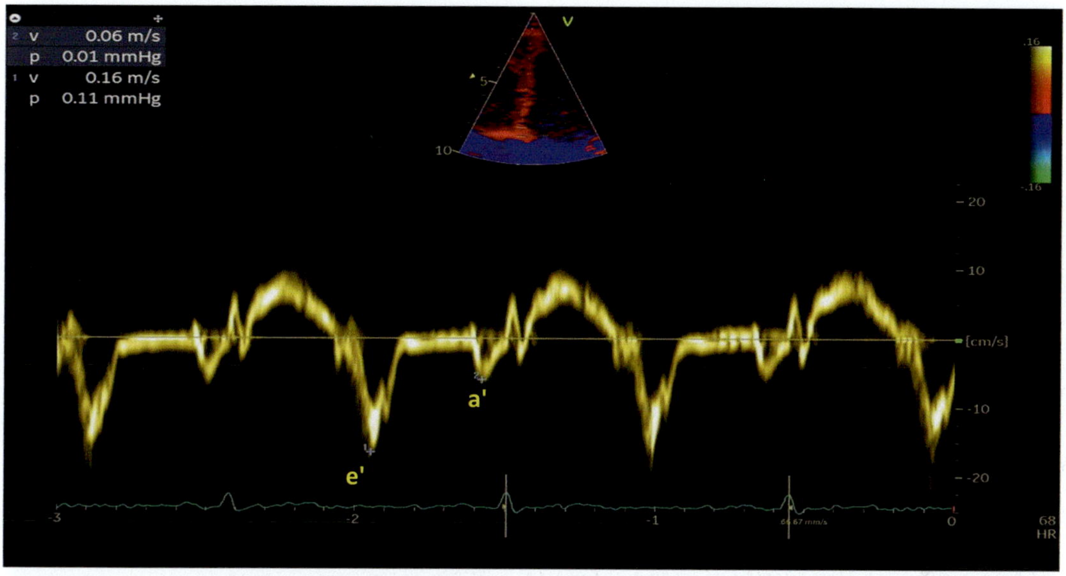

Fig. 3.4 e′, a′ measurement with tissue Doppler echocardiography t the level of interventricular basal septum

- The S/D ratio (Fig. 3.5).
- Peak atrial reversal (AR) velocity—represents the pump function and corresponds temporarily to the mitral inflow A velocity

AR velocity is influenced by atrial preload, LA contractility, and LVEDP and is relatively age – age-independent.

The time duration of AR velocity (msec)-represents the time interval from AR-wave onset to the end of AR at zero baseline (Fig. 3.5)

- AR-A duration: the time difference between AR duration and mitral A duration (Kossaify and Nasr 2019; Fukuta and Little 2008) AR-A duration> 30 ms is highly predictive of increased LVFP.

LAVi (ml/BSA) measurement:

- method of disks or area-length method and correct for BSA
- apical four- and two-chamber view
- 1–2 frames before MV opening will be acquired
- LA volume should be measured in dedicated views that maximize LA length and transverse diameters. The measurement will not include LA appendage or pulmonary veins in LA tracings.

LAVI—cutoff value is < 34 mL/m^{2} [7] (Fig. 3.6).

TR systolic jet velocity (m/s) will be evaluated:

- by CW Doppler, measuring the peak modal velocity during systole at the leading edge of the spectral waveform
- parasternal and apical four-chamber view with color flow imaging to obtain the best Doppler velocity alignment
- gain and contrast must be set to display a complete spectral envelope with no signal spikes or feathering
- TRpV—cutoff value: > 2.8 m/s (Chiladakis et al. 2007) (Fig. 3.7)

Specific conditions need *additional parameters*:

- IVRT: the time between aortic valve closure and mitral valve opening (Fig. 3.8), measured from the apical long-axis or five-chamber view, with PW Doppler sample placed in LVOT simultaneously displaying the end of

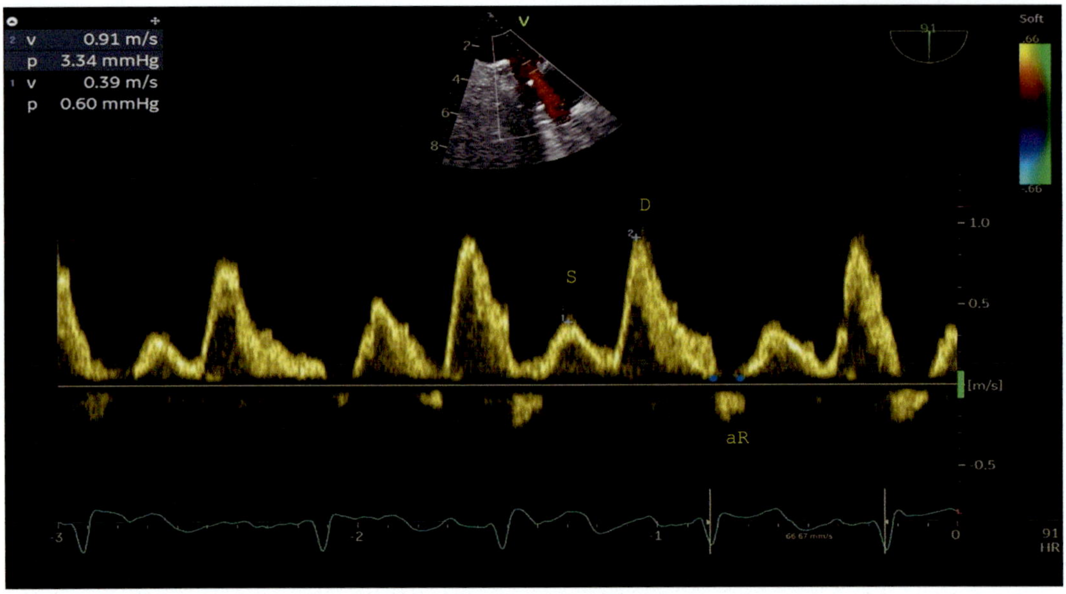

Fig. 3.5 Pulmonary venous flow components recording by transesophageal echocardiography at the level of the left superior pulmonary vein

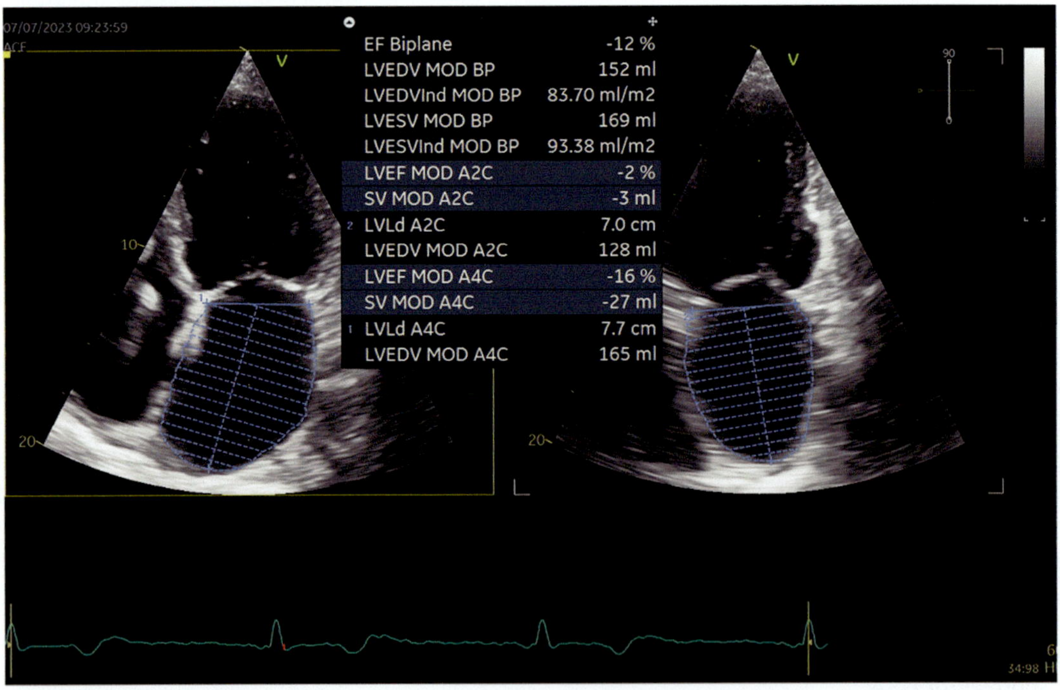

Fig. 3.6 Left atrium volume index measurement

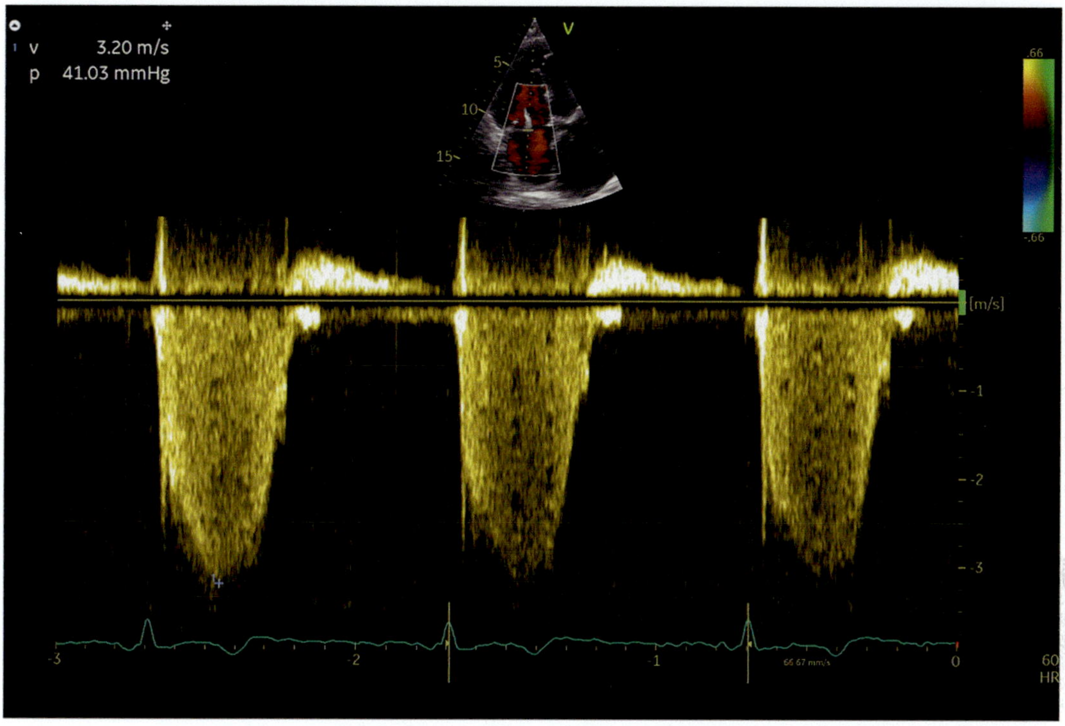

Fig. 3.7 Tricuspid regurgitation systolic jet velocity measurement by CW Doppler from apical four-chamber view

aortic ejection and the beginning of mitral inflow, at a sweep speed of 100 mm/s (Fukuta and Little 2008; Nagueh et al. 2016). A short IVRT is a high LV end-diastolic pressure indicator (Henein and Lindqvist 2020) (Fig. 3.8).

- TE-e′- Represents the difference between two intervals measured from the apical four-chamber view at a sweep speed of 100 mm/sec. First is the time interval between the peak of the R wave and the onset of mitral E velocity, and the second is the time interval between the QRS complex and the onset of e′ velocity. RR intervals should be matched and should avoid high gain and filter settings (Fukuta and Little 2008; Nagueh et al. 2016).
- IVRT/TE-e′
- L wave (during diastasis): is an abnormal wave representing an LV filling in mid-diastole (Fig. 3.9) Valsalva maneuver - represents the change in MV E velocity and E/A ratio during forced expiration. The recording will be obtained continuously through peak inspiration followed by forced expiration for 10 s with mouth and nose closed (Fukuta and Little 2008; Nagueh et al. 2016) (Fig. 3.10). A decrease in the E/A ratio of $\geq 50\%$ is highly specific for increased LV filling pressures.
- *Color M-mode Vp* (cm/s)—represents the slope of inflow from the MV plane into the LV chamber during early diastole, and assesses LV relaxation

Indications for flow velocity—vp by color M-mode of the mitral inflow recording are:

- M-mode cursor placed in the direction of the mitral inflow jet
- A4c view
- a narrow color flow sector
- the gain setting to reduce the noise
- color flow baseline shifted below the Nyquist limit until the highest velocity becomes blue
- the slope method measures the slope of the line of the first aliasing velocity during early

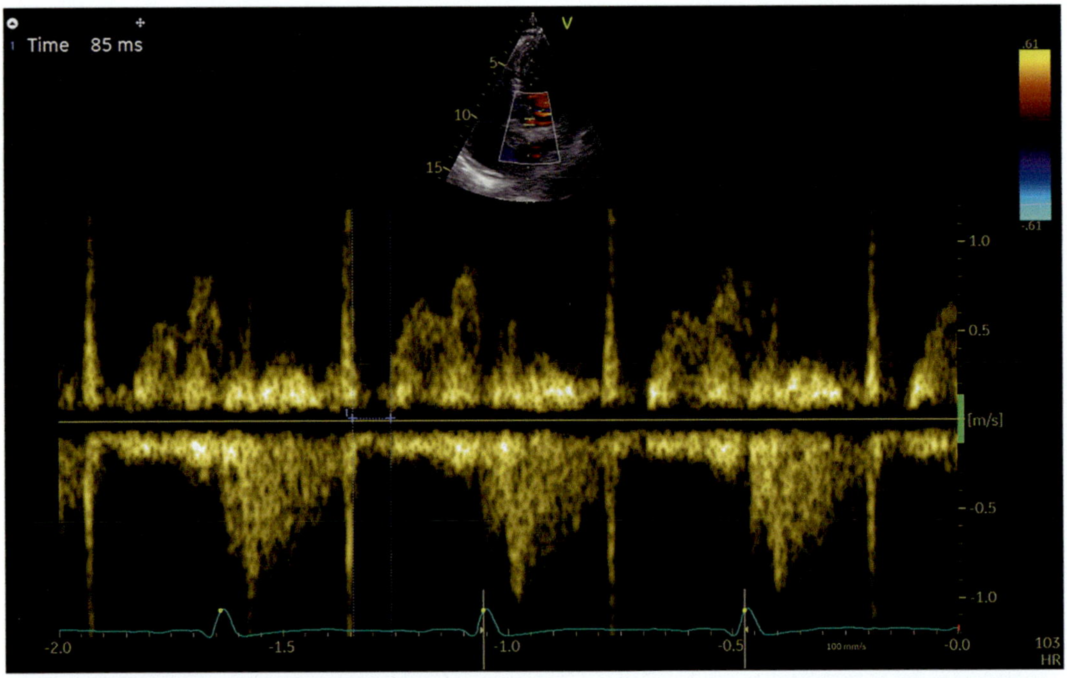

Fig. 3.8 Isovolumic relaxation time measurement by PW Doppler

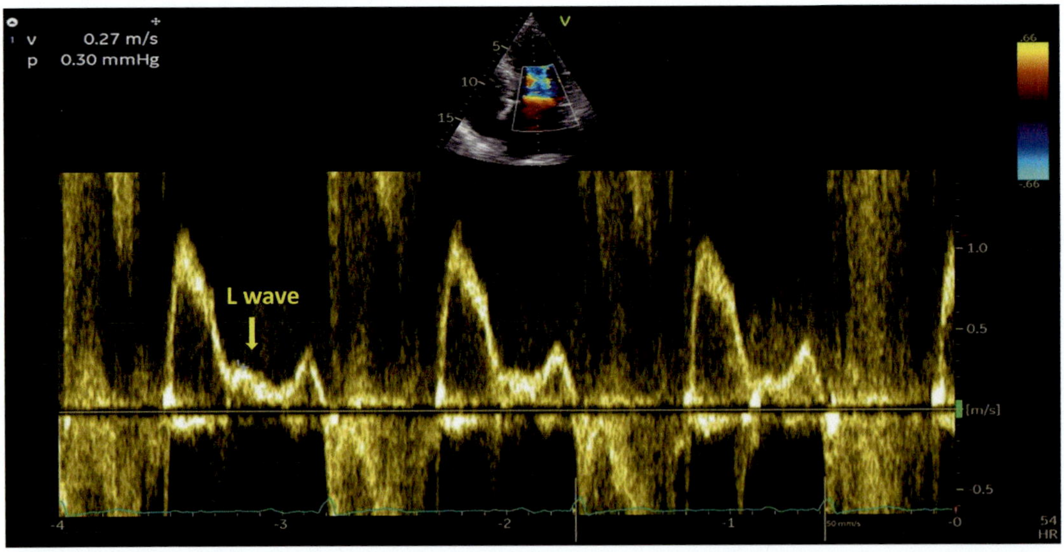

Fig. 3.9 L wave measurement during diastasis on mitral valve diastolic inflow in a patient with increased left ventricle filling pressure

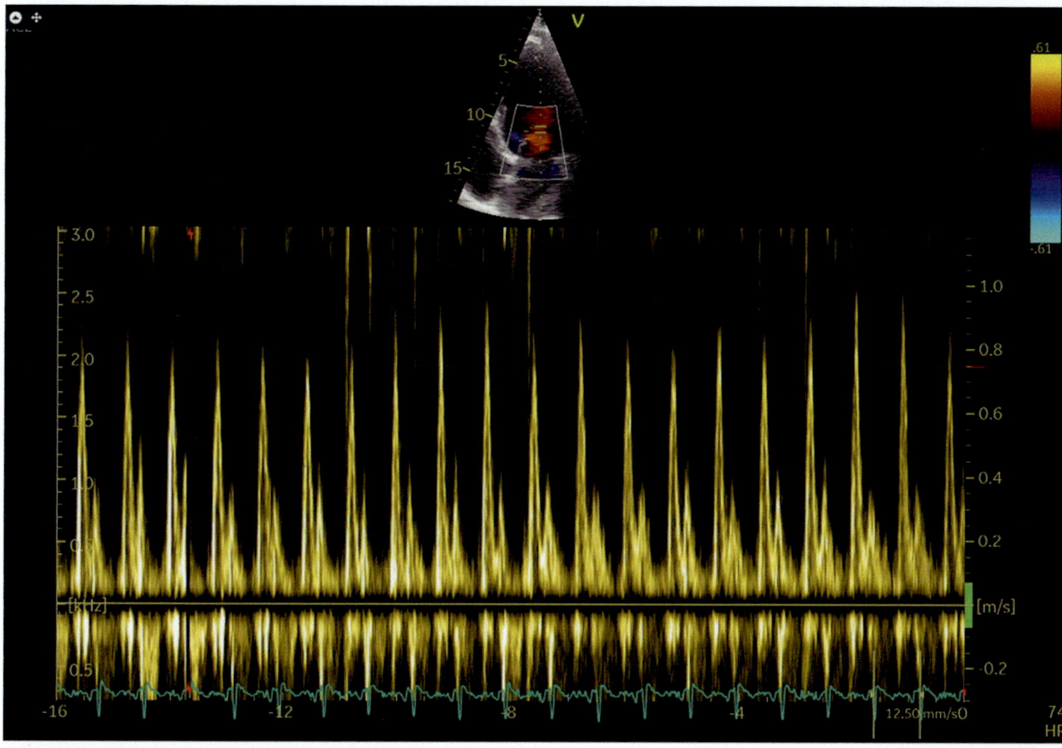

Fig. 3.10 Valsalva maneuver

filling, from the MV plane to approximately 4 cm distal into the LV cavity (Fig. 3.11) Normal Vp value is>55 cm/s(Xiao et al. 1992) (Fig. 3.5)

- E/vp ratio estimates LV filling pressure (Kossaify and Nasr 2019; Fukuta and Little 2008; Nagueh et al. 2016).

The initial step in diastolic function evaluation consists of the identification of the presence of DD by measuring *four parameters*: e′ (septal<7 cm/s, lateral e<10 cm/s), average E/e′ ratio>14, LA,>34 mL/m2, and peak TR velocity>2.8 m/s (Kossaify and Nasr 2019; Nagueh et al. 2016).

The second step is mitral inflow pattern identification (Kossaify and Nasr 2019; Nagueh et al. 2016).

The probability of normal diastolic function in patients with CRT or right ventricular (RV) pacing is low. Patients with a pacemaker (PM) or cardiac resynchronization therapy (CRT) usually present structural heart disease and we aspect of having some degree of DD. The approach in this situation is the second step: DD grading and filling pressure evaluation. According to the current guidelines, in patients with preserved LVEF, one should evaluate four variables: e′, E/e′ ratio, LAVI, and TRpV. If three are abnormal, there is DD; if two are abnormal and two are normal, the diastolic function cannot be assessed; and if three are normal, the diastolic function is normal (Nagueh et al. 2016). In patients with reduced LVEF or patients with normal LVEF but with myocardial disease, it is essential to DD grade and filling pressure estimate (Nagueh et al. 2016).

E/A ratio ≤ 0.8, and a peak E velocity ≤ 50 cm/s in patients with LVEF reduced and in patients with LVEF normal but with myocardial disease, represents grade I of DD (delayed relaxation), and LAP is normal (Nagueh et al. 2016) (Fig. 3.3). E/A ratio is>2 in patients with reduced LVEF and in patients with normal

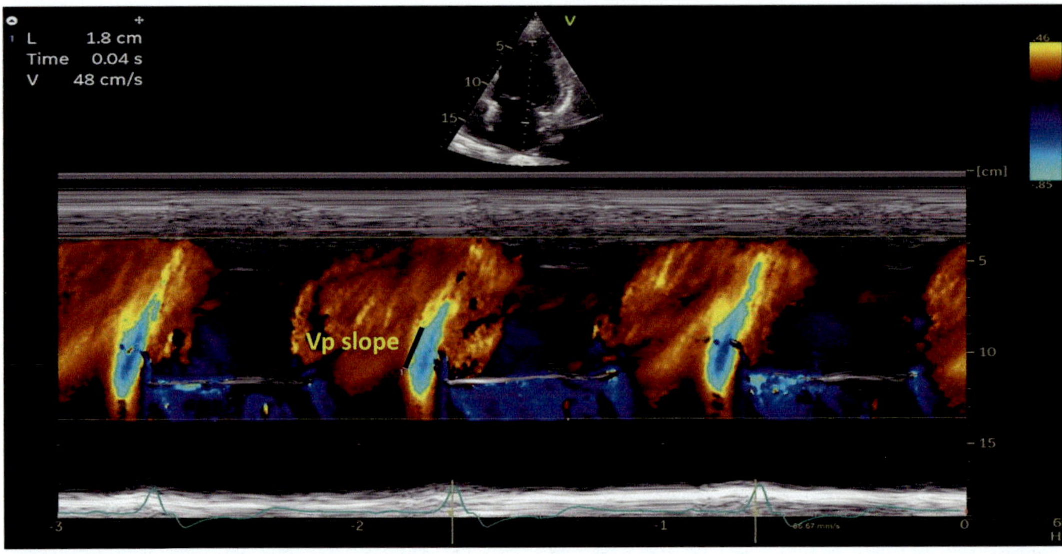

Fig. 3.11 Flow velocity propagation measurement by Color M-mode

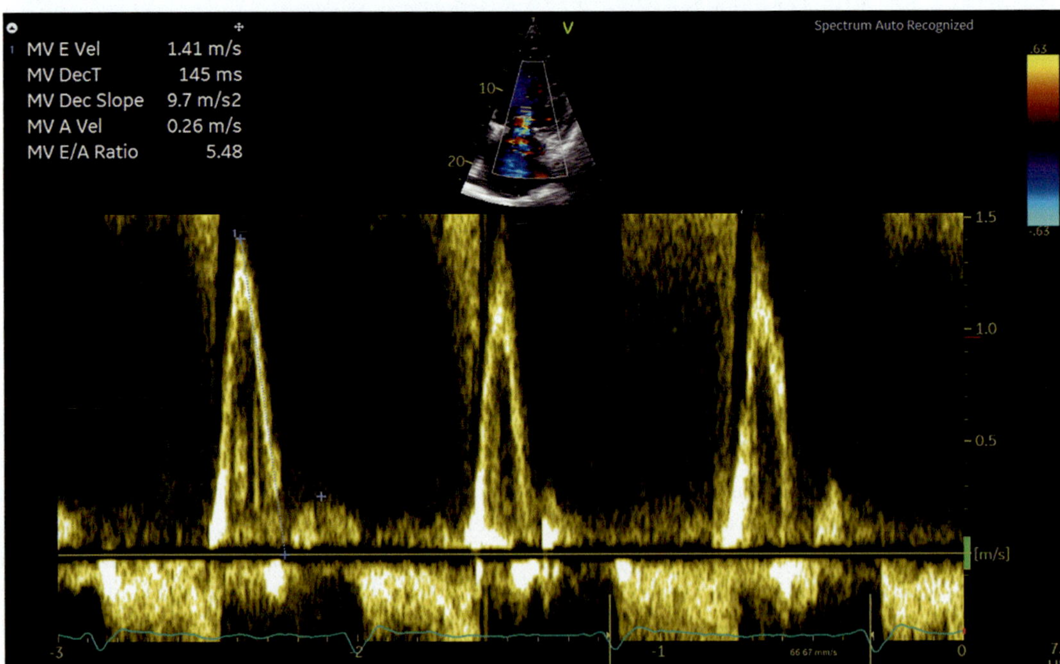

Fig. 3.12 Restrictive filling pattern of mitral valve diastolic inflow

LVEF but with myocardial disease, represents grade III of DD (restrictive) with decreased LV compliance and elevated filling pressures (Nagueh et al. 2016) (Fig. 3.12).

When E/A is>8 and E</50 cm/s, additional parameters will be used: average E/e′, TRpV, and LAVI. If two or three of these parameters are positive, DD is grade II, and filling pressures are

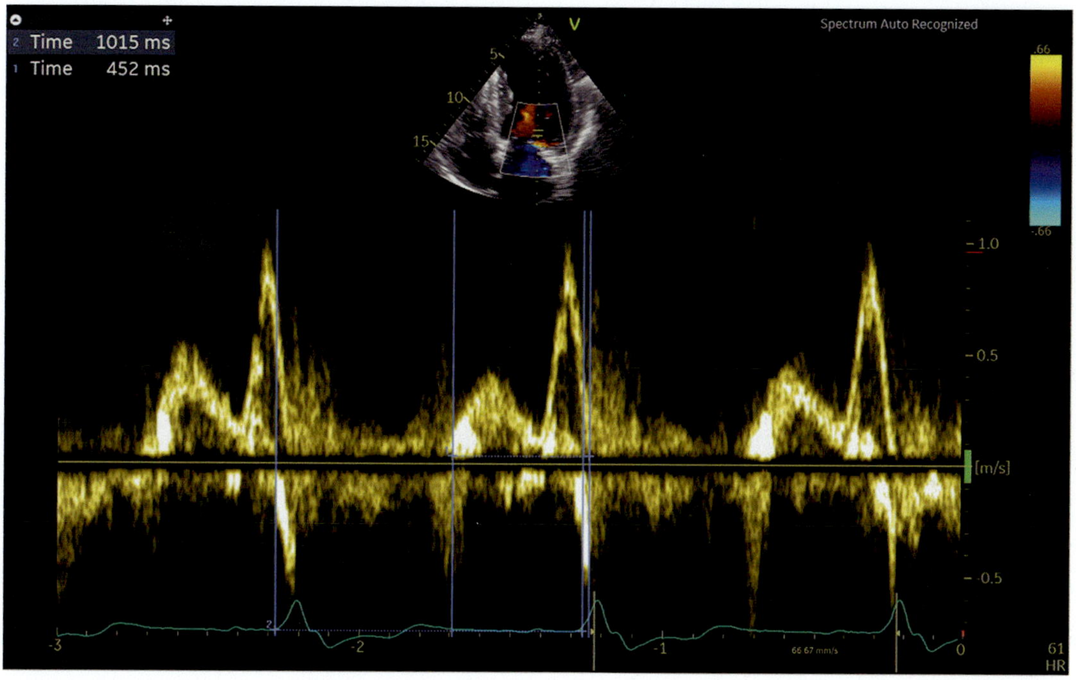

Fig. 3.13 Shortened early diastolic left ventricular filling in a patient with right ventricle lead

elevated; if two or three are negative, DD is grade I with normal filling pressure; if one is positive and one negative, pulmonary vein flow pattern will be evaluated if S/D < 1, DD is grade II with increased LV stiffness and filling pressure (Nagueh et al. 2016). In patients with reduced LVEF, a pulmonary vein S/D ratio may be used if one of the three main parameters is unavailable. A ratio < 1 reveals an increased LAP (Nagueh et al. 2016).

The more advanced diastolic dysfunction, the more increased LV filling pressure (Nagueh et al. 2009; Paulus et al. 2007). Because there are no specific indications for DD evaluation in patients with implanted devices, generally, the last guidelines may be used mainly for grading DD, considering the accuracy of presented parameters in this situation. Compared with patients without intracardiac devices, patients with implanted devices will present some inconvenience in DD evaluation linked to dyssynchrony due to RV lead presence and atrioventricular interval optimization. Small studies on short and long-term patients with RV pacing and CRT provide some information about DD parameters in these patients.

Particularities of diastolic dysfunction parameters in patients with RV pacing and CRT

In the normal heart, sinus node depolarization arrives at the atrioventricular (AV) node at 200 ms. A properly timed atrial contraction contributes 25–30% of cardiac output. The electrical impulse travels through the specialized cardiac conduction system and activates both ventricles simultaneously.

Abnormities of the cardiac conduction system due to pacing, adversely affect AV synchrony and synchronous LV contraction and relaxation, altering both LV systolic and diastolic function, making the variables used to assess diastolic function less accurate (Nagueh et al. 2016). Diastolic phases depend on the electrical pattern of LV activation. QRS broadening in patients with RV pacing associates delayed activation and delayed septal inward motion, with post-ejection shortening. This process will result in delayed onset with shortened early diastolic LV filling (Xiao et al. 1992) (Fig. 3.13).

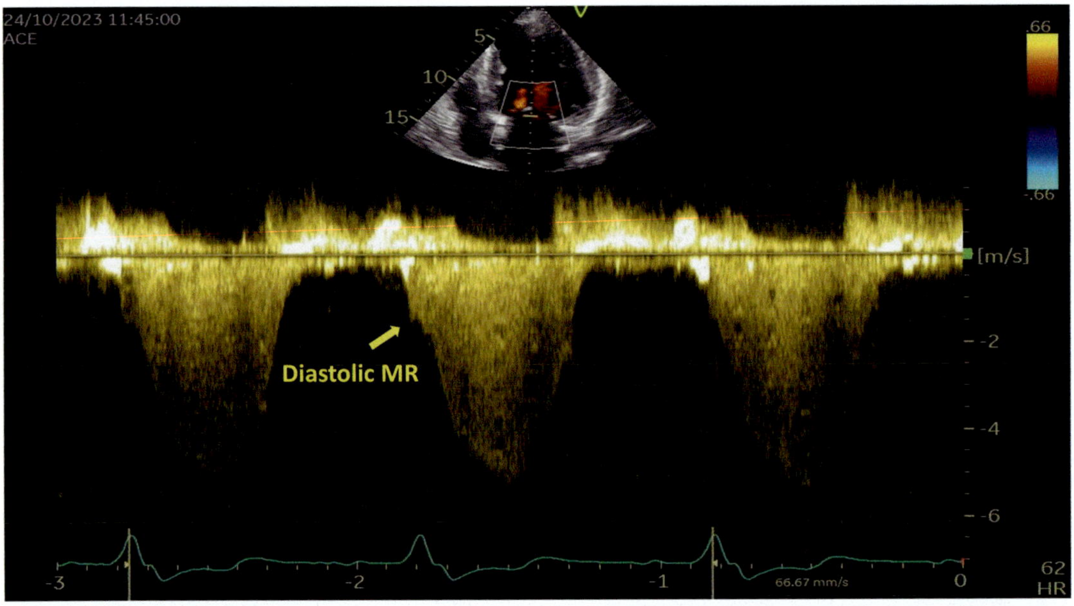

Fig. 3.14 Diastolic mitral regurgitation in a patient with a too-long atrioventricular delay

Chronic RV pacing induces LV dyssynchrony, reduction in LVEF, impaired LV filling and increased incidence of AF (Tops et al. 2006).

Patients with atrial pacing with rare RV pacing seem to have no alterations in systolic and diastolic function. In patients with AV delay, *a long AV delay* in pacemaker settings produces fusion or native QRS beats to minimize RV pacing. Sometimes these settings require a very long PR interval, followed by E and A velocities fusion and diastolic MR (Nagueh et al. 2016) (Fig. 3.14). In this situation, MV inflow and pv flow variables are inaccurate for diastolic function assessment and LVFP evaluation (Nagueh et al. 2016). The E/A ratio will not measure reliably diastolic function in patients with a paced rhythm (Nagueh et al. 2016). As long as no fusion of mitral E and A velocities occurs, the echocardiographic parameters recommended for the diastolic function and filling pressures evaluation remain valid in the pacing setting (Chan et al. 2023).

The accuracy of mitral annular velocities and E/e′ ratio are less in the presence of RV pacing and in patients who have received CRT (Nagueh et al. 2016; D'Souza et al. 2005).

LV dyssynchrony may suppress early diastolic filling in severe cases. If only mitral A velocity is present, only TR peak velocity (>2.8 m/s) can be used to indicate LV filling pressures (Nagueh et al. 2016).

Sub-optimal LA emptying increases cavity pressure and causes an enlarged left atrium with subsequent atrial arrhythmias (Henein and Lindqvist 2020). LAVI > 34 ml/m2 and TR peak velocity > 2.8 m/s remain applicable cut-off values for elevated LVFP estimation. LAVI may be less accurate in cases of reduced LVEF, and in these patients, LARS is recommended (Nagueh et al. 2016). Studies have shown that LA myocardial strain and strain rate plays an important role in estimating cavity pressure (Fig. 3.15). LA systolic strain < 19% is a very accurate marker for estimating raised pulmonary capillary wedge pressure of > 15 mm (Henein and Lindqvist 2020). In patients with AF, E/e′, a short DT and an increased LA volume have diagnostic values for increased LA pressure (Henein and Lindqvist 2020).

In conclusion, the evaluation of diastolic function in the setting of implanted devices needs a specific approach because of the impact of conduction delay on the cardiac cycle phases.

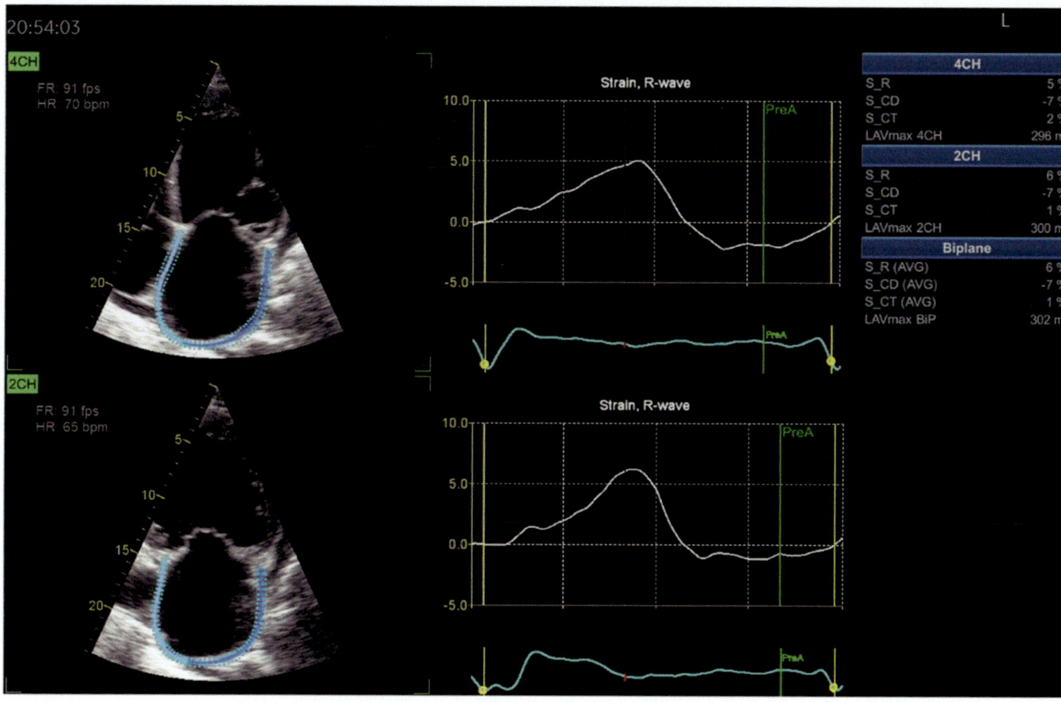

Fig. 3.15 Left atrium strain measurement by speckle tracking echocardiography

Electromechanical dyssynchrony impacts the atrial and ventricular filling mechanics, and the echocardiographic parameters used for the DD evaluation can be less accurate. The studies also revealed a reduced diastolic filling time in patients with ventricular pacing (Chan et al. 2023; Egnaczyk and Chung 2014).

Effect of RV pacing on DD

In patients with preserved EF, RVA pacing is associated with the deterioration of both LV diastolic and systolic functions, which is particularly obvious in those with pre-existing LV diastolic dysfunction and V-pace-induced systolic dyssynchrony (Fang et al. 2011).

The stimulation from a ventricular rather than supraventricular focus produces a reduced pulse pressure and prolongation of both isovolumetric contraction and systolic ejection time in normal hearts (Wiggers 1952). Consequently, the systolic function will influence the diastolic function (Xiao et al. 1992).

Electromechanical delay in systole owing to RVA pacing-induced LBBB pattern harms diastolic function, damaging early diastolic filling, and recoil (Yip et al. 2009). The negative effect of pacemaker stimulation on LV diastolic function is well-known (Wang et al. 2009; Ha and Oh 2009).

Pacemaker stimulation from the RV outflow tract (RVOT), but not in RV apex (RVA), leads to the progression of diastolic dysfunction in patients with preserved LVEF (Mitov et al. 2013). The LV dyssynchrony caused by RVA pacing slows LV relaxation and prolongs the isovolumetric relaxation time, which leads to decreased E′. The delayed LV relaxation and the increased LV filling pressure results in left atria compensatory contraction (Wang et al. 2009; Chiladakis et al. 2007).

Effects of CRT on DD

Studies have demonstrated discordant results in the improvement of LV diastolic dysfunction parameters parallel with reverse remodeling after CRT.

In the short term, CRT improved diastolic filling and lowered filling pressures in patients with an acute decrease in LV volumes and EF. The LA–LV pressure gradient (mitral E wave velocity) improved, the E/A ratio decreased, and the DT and LV DFT increased (Waggoner et al. 2005a). The improvement of E/e′ septal and E/vp velocity ratios confirmed that LV filling pressures decreased in patients with pseudonormalized or restrictive filling (Waggoner et al. 2005a). No significant changes in LV relaxation indices IVRT, E′, or vp velocities were obtained in acute states (Waggoner et al. 2005a). It is also possible that recovery of LV relaxation is delayed after CRT and was not evident in short-term follow-up studies of four months (Xiao et al. 1992; Waggoner et al. 2005b). Conversely, in some studies, only IVRT increased significantly (Shanks et al. 2011). The myocardial scar may reduce the beneficial effects of CRT on LV relaxation and LV filling pressures (Shanks et al. 2011).

Diastolic function improvement seems to depend on the LV filling patterns prior to CRT (Waggoner et al. 2005a). Significant changes in PWD-derived measurements of LV diastolic function after CRT were only observed for patients with a mitral E/A ratio > 1. Patients with pseudo normal and restrictive filling patterns decreased in E wave velocity and improved in indices of diastolic filling (E wave duration, DFT, and DT). Patients with a pre-CRT mitral E/A < 1.0 did not have changes in PWD-derived measurements of LV diastolic function (Waggoner et al. 2005a).

CRT increased DFT in the responder's group in all studies (Lau et al. 2000; Porcianai et al. 2000; Yu et al. 2002a, 2002b; St. John Sutton M, Plappert T, Abraham WT,, et al. 2003; Doltra, et al. 2013), but the effects on LV filling (E-wave, E/A ratio, and DT) have been variable in different studies (Ha and Oh 2009; Lau et al. 2000; Porcianai et al. 2000; Yu et al. 2002a, 2002b; St. John Sutton et al. 2003; Garrigue et al. 2001; Alksoy et al. 2010). Similarly, increases in mitral DT after CRT have been observed in some studies (Garrigue et al. 2001) but not in others (Porcianai et al. 2000; Yu et al. 2002a, 2002b; John Sutton et al. 2003) The increase in DT was observed in those patients with positive responses after CRT Alksoy et al. (2010). Some authors suggested that increases in DT after CRT may reflect improvements in LV compliance (Lisauskas et al. 2001; Myreng et al. 1990).

Parameters reflecting increased filling pressure: E/e′, E/vp, were observed at short-term follow-up (3 months) (Jansen et al. 2007) and 4 months follow-up (Waggoner et al. 2005a). Decreased filling pressures at long-term follow-up linked to LV reverse remodeling (Waggoner et al. 2005b; Jansen et al. 2007). Some studies suggest improvement in left ventricular (LV) filling pressures in responder patients (Doltra, et al. 2013), whereas in other studies, this effect was less clear (Saxon et al. 2002; Yu et al. 2006).

Part of the hemodynamic benefit induced by CRT may be obtained by optimization of cardiac time intervals. DFT increases after CRT (Waggoner et al. 2005a; John Sutton et al. 2003; Penicka et al. 2004) However, CRT's cardiac time interval optimization alone is insufficient to improve diastolic function (Jansen et al. 2007). As CRT reduces MR in patients with reverse remodeling, we expect an improved early LV relaxation, as determined by preload-independent parameters such as tissue Doppler E′ and color M-mode Vp (Jansen et al. 2007).

Using new DD parameters, some studies showed that neither relaxation parameters (E′ and SRivr) nor filling pressure parameters (E/E′ and E/SRIVR) showed statistically significant improvements (Shanks et al. 2011; Facchini et al. 2014). Other studies identified LV myocardial relaxation assessed with SRIVR and LV filling pressures assessed with E/SRIVR improving in the responder and the non-ischemic group (Shanks et al. 2011).

Researchers described a particular group of patients, most with ischemic cardiomyopathy and NYHA class IV of HF, without significant reverse remodeling but with a positive clinical response. This group showed a decrease in E wave velocity and an increase in DT values but nonsignificant improvement in the degree of DD, SPAP, E/A, S/D, and filling time (Doltra, et al. 2013). SPAP decreased at more than one year follow-up in patients with clinical and echocardiographic response and patients with the only clinical response at CRT, identifying a subgroup of patients with a better prognosis (Doltra et al. 2013).

The patients with favorable CRT response also present a decreased LA pressure and reverse atrial remodeling (Doltra, et al. 2013; Yancy et al. 2017).

Left atrium

In normal conditions, during the reservoir phase, which corresponds to LV synchronized longitudinal contraction, the LA wall stretches, and the blood enters from pv into the atria (Matsumoto et al. 2014). The blood passes from the LA to the LV during the conduit phase which corresponds to early ventricular diastole. The LA contractile pump assures 15% to 30% of the LV filling (Rosca et al. 2011) (Fig. 3.16). LA enlargement is a marker of the severity and chronicity of diastolic dysfunction and serves at LA pressure elevation (Tsang et al. 2002; Guron et al. 2005).

LA size should be measured at the end of LV systole, and end of ECG T wave when its volume is the largest (Lang et al. 2015). Dedicate acquisition, from A4ch and A2ch views, should provide the largest size of the LA base, avoiding foreshortening. This approach indicates that the imaging plane passes through the maximal short-axis area. With the biplane disk summation method, the lengths of the long axes measured in the two- and four-chamber views should be equal (Thomas et al. 2002). When tracing the borders of the left atrium, the confluences of the pulmonary veins, and the LA appendage should be excluded from the measurement. The atrioventricular interface should be represented by the mitral annulus plane (Lang et al. 2015) (Fig. 3.6).

3DE also provides some parameters of LA morphology and function, without geometric assumption, using automated quantification software (LAQ): volumes, ejection fraction, and strain during the reservoir, conduct, and contraction phase (Fig. 3.17). LA volume has a prognostic value in cardiac disease (Barnes et al. 2004; Beinart et al. 2004; Moller et al. 2003; Sabharwal et al. 2004; Gottdiener et al. 2006; Takemoto et al. 2005; Tsang et al. 2006).

Two-dimensional echocardiographic LA volumes are smaller compared with computed tomography or CMR (Maceira et al. 2010; Stojanovska et al. 2011; Ujino et al. 2006). Three-dimensional echocardiography LA volume correlates with cardiac computed tomography (Miyasaka et al. 2011; Rohner et al.

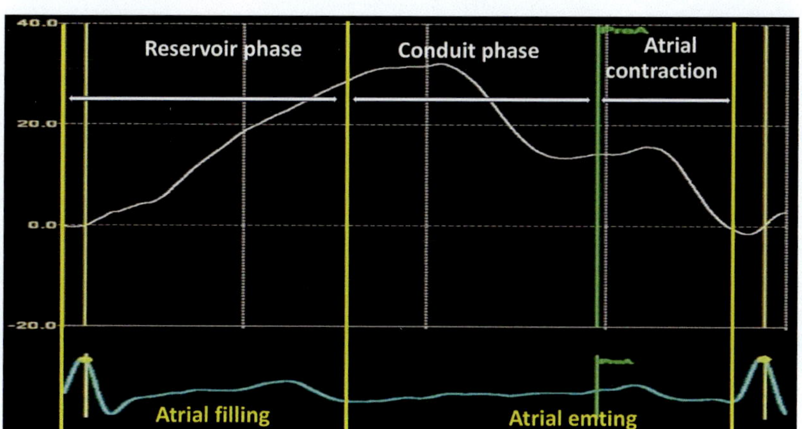

Fig. 3.16 Left atrium function

2011) and magnetic resonance imaging (Artang et al. 2009; Mor-Avi et al. 2012) and has superior prognostic value (Caselli et al. 2010; Suh et al. 2008). Three-dimensional echocardiographic LA volumes are larger than 2D echocardiographic volumes (Maddukuri et al. 2006) (Fig. 3.17).

Mechanisms of LA changes in HF patients:

- elevated LV filling pressures, which increase LA afterload
- impaired LA reservoir function (Dokuni et al. 2020)
- functional MR with additional volume overload on the thin-walled LA, leading to LA structural remodeling, (Dokuni et al. 2020) interstitial fibrosis of the atrial wall, and reduced LA compliance.
- LA electrical and structural remodeling with enhanced risk of atrial fibrillation (Stassen et al. 2022)

These abnormalities improved after CRT only in the responders' group (Dokuni et al. 2020). In CRT-responders reducing functional MR severity (Bijl et al. 2019), diastolic function improvement (Waggoner et al. 2005b; Jansen et al. 2007) may lead to LA reverse remodeling (Yu et al. 2007; Valzania et al. 2016). In 3 months, follow-up, E wave velocity reduction, and mitral inflow diastolic pattern optimization correlated with LAV volume decrease in CRT responders. This positive short-term LA volume response was followed by a positive response in long-term, at 30 months follow-up of LV volume and function. This observation suggested a link between LA remodeling and long-term LV reverse remodeling (Cho et al. 2020). In MADIT-CRT trial, CRT was associated with a significant reverse remodeling of LA (Kuperstein et al. 2014). The authors also observed an ineffective reverse LA remodeling after severe LA enlargement and suggested

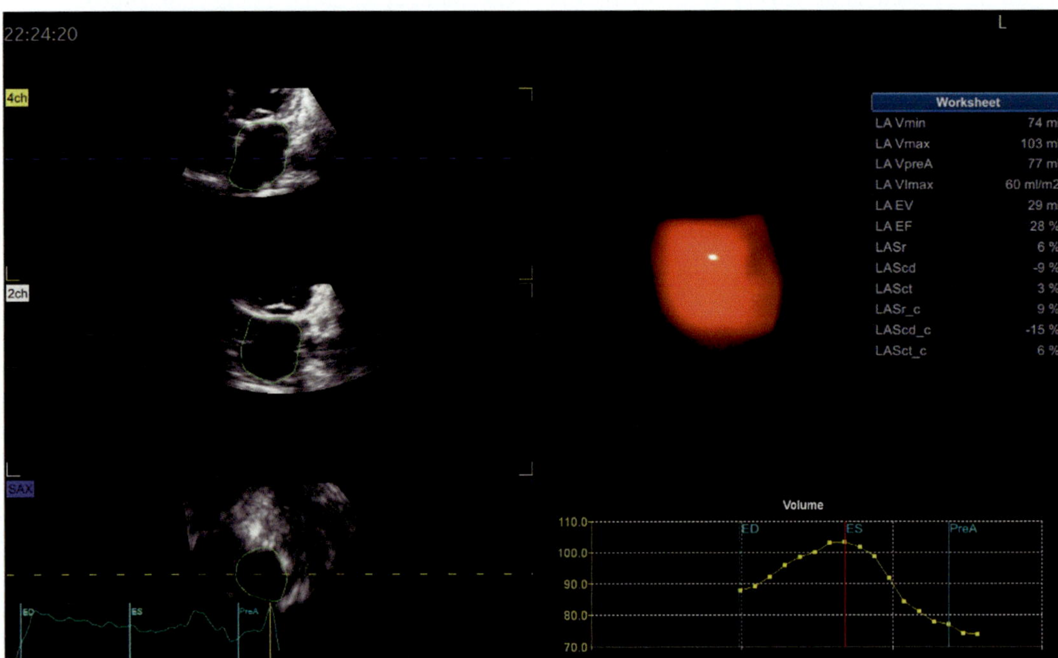

Fig. 3.17 Left atrium morphology and function evaluation by tridimensional echocardiography, using an automated quantification software

initiation of CRT at the appropriate time (Rossi et al. 2013). 6 months follow-up, CRT responders presented improvement in maximum LA area and volume and the LA emptying fraction (Donal et al. 2009). Other studies revealed both volumetric and LA functions in CRT responders (Yu et al. 2007; Valzania et al. 2016; Fung et al. 2008).

- In the CRT responders, LAA-EF increased, and LA size area and volume decreased before and after atrial systole (Yu et al. 2007) Novel markers.
- LARS is a functional parameter that correlates well with atrial fibrosis and LA compliance. Studies on speckle tracking in patients with CRT considered positive response a LARS increase>_5% at 6-month follow-up (Stassen et al. 2022) 3-months follow-up echocardiograms after CRT implantation revealed an increase in LARS (Bijl et al. 2019; Bouwmeester et al. 2022) LARS improved in CRT responders, parallel with LV systolic and diastolic function improvement (Dokuni et al. 2020).
- significant reduction in the risk of atrial arrhythmias (Brenyo et al. 2011).

In the MADIT-CRT study, reverse remodeling of the LA with CRT-D therapy was associated with a significant reduction in risk of subsequent AT (atrial fibrillation, atrial flutter, atrial tachycardia, and supraventricular tachyarrhythmias) in patients enrolled (Brenyo et al. 2011). LA mechanical dyssynchrony was defined as the maximal difference of time-to-peak strain (LA time-dif). Six months follow-up LA-GLS significantly improved, and LA time-dif was reduced in CRT responders (Dokuni et al. 2020).

The studies showed that CRT patients had impaired LA reservoir function, more pronounced as the QRS complex broadens. These observations sustain LV and LA dysfunction as an ideal candidate for CRT. In conditions with altered LA reservoir function associated with LV dyssynchrony, CRT might improve LV dyssynchrony and, subsequently, LA dyssynchrony (Dokuni et al. 2020).

3.1 Conclusions

The evaluation of diastolic function in the setting of implanted devices needs a specific approach because of the impact of conduction abnormalities on the cardiac cycle phases.

RVA pacing is usually associated with the deterioration of LV diastolic functions. The studies about CRT on DD response had variable results because of the criteria chosen for LVEF and LVV reverse remodeling, the method used for diastolic function evaluation, and the follow-up time.

Because of the tight correlation between systolic and diastolic function, a favorable effect of CRT on DD is expected in the responders' group.

References

AlksoyH, Okutucu S, Kaya EB, Deveci OS, Evranos B et al, Clinical and echocardiographic correlates of improvement in left ventricular diastolic function after cardiac resynchronization therapy Europace 2010;12:1256–1261.

Artang R, Migrino RQ, Harmann L, Bowers M, Woods TD. Left atrial volume measurement with automated border detection by 3-dimensional echocardiography: comparison with Magnetic Resonance Imaging. Cardiovasc Ultrasound. 2009;7:16.

Barnes ME, Miyasaka Y, Seward JB, Gersh BJ, Rosales AG, Bailey KR, et al. Left atrial volume in the prediction of first ischemic stroke in an elderly cohort without atrial fibrillation. Mayo Clin Proc. 2004;79:1008–14.

Beinart R, Boyko V, Schwammenthal E, Kuperstein R, Sagie A, Hod H, et al. Longterm prognostic significance of left atrial volume in acute myocardial infarction. J Am Coll Cardiol. 2004;44:327–34.

Bouwmeester S, Mast TP, Keulards DCJ, de Lepper AGW, Herold IHF, et al. Left atrial reverse remodeling predicts long-term survival after cardiac resynchronization therapy. J Echocardiography. 2022;20:115–23.

Brenyo A, Link MS, Barsheshet A, Moss AJ, Zareba W, Wang PJ et al. Cardiac resynchronization therapy reduces left atrial volume and the risk of atrial tachyarrhythmias in MADIT-CRT (Multicenter Automatic Defibrillator Implantation Trial with Cardiac Resynchronization Therapy). J Am Coll Cardiol. 2011;58:1682–9.Defibrillator Implantation Trial with Cardiac Resynchronization Therapy), J Am Coll Cardiol. 2011;58:1682–1689.

Brutsaert DL, Sys SU, Gillebert TC. Diastolic failure: pathophysiology and therapeutic implications. J Am Coll Cardiol. 1993;22:318–25.

Caselli S, Canali E, Foschi ML, Santini D, Di Angelantonio E, Pandian NG, et al. Longterm prognostic significance of three-dimensional echocardiographic parameters of the left ventricle and left atrium. Eur J Echocardiogr. 2010;11:250–6.

Chan N, Wang TKM, Anthony C, Hassan OA, Chetrit M, et al. Echocardiographic evaluation of diastolic function in special populations. Am J Cardiol. 2023;202:131–43.

Chiladakis JA, Koutsogiannis N, Kalogeropoulos A, et al. Unfavourable effects of continuous, atrial-synchronised ventricular pacing on ventricular systolic and diastolic function in patients with normal left ventricular EjectionFraction: usefulness of tissue and colour doppler echocardiography. Hellenic J Cardiol. 2007;48:335–40.

Cho I-J, Uhm J-S, Oh J, Nam J-H, Yu HT, et al. Left ventricular response after cardiac resynchronization therapy is related to early left atrial volume reduction. Korean J Intern Med. 2020;35:1125–35.

D'Souza KA, Mooney DJ, Russell AE, MacIsaac AI, Aylward PE, Prior DL. Abnormal septal motion affects early diastolic velocities at the septal and lateral mitral annulus, and impacts on estimation of the pulmonary capillary wedge pressure. J Am Soc Echocardiogr. 2005;18:445–53.

Dokuni K, Matsumoto K, Tatsumi K, et al. Cardiac resynchronization therapy improves left atrial reservoir function through resynchronization of the left atrium in patients with heart failure with reduced ejection fraction. Int J Cardiovasc Imaging. 2020;36:1203–2121.

Doltra A, Bart Bijnens B, Tosolana JM, Gabrielli L, Castel MA, et al. Effect of cardiac resynchronization therapy on left ventricular diastolic function: implications for clinical outcome. J Cardiac Fail 2013;19:795–801.

Donal E, Kannika Tan, Christophe Leclercq C, Ollivier R, Genevieve Derumeaux G. et al. Left atrial reverse remodeling and cardiac resynchronization therapy for chronic heart failure patients in sinus Rhythm. J Am Soc Echocardiogr 2009;22:1152–8.

Egnaczyk GF, Chung ES. The Relationship between cardiac resynchronization therapy and diastolic function. Curr Heart Fail Rep. 2014;11:64–9.

Facchini E, Varalda M, Sartori C, Burkhoff D, Marino PN. Systolic heart failure and cardiac resynchronization therapy: a focus on diastole. Int J Cardiovasc Imaging. 2014;30:897–905.

Fang F, Zhang O, Chan JYS, Xie J-M, Fung JWH, et al. Deleterious effect of right ventricular apical pacing on left ventricular diastolic function and the impact of pre-existing diastolic disease. Eur Heart J. 2011;32:1891–9.

Fukuta H, Little WC. The cardiac cycle and the physiological basis of left ventricular contraction. Ejection, Relaxation, and Filling, Heart Fail Clin. 2008;4(1):1–11.

Fung JW, Yip GW, Zhang Q, Fang F, Chan JY, Li CM, Wu LW, Chan GC, Chan HC, Yu CM. Improvement of left atrial function is associated with lower incidence of atrial fbrillation and mortality after cardiac resynchronization therapy. Heart Rhythm. 2008;5:780–6.

Garrigue S, Jais P, Espil G, et al. Comparisons of chronic biventricular pacing between epicardial and endocardial left ventricular stimulation using Doppler tissue imaging in patients with heart failure. Am J Cardiol. 2001;88:858–62.

Gottdiener JS, Kitzman DW, Aurigemma GP, Arnold AM, Manolio TA. Left atrial volume, geometry, and function in systolic and diastolic heart failure of persons >= 65 years of age (The Cardiovascular Health Study). Am J Cardiol. 2006;97:83–9.

Guron CW, Hartford M, Rosengren A, Thelle D, Wallentin I, Caidahl K. Usefulness of atrial size inequality as an indicator of abnormal left ventricular filling. Am J Cardiol. 2005;95:1448–52.

Ha JW, Oh JK. Therapeutic strategies for diastolic dysfunction: a clinical perspective. J Cardiovasc Ultrasound. 2009;17:86–95.

Henein MY, Lindqvist P. Diastolic function assessment by echocardiography: a practical manual for clinical use and future applications. Echocardiography. 2020;37:1908–18.

Jansen AHM, van Dantzig JM, Bracke F, Peels KH, Koolen JJ, et al. Improvement in diastolic function and left ventricular filling pressure induced by cardiac resynchronization therapy. Am Heart J. 2007;153:84329.

Kossaify A, comNasr M. Diastolic dysfunction and the new recommendations for echocardiographic assessment of left ventricular diastolic function: summary of guidelines and novelties in diagnosis and grading. J Diagn Med Sonogr. 2019;35(4):317–25.

Kossaify A, Nasr M. Diastolic dysfunction and the new recommendations for echocardiographic assessment of left ventricular diastolic function: Summary of guidelines and novelties in diagnosis and grading. J Diagnostic Med Sonography. 2019;354:317–25.

Kuperstein R, Goldenberg I, Moss AJ, Solomon S, Bourgoun M, Shah A, McNitt S, Zareba W, Klempfner R. Left atrial volume and the benefit of cardiac resynchronization therapy in the MADIT-CRT trial. Circ Heart Fail. 2014;7:154–60.

Lang RM, Badano LP, Mor-Avi V, et al. Recommendations for cardiac chamber quantification by echocardiography in adults: an update from the American society of echocardiography and the european association of cardiovascular imaging. Europ Heart J Cardiovascular Imaging. 2015;16:233–71.

Lau CP, Yu CM, Chau E, et al. Reversal of left ventricular remodeling by synchronous biventricular pacing in heart failure. Pacing Clin Electrophysiol. 2000;23:1722–5.

Lisauskas JB, Singh J, Bowman AW, Kovacs SJ. Chamber properties from transmitral flow: prediction of average and passive left ventricular diastolic stiffness. J Appl Physiol. 2001;91:154–62.

Maceira AM, Cosin-Sales J, Roughton M, Prasad SK, Pennell DJ. Reference left atrial dimensions and volumes by steady state free precession cardiovascular magnetic resonance. J Cardiovasc Magn Reson. 2010;12:65.

Maddukuri PV, Vieira ML, DeCastro S, et al. What is the best approach for the assessment of left atrial size? Comparison of various unidimensional and two-dimensional parameters with three-dimensional echocardiographically determined left atrial volume. J Am Soc Echocardiogr. 2006;19:1026–32.

Matsumoto K, Tanaka H, Imanishi J, et al. Preliminary observations of prognostic value of left atrial functional reserve during dobutamine infusion in patients with dilated cardiomyopathy. J Am Soc Echocardiogr. 2014;27:430–9.

Mitov V, Perišić Z, Jolić A, Adamović D, Zastranović L, et al. The effect of right ventricle pacemaker lead position on diastolic function in patients with preserved left ventricle ejection fraction. Hell J Nucl Med. 2013;16(3):204–8.

Miyasaka Y, Tsujimoto S, Maeba H, Yuasa F, Takehana K, Dote K, et al. Left atrial volume by real-time three-dimensional echocardiography: validation by 64-slice multidetector computed tomography. J Am Soc Echocardiogr. 2011;24:680–6.

Moller JE, Hillis GS, Oh JK, Seward JB, Reeder GS, Wright RS et al. Left atrial volume—A powerful predictor of survival after acute myocardial infarction. Circulation 2003;107:2207–12.

Mor-Avi V, Yodwut C, Jenkins C, Kuhl H, Nesser HJ, Marwick TH, et al. Real-time 3D echocardiographic quantification of left atrial volume: multicenter study for validation with CMR. JACC Cardiovasc Imaging. 2012;5:769–77.

Myreng Y, Smiseth OA, Risoe C. Left ventricular filling at elevated diastolic pressures: relationship between transmitral Doppler flow velocities and atrial contribution. Am Heart J. 1990;119:620–6.

Nagueh SF, Appleton CP, Gillebert TC, et al. Recommendations for the evaluation of left ventricular diastolic function by echocardiography. J Am Soc Echocardiogr. 2009;22:107–33.

Nagueh SF, Smiseth OA, Appleton CP, Byrd BF, Dokainish H, et al. Recommendations for the evaluation of left ventricular diastolic function by echocardiography: an update from the American society of echocardiography and the European association of cardiovascular imaging. J Am Soc Echocardiogr. 2016;29:277–314.

Paulus WJ, Tschope C, Sanderson JE, et al. How to diagnose diastolic heart failure: a consensus statement on the diagnosis of heart failure with normal left ventricular ejection fraction by the heart failure and echocardiography associations of the European society of cardiology. Eur Heart J. 2007;28:2539–50.

Penicka M, Bartunek J, De Bruyne B, et al. Improvement of left ventricular function after cardiac resynchronization therapy is predicted by tissue Doppler imaging echocardiography. Circulation. 2004;109:978–83.

Popović ZB, Sato K, Desai MY. Is universal grading of diastolic function by echocardiography feasible? Cardiovasc Diagn Ther. 2018;8(1):18–28.

Porcianai MC, Puglisi A, Colella A, et al. Echocardiographic evaluation of the effect of biventricular pacing: the In-Sync Italian Registry. Eur Heart J 2000;(Suppl) J:J23–30.

Rohner A, Brinkert M, Kawel N, Buechel RR, Leibundgut G, Grize L, et al. Functional assessment of the left atrium by real-time three-dimensional echocardiography using a novel dedicated analysis tool: initial validation studies in comparison with computed tomography. Eur J Echocardiogr. 2011;12:497–505.

Rosca M, Lancellotti P, Popescu BA, Pierard LA. Left atrial function: pathophysiology, echocardiographic assessment, and clinical applications. Heart. 2011;97:1982–9.

Rossi L, Malagoli A, Piepoli M, et al. Indexed maximal left atrial volume predicts response to cardiac resynchronization therapy. Int J Cardiol. 2013;168:3629–33.

Sabharwal N, Cemin R, Rajan K, Hickman M, Lahiri A, Senior R. Usefulness of left atrial volume as a predictor of mortality in patients with ischemic cardiomyopathy. Am J Cardiol. 2004;94:760–3.

Saxon LA, de Marco T, Schafer J, Chatterjee K, Kumar UN, Foster E. Effects of long-term biventricular stimulation for resynchronization on echocardiographic measures of remodeling. *Circulation* 2002;105:1304e10.

Schirmer H, Lunde P, Rasmussen K. Mitral flow derived Doppler indices of left ventricular diastolic function in a general population—The Tromso study. Eur Heart J. 2000;21:1376–86.

Shanks M, Antoni L, Hoke U, Bertini M, Ng ACT, et al. The effect of cardiac resynchronization therapy on left ventricular diastolic function assessed with speckle-tracking echocardiography. Eur J Heart Fail. 2011;13:1133–9.

St. John Sutton M, Plappert T, Abraham WT et al. Effect of cardiac resynchronization therapy on left ventricular size and function in chronic heart failure. Circulation 2003;107:1985–1990.

Stassen J, Galloo X, Chimed S, Hirasawa K, Marsan NA, et al. Clinical implications of left atrial reverse remodelling after cardiac resynchronization therapy. Europ Heart J- Cardiovascular Imaging. 2022;23:730–40.

Stojanovska J, Cronin P, Patel S, Gross BH, Oral H, Chughtai K, et al. Reference normal absolute and indexed values from ECG-Gated MDCT: left atrial volume, function, and diameter. Am J Roentgenol. 2011;197:631–7.

Suh IW, Song JM, Lee EY, Kang SH, Kim MJ, Kim JJ, et al. Left atrial volume measured by real-time 3-dimensional echocardiography predicts clinical outcomes in patients with severe left ventricular dysfunction and in sinus rhythm. J Am Soc Echocardiogr. 2008;21:439–45.

Takemoto Y, Barnes ME, Seward JB, Lester SJ, Appleton CA, Gersh BJ, et al. Usefulness of left atrial volume in predicting first congestive heart failure in patients >= 65 years of age with well-preserved left ventricular systolic function. Am J Cardiol. 2005;96:832–6.

Thomas JD, Newell JB, Choong CY, et al. Physical and physiological determinants of transmitral velocity: numerical analysis. Am J Physiol. 1991;260:H1718–31.

Thomas JD, Zhou J, Greenberg N, et al. Physical and physiological determinants of pulmonary venous flow: numerical analysis. Am J Physiol. 1997;272:H2453–65.

Thomas L, Levett K, Boyd A, Leung DYC, Schiller NB, Ross DL. Compensatory changes in atrial volumes with normal aging: Is atrial enlargement inevitable? J Am Coll Cardiol. 2002;40:1630–5.

Tops LF, Schalij MJ, Holman ER, van Erven L, van der Wall EE, Bax JJ. Right ventricular pacing can induce ventricular dyssynchrony in patients with atrial fibrillation after atrioventricular node ablation. J Am Coll Cardiol. 2006;48:1642–8.

Tsang TSM, Barnes ME, Gersh BJ, Bailey KR, Seward JB. Left atrial volume as a morphophysiologic expression of left ventricular diastolic dysfunction and relation to cardiovascular risk burden. Am J Cardiol. 2002;90:1284–9.

Tsang TS, Abhayaratna WP, Barnes ME, Miyasaka Y, Gersh BJ, Bailey KR, et al. Prediction of cardiovascular outcomes with left atrial size—is volume superior to area or diameter? J Am Coll Cardiol. 2006;47:1018–102.

Ujino K, Barnes ME, Cha SS, Langins AP, Bailey KR, Seward JB, et al. Two-dimensional echocardiographic methods for assessment of left atrial volume. Am J Cardiol. 2006;98:1185–8.

Valzania C, Gadler F, Boriani G, Rapezzi C, Eriksson MJ. Effect of cardiac resynchronization therapy on left atrial size and function as expressed by speckle tracking 2-dimensional strain. Am J Cardiol. 2016;118:237–43.

van der Bijl P, Khidir M, Ajmone Marsan N, Delgado V, Leon MB, Stone GW, et al. Effect of functional mitral regurgitation on outcome in patients receiving cardiac resynchronization therapy for heart failure. Am J Cardiol. 2019;123:75–83.

Waggoner AD, Bierig SM. Tissue Doppler imaging: a useful echocardiographic method for the cardiac sonographer to assess systolic and diastolic left ventricular function. J Am Soc Echocardiogr. 2001;14:1143–52.

Waggoner AD, Faddis MN, Gleva MJ, de Las FL, Osborn J, et al. Cardiac resynchronization therapy acutely improves diastolic function. J Am Soc Echocardiogr. 2005a;18:216–20.

Waggoner AD, Faddis MN, Gleva MJ, de las Fuentes L, Dávila-Román VG. Improvements in left ventricular diastolic function after cardiac resynchronization therapy are coupled to response in systolic performance. J Am Coll Cardiol. 2005;46:2244–9.

Wang YC, Lin YH, Iu YB. The immediate effects of pacemaker related electric remodelling on left ventricular function in patients with sick sinus syndrome. *Europace* 2009;11

Wiggers CJ. Dynamics of ventricle contraction under abnormal conditions. Circulation. 1952;5:321–48.

Xiao HB, Brecker SJ, Gibson DG. Effects of abnormal activation on the time course of the left ventricular pressure pulse in dilated cardiomyopathy. Br Heart J. 1992;68(4):403–7.

Yancy CW, Jessup M, Bozkurt B et al. ACC/AHA/HFSA focused update of the 2013 ACCF/AHA guideline for the management of heart failure: a report of the American College of Cardiology/American Heart Association task force on clinical practice guidelines and the Heart Failure Society of America. Circulation. 136:e137–61.

Yip GW, Frenneaux M, Sanderson JE. Heart failure with a normal ejection fraction: new developments. Heart. 2009;95:1549–52.

Yu C, Chau E, Sanderson JL, et al. Tissue Doppler echocardiographic evidence of reverse remodeling and improved synchronicity by simultaneously delaying regional contraction after biventricular pacing therapy in heart failure. Circulation. 2002a;105:438–45.

Yu C, Fung W, Lin H, Zhang Q, Sanderson JE, Lau C. Predictors of left ventricular reverse remodeling after cardiac resynchronization therapy for heart failure secondary to idiopathic dilated or ischemic cardiomyopathy. Am J Cardiol. 2002b;91:684–8.

Yu CM, Zhang Q, Yip GW et al. Are left ventricular diastolic function and diastolic asynchrony important determinants of response to cardiac resynchronization therapy? Am J Cardiol. 2006;98:1083e7.

Yu C-M, Fang F, Zhang Q, Yip GWK, Li CM, Chan JY-S et al. Improvement of atrial function and atrial reverse remodeling after cardiac resynchronization therapy for heart failure. J Am Coll Cardiol. 2007;50:778–785.

4 Lead Position Evaluation in Patients with Implanted Devices

Abstract

Patients with CRT have an epicardial lead for LV and two endocardial leads, one in the right ventricle and one in the right atrium. Patients with dual chamber pacemakers have an electrode in the right ventricle and another in the right atrium. Patients with a single-chamber pacemaker present a lead at the level of the right ventricle. Patients with ICD with or without pacemaker represent another category. Echocardiography is essential for right ventricle lead position identification, especially before a planned upgrade. In CRT patients, the lead must be implanted far from the fibrosis area and will be evaluated in non-responders. The right atrial lead position usually necessitates transesophageal echocardiography.

Patients with cardiac resynchronization therapy (CRT) have an epicardial lead for left ventricle (LV) and two endocardial leads, one in the right ventricle (RV) and one in the right atrium (RA). Patients with dual chamber pacemakers have an electrode in the RV and another in the RA. Patients with a single chamber pacemaker present a lead at the RV level. Another category of patients is those with implanted cardio defibrillator (ICD) with or without a pacemaker.

Echocardiography is an essential imaging tool for identifying lead positions in implanted patients (Kydd et al. 2012; Smiseth et al. 2012). Some studies indicated echocardiography in guiding RV septal lead deployment, but this approach is still under research. RV lead might be responsible for LV dyssynchrony in patients with a single or dual-chamber pacemaker. This group necessitates three- and six-month reevaluations after the implantation, using tissue Doppler and Speckle tracking echocardiography, to identify LV subclinical dysfunction or HF and decide the moment of CRT upgrading (Kydd et al. 2012; Smiseth et al. 2012).

Echocardiography in patients with CRT is essential in identifying the best site for a lead position.

- For LV lead—LV fibrosis and scar area identification
- LV area with the latest activation identification
- For the RV lead—the best-recommended position is at the septum level (Fig. 4.1, Supplementary material 1), avoiding the RV apex (Kydd et al. 2012) (Fig. 4.2, Supplementary material 2).

Supplementary Information The online version contains supplementary material available at https://doi.org/10.1007/978-3-031-64079-7_4.

D.-M. Toader, *Echocardiographic Evaluation of Patients with Implanted Devices*, https://doi.org/10.1007/978-3-031-64079-7_4

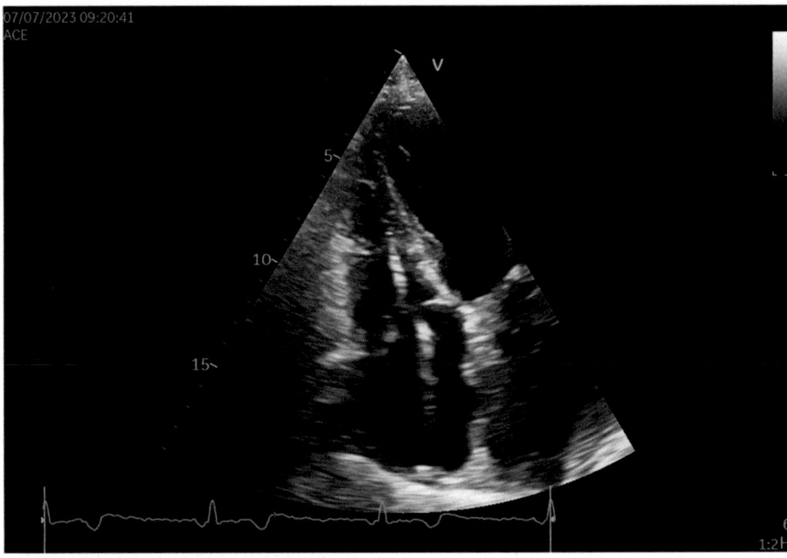

Fig. 4.1 Apical four-chamber view right ventricle focused in a patient with CRT and right ventricle lead at the septum level

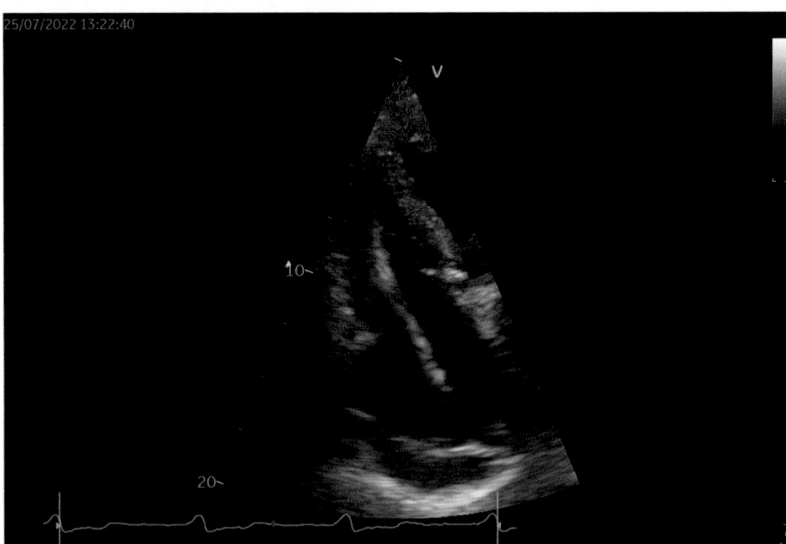

Fig. 4.2 Apical four-chamber view right ventricle focused in a patient with CRT and right ventricle lead at the apex

Echocardiography for LV lead positioning identifying in patients with CRT

Patients with typical left bundle branch block (LBBB) present an abnormal sequence of mechanical activation. The early septum contraction, named septal flush (Fig. 4.3, arrow 1), is concomitant with the passive stretch of the infero-lateral wall. (Fig. 4.3, arrow 2) This movement is followed by inferolateral wall contraction (Fig. 4.3, arrow 3) and is concomitant with passive septal stretch. (Fig. 4.3, arrow 4) This sequence of contraction results in apical rocking (Supplementary material 3) and an inefficient contraction (Kydd et al. 2012).

Mechanical dyssynchrony can be present because of coronary artery disease with

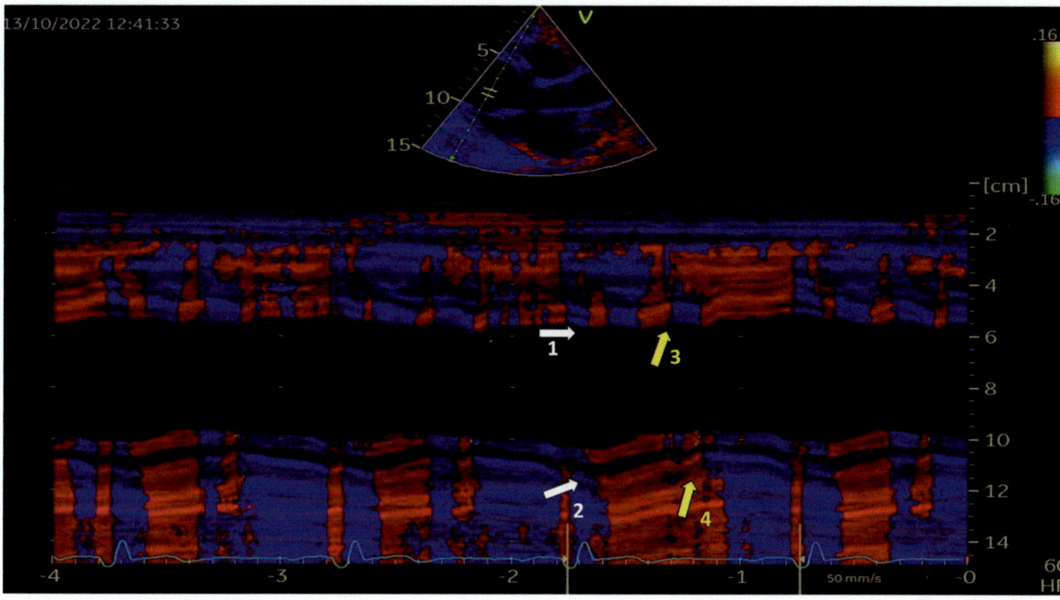

Fig. 4.3 Abnormal motion in a patient with dilated cardiomyopathy and left ventricle branch block: arrow 1: septal flush, arrow 2: concomitant with passive stretch of infero-lateral wall, arrow 3: infero-lateral wall contraction, arrow 4: concomitant with passive septal stretch

myocardial stunning or hibernation, scar, or fibrosis. (2) Intraventricular dyssynchrony produces abnormal LV loading, capable of metabolic changes that may exacerbate the syndrome of heart failure.(Chakir et al. 2008)

Correcting mechanical dyssynchrony is the key mechanism of benefit from CRT.(Kass 2009; Aiba et al. 2009; Gorcsan et al. 2012)

Depending on the coronary venous anatomy, the LV pacing lead is placed in an epicardial location via a transvenous approach (Kass 2009; Aiba et al. 2009). The optimum LV lead position is at the site of maximal mechanical dyssynchrony and away from the transmural scar (Ypenburg et al. 2007).

The LV lead position is an essential determinant of CRT response (Ypenburg et al. 2007; Khan et al. 2009; Thebault et al. 2012; Adelstein et al. 2014). For a good CRT response rate and survival benefit, optimal LV lead position must be achieved (Delgado et al. 2011). Pacing the segments with late contraction in patients with LBBB results in earlier electrical stimulation, an earlier mechanical activation, and an efficient LV contraction (Kydd et al. 2012). Important determinants of reverse remodeling after CRT are the extent of myocardial scar tissue and the position of the LV lead (Ypenburg et al. 2008).

Identification of LV Area of Scar

The presence of a large LV scar is a strong independent predictor of poor clinical outcome and lack of CRT response. Identifying the presence and localization of the scar area is essential because patients with ischemic heart disease have a poor response to CRT (Delgado et al. 2011; Ypenburg et al. 2008).

LV systolic strain measured by speckle tracking echocardiography (STE) is an imaging technique useful for areas of scar identification (Delgado et al. 2011; Bleeker et al. 2006; Becker et al. 2011). The scar position is also important in CRT response prediction (Becker et al. 2006; Shanks et al. 2011; Molhoek et al. 2004).

This method uses offline analysis by frame-by-frame tracking of speckles within the myocardium (Suffoletto et al. 2006; Voight et al. 2015). The semi-automated process requires the manual definition of the myocardium. The region of interest must incorporate the total thickness of the myocardial wall. After tracking results, the time-strain curve (Fig. 4.4). Strain describes the deformation or fractional change in the length of a myocardial segment and is expressed as percentages. Strain is positive when it reflects the lengthening or thickening and is negative when it reflects the shortening or thinning. (Fig. 4.5) The strain rate describes the speed of deformation (Suffoletto et al. 2006; Voight et al. 2015) (Fig. 4.6).

Echocardiographic reverse remodeling is significant in patients with nonischemic heart failure. (Woo et al. 2005) Pacing an LV segment containing transmural scar is associated with higher mortality, hospital admissions for heart failure, and reduced LV reverse remodeling (Ypenburg et al. 2007; Khan et al. 2009; Bleeker et al. 2006; Wikstrom et al. 2009; Ghio et al. 2009).

The precise mechanisms underlying scar formation in patients without coronary artery disease are unclear, although distinct patterns are recognized. The scar pattern is subendocardial or transmural in patients with coronary artery disease. The scar is located in the midwall or subepicardium in patients with nonischemic cardiomyopathies. The impact of patterns of fibrosis on outcomes in CRT is not yet established (Kydd et al. 2012).

High values of the peak strain identify viability in animal models (Popovic et al. 2007; Adelstein and Saba 2007). In patients with prior myocardial infarction, with preserved ejection fraction, segmental longitudinal strain identified a cutoff value of −13% for transmural infarction (sensitivity 80%; specificity 83% Gjesdal et al. 2007; Duckett et al. 2012) Exercise-related changes in longitudinal strain may indicate the presence of contractile reserve and therefore predict reverse remodeling following CRT but studies to demonstrate this approach are awaited (Lancellotti et al. 2009; Becker et al. 2009).

The two-dimensional (2D) circumferential and radial strain has also been used to identify segments with a transmural scar and predict

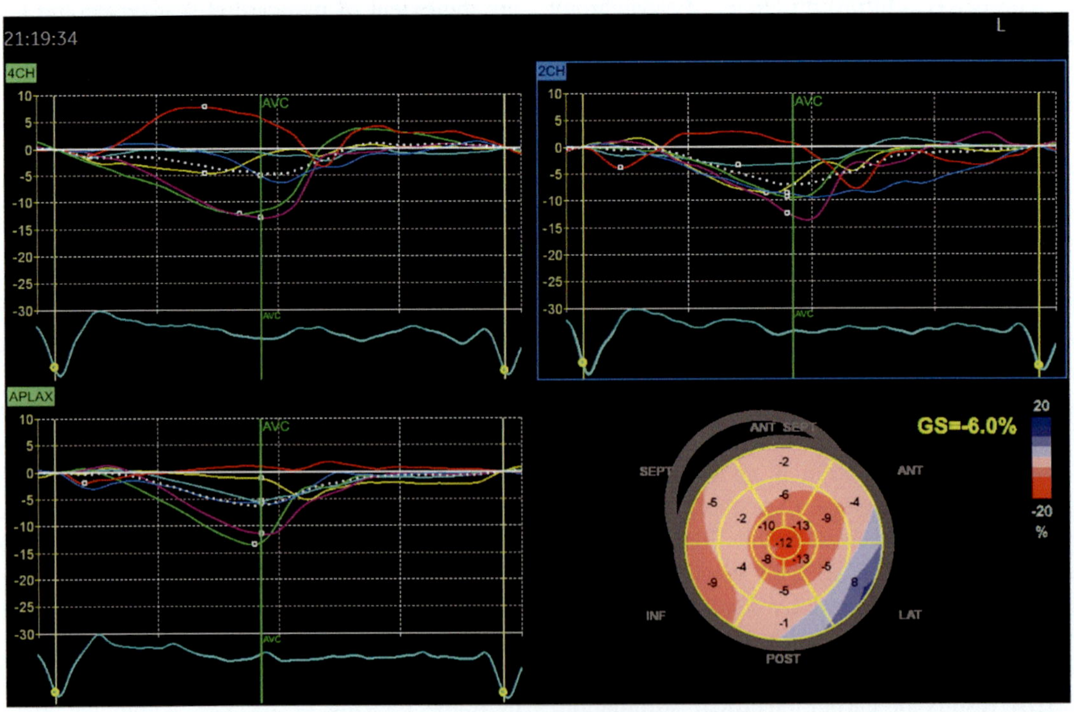

Fig. 4.4 Bullseye display representation obtained by speckle tracking echocardiography: posterolateral scar (blue) in a patient with dilated cardiomyopathy, CRT, and posterolateral old myocardial infarction

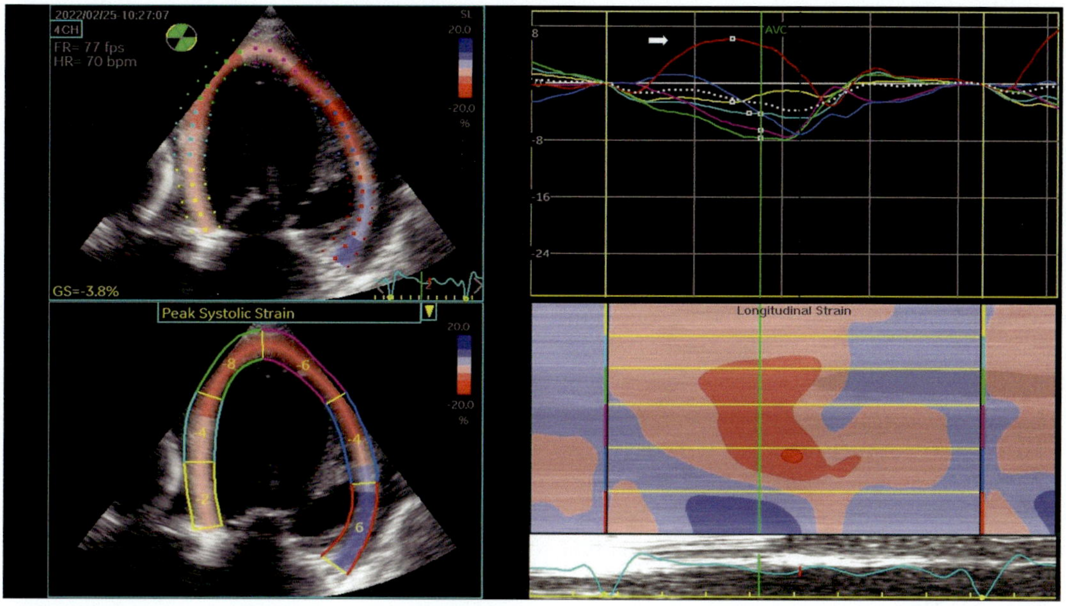

Fig. 4.5 Longitudinal strain obtained with 2D speckle tracking echocardiography in apical four-chamber view in a patient with dilated cardiomyopathy and CRT; dyssynchronous aspect of the red curve, which corresponds to the anterolateral basal segment of the left ventricle. (arrow)

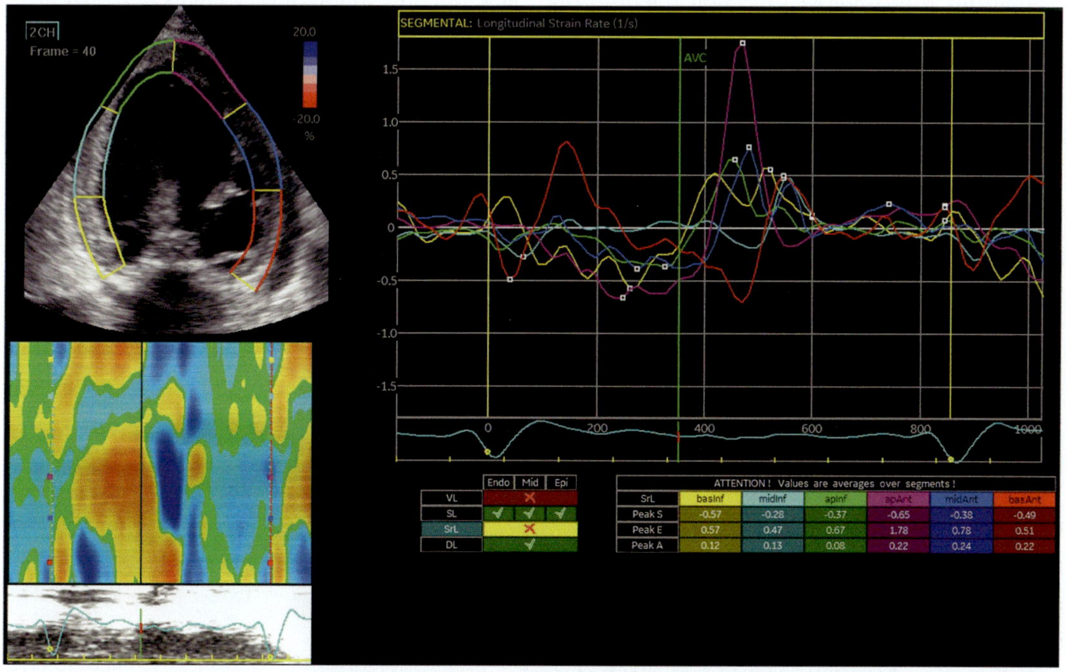

Fig. 4.6 Strain rate obtained with 2D speckle tracking echocardiography in apical four-chamber view of a patient with dilated cardiomyopathy and CRT

CRT outcome (Kydd et al. 2012) (Fig. 4.7). The placement of LV lead away from segments of scar, identified by low amplitude **radial strain**, has a positive impact on LV remodeling following CRT (Kydd et al. 2012). A regional radial strain < 5% (Delgado et al. 2011; Bleeker et al. 2006; Becker et al. 2011) and a peak systolic radial strain < 16.5% (Delgado et al. 2011) by speckle tracking echocardiography identifies the presence of a myocardial scar and may help the lead placement away from this area (Delgado et al. 2011; Bleeker et al. 2006; Becker et al. 2011, 2006).

With **three-dimensional (3D) STE,** the deformation or strain can be performed in multiple planes, and all the segments can be assessed simultaneously with single-beat acquisition, without beat-to-beat variability or out-of-plane motion, with the sequential assessment of basal, mid, and apical regions (Nesser et al. 2009; Bordachar et al. 2010) (Fig. 4.8).

A greater scar density in segments immediately adjacent to the LV lead tip has an inverse relationship with improved ejection fraction following CRT (Adelstein and Saba 2007; Becker et al. 2007). The septal scar in patients with ischemic cardiomyopathy is associated with a poor response to CRT, both acutely and at six months (Duckett et al. 2012; Boogers et al. 2011).

Peak radial strain imaging at the mid myocardial level in ischemic and nonischemic HF patients > 9.8% indicates the absence of transmural scar. Guided lead placement to either targeted or adjacent segments is followed by a positive response to CRT, a 15% reduction in LV end-systolic volumes, improved functional class, and reduced mortality or heart failure hospitalization (Khan et al. 2009).

Circumferential strain may offer an alternative to radial strain in patients with significant scar. The utility of speckle tracking to guide CRT is still under research (Kydd et al. 2012). In patients with ischemic disease, the epicardial circumferential strain could distinguish transmural from nontransmural scar better than full-thickness circumferential strain (Becker et al. 2009; Singh et al. 2011) (Fig. 4.9) Peak systolic circumferential strain > −11.1% by STE identified transmural scar for the LV lead position. The absence of transmural scar at the LV lead position resulted in significantly greater LV, reverse remodeling, and functional improvement at 12 months follow-up (Delgado et al. 2011).

The pacing of a scarred area produces an electrical capture, and similar sensing and pacing thresholds may be present in patients with and without scar but without mechanical capture and myocardial thickening. This is followed

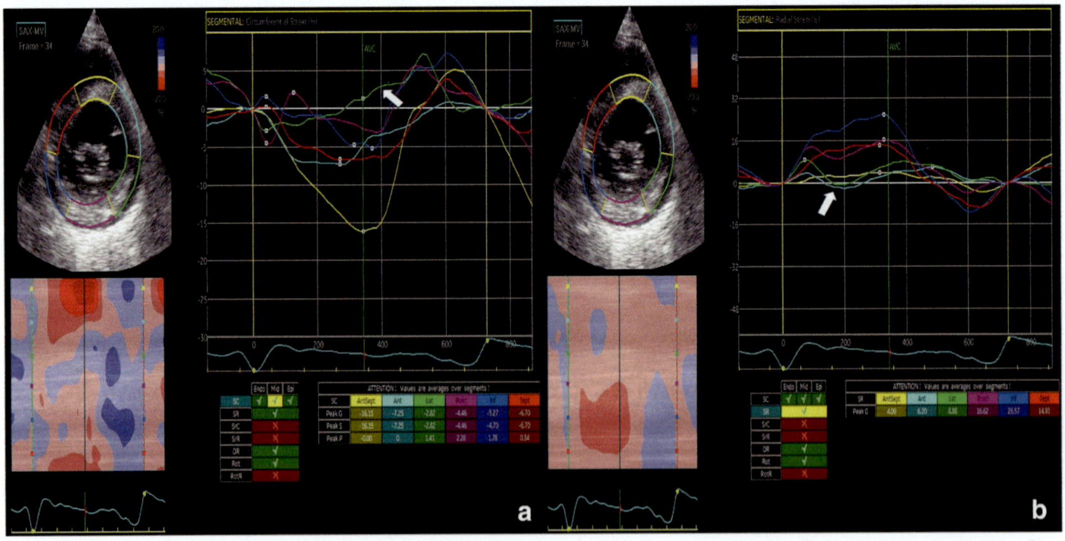

Fig. 4.7 Abnormal curves of CS (**a**) and RS (**b**) in a patient with old lateral infarction and CRT. (arrows)

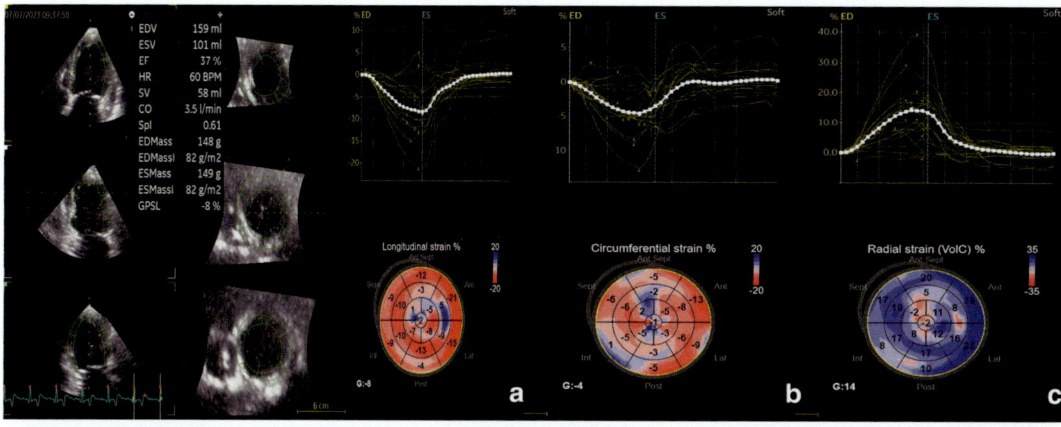

Fig. 4.8 3D echocardiography strain measurement: longitudinal strain (**a**), circumferential strain (**b**), radial strain (**c**), in a patient with dilated cardiomyopathy and CRT

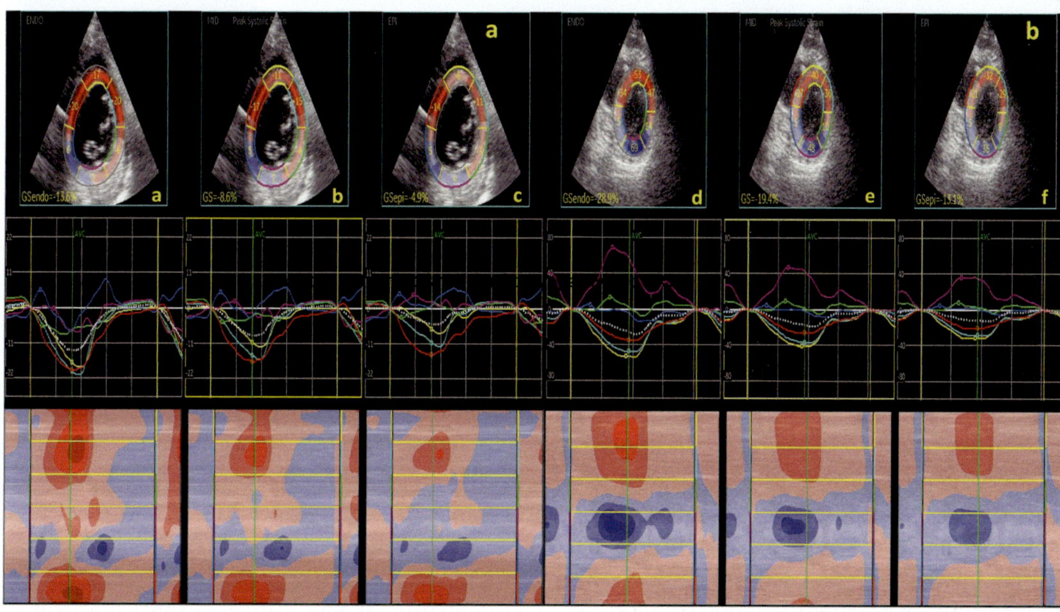

Fig. 4.9 Layer-specific strain analysis: decrease circumferential strain at all myocardium levels in a patient with dilated cardiomyopathy, CRT, and myocardial infarction **a**: endocardial (a), mid-level (b), epicardial (c), versus normal values **b**: endocardial (d), mid-level (e), epicardial (f)

by dyssynchrony and no LV hemodynamic improvement after CRT (Lambiase et al. 2004; Ansalone et al. 2002).

Myocardial areas without viability are akinetic or dyskinetic. CRT response will be harmful if the LV lead is placed in a nonviable segment. The LV lead position remote from the area of the latest mechanical activation will not improve the dyssynchrony or symptoms (Veire et al. 2006; Murphy et al. 2006).

Longitudinal systolic strain dyssynchrony index (SDI) represents the difference between peak end-systolic longitudinal strain for each segment and is linked to wasted energy (Fig. 4.10). Delayed segments, with maximum contraction after aortic valve closure

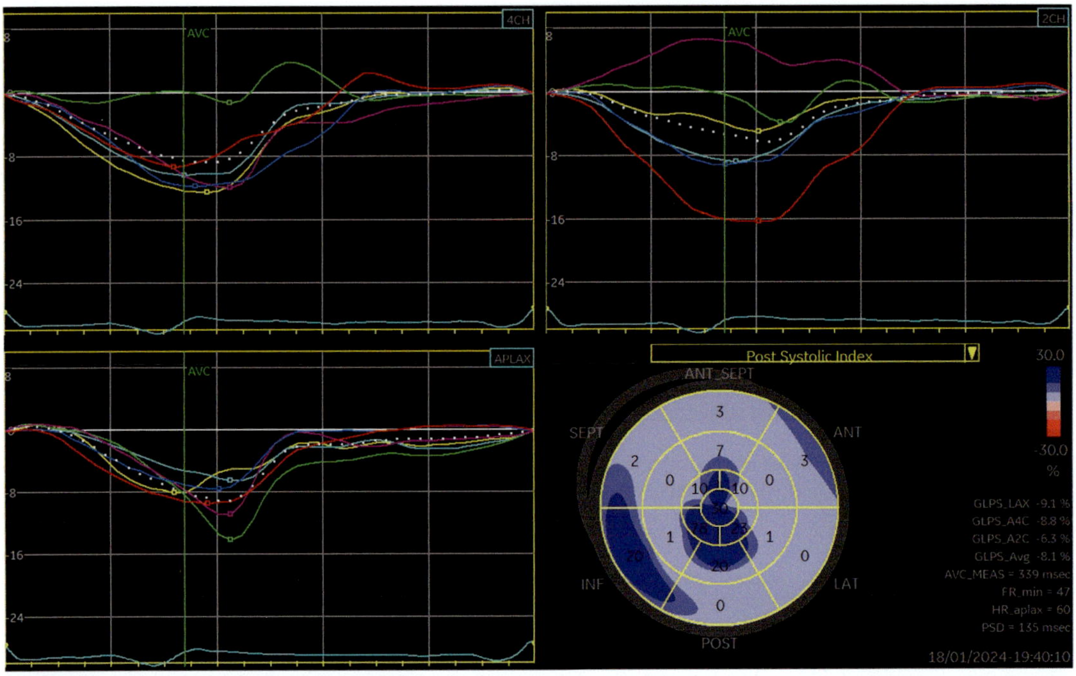

Fig. 4.10 Systolic dyssynchrony index obtained by speckle tracking echocardiography in a patient with dilated cardiomyopathy and CRT

(post systolic), do not fully contribute to ejection. The extent of wasted energy is higher in segments with preserved contractility, which can contribute to ejection, and is decreased in segments with minimal or no contractility but similar degrees of delay in timing (Fig. 4.11). A cutoff value of SI > 25% predicts the response to CRT (sensitivity 92%; specificity 65%) (Lim et al. 2011; Mele et al. 2017).

Echocardiographic optimization of LV lead with an adjacent position will produce the best increase in cardiac output, compared with optimally or remotely placed lead. An alternative technique may be required if this LV lead cannot be achieved via a standard transvenous approach (Khan et al. 2009).

In patients with implanted LV lead without symptomatic or LV remodeling response and with suboptimal lead position, either remote from the site of the latest mechanical activation or overlying a region of scar, the lead repositioning should be considered (Uebleis et al. 2011; Bordachar et al. 2010; Morgan and Delgado 2009; Sogaard et al. 2002).

The site of LV with the latest mechanical activation identification

Stimulating the segment with the latest activation earlier will synchronize the septum and LV-free wall and improve hemodynamic response (Becker et al. 2007; Tanaka et al. 2010). Echocardiographic Doppler methods are essential in identifying the anatomic site of the latest mechanical activation.

LV lead placement concordant with the site of the latest velocity activation associates a more favorable response to CRT. The inferior or posterolateral wall is the location of most patients' latest mechanical activation (Adelstein and Saba 2007; Becker et al. 2007; Boogers et al. 2011; Tanaka et al. 2010; Yu et al. 2005). The apical LV lead position seems also to be associated with a significantly increased risk of heart failure or death. Usually, the basal or midventricular position, without diaphragmatic capture, is preferred (Singh et al. 2011; Bommel et al. 2011).

The selective LV lead placement at the site of the latest LV mechanical activation detected by

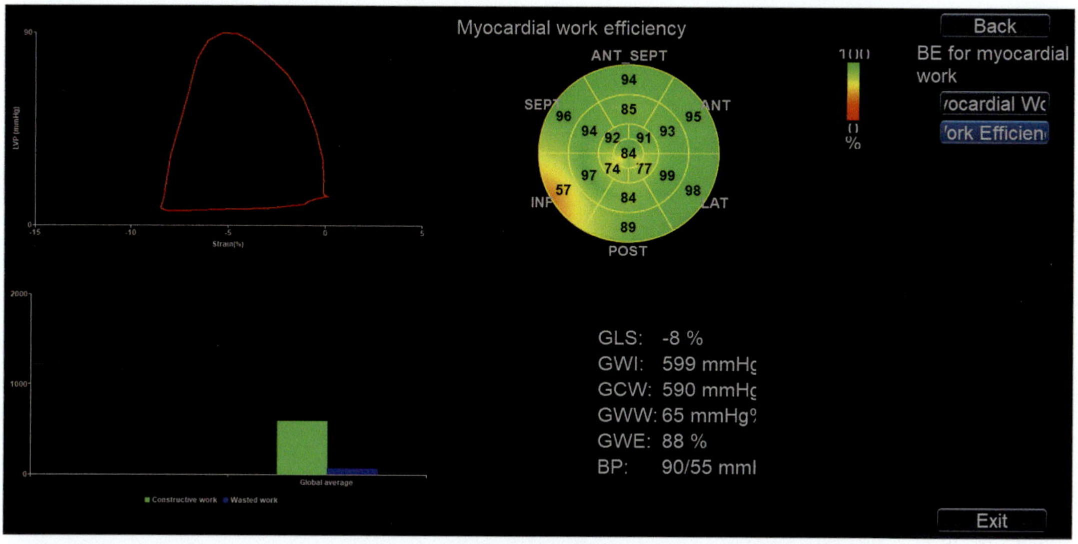

Fig. 4.11 Global Waste Energy calculation obtained by speckle tracking echocardiography and arterial pressure measurement during the examination, in a patient with dilated cardiomyopathy and CRT

STE was followed by a more significant proportion of responders and a lower rate of death and heart failure-related hospitalization (Khan et al. 2009; Adelstein et al. 2014).

The imaging techniques that identify this area are:

- tissue Doppler echocardiography - the color-coded time-to-peak velocities (Murphy et al. 2006) (Fig. 4.12)
- strain analysis by 2D STE: longitudinal (Fig. 13a), circumferential (Fig. 13b), and radial (Fig. 13c)
- strain analysis by 3D STE (Fig. 13d)

LV lead at the latest site of activation results in more significant clinical benefits and improvement in LV performance and survival (Ypenburg et al. 2008; Lambiase et al. 2004; Ansalone et al. 2002; Murphy et al. 2006; Bai et al. 2011). STE allows the assessment of both magnitude and delay of segmental contraction on the same regional strain curves and thus identifies the stimulating site (Mele et al. 2017; Chan and Choy 2010).

STE radial strain at the mid-myocardial level identifies the latest site of activation (Ypenburg et al. 2008) the most commonly at the posterior (36%) or lateral (33%) LV wall.

The viable myocardium is the best place for LV pacing, showing the most delayed contraction**.** (Morgan and Delgado 2009; Jacob et al. 2009) It is essential to identify this point because it influences the CRT response. This site is usually located at the level of the postero-lateral wall but depends on the etiology of the cardiomyopathy (Sogaard et al. 2002; Becker et al. 2010) and must be determined in the individual patient. To this purpose, various echocardiographic methods have been suggested over the years (Becker et al. 2007, 2010; Murphy et al. 2006; Sogaard et al. 2002; Tanaka et al. 2010; Yu et al. 2005; Bakos et al. 2014; Bai et al. 2011; Derval et al. 2010; Mele et al. 2013; Lim et al. 2007; Sénéchal et al. 2010). This site can be identified in intraprocedural, in the operating room with the use of intracardiac (Bai et al. 2011; Khan et al. 2010) or even transthoracic echocardiography (Chan and Choy 2010; Jacob et al. 2009; Becker et al. 2010; Derval et al. 2010; Norisada et al. 2010; Khan et al. 2012; Kydd et al. 2014; Daya et al. 2014). The most appropriate method is to determine the optimal site of LV pacing before the CRT implant. (Mele et al. 2017; Chan and Choy 2010). It is essential to identify the viable myocardium by 2D transthoracic echocardiography (Mele et al. 2013,

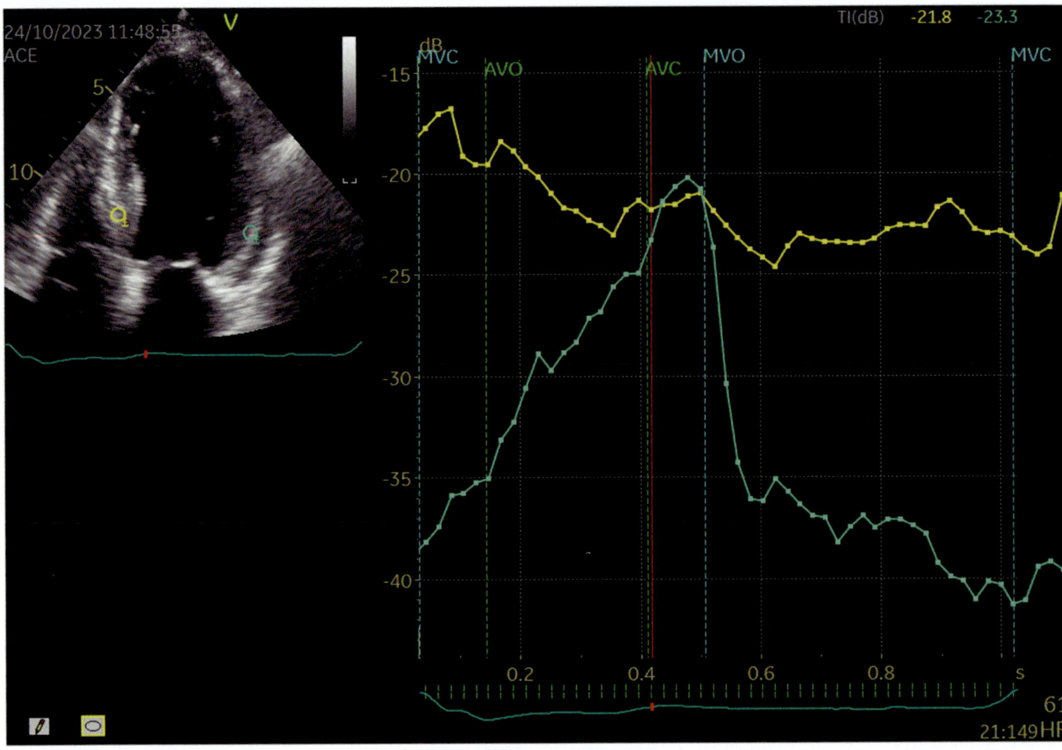

Fig. 4.12 Tissue Doppler echocardiography in a patient with dual chamber pacemaker before upgrade: curves feature at the level of interventricular septum vs lateral wall

2017) stress echocardiography (Ypenburg et al. 2007; Lim et al. 2007; Sénéchal et al. 2010; Hussain et al. 2015; Cano et al. 20178) or STE (Ypenburg et al. 2007; Delgado et al. 2011; Becker et al. 2011; Khan et al. 2010, 2012; Norisada et al. 2010; Domenichini et al. 2012; Glikson et al. 2021; Bongiorni et al. 2013) 2D STE measures radial strain from short-axis views of the LV. The optimal site of pacing was defined as the latest radial strain peak with an amplitude of strain ≥ 10% (Adelstein et al. 2014; Kydd et al. 2014; Daya et al. 2014; Hussain et al. 2015; Cano et al. 2017). Longitudinal strain by 2D STE can also be used to guide the position of the LV lead (Mele et al. 2017; Biffi et al. 2018).

Right Ventricular Lead

The clinical benefit of RV non-apical pacing, such as the RVOT, septum or mid-septum needs to be clarified (Shimony et al. 2012; Ali et al. 2022). The RV anterior free wall lead position is associated with adverse outcomes (Ng et al. 2009; Domenichini et al. 2012; Glikson et al. 2021; Merchant and Mittal 2018; Tops et al. 2007; Zhang et al. 2020). The most used position is the right ventricular apex (RVA), followed by the interventricular septum and the outflow tract (Bongiorni et al. 2013; Ypenburg et al. 2009).

The right ventricular apex—is a traditional place due to ease of positioning and the presence of the trabeculae for anchoring passive leads. Heart failure and death are the long-term deleterious effects of RVA pacing (Shimony et al. 2012; Hussain et al. 2015; Ali et al. 2022; Manolis 2006). An apical lead position was independently associated with cardiac perforation in patients with a pacemaker or ICD (Cano et al. 2017; Tops et al. 2006). Active-fixation pacing and defibrillation leads are predictors

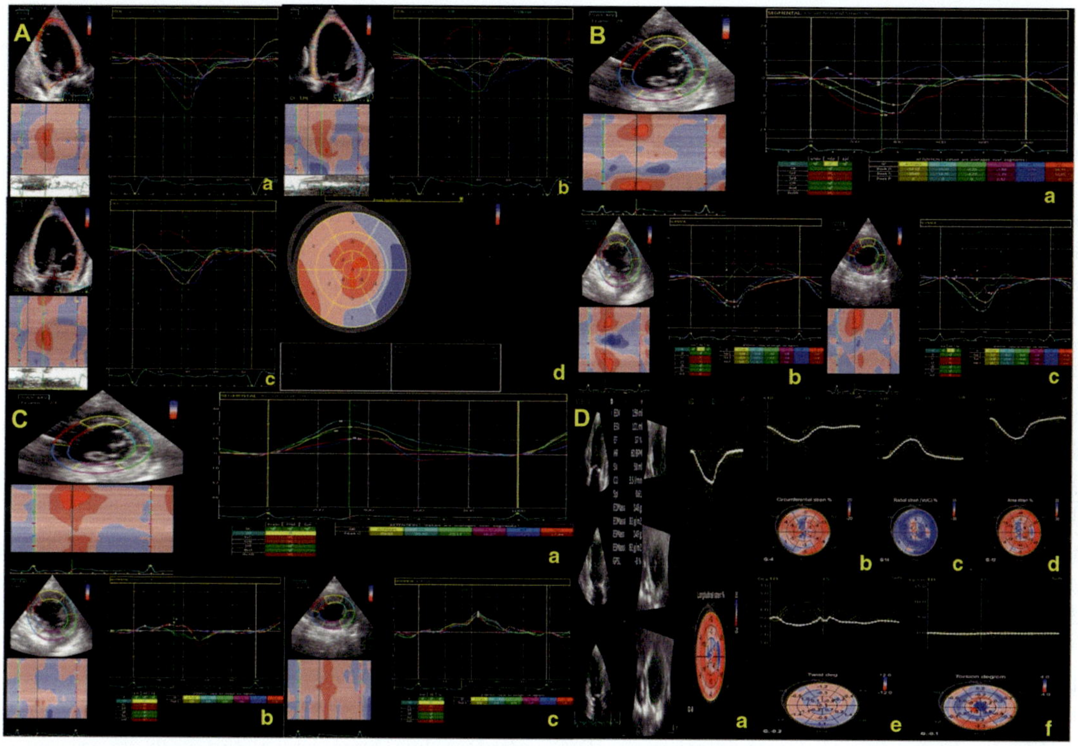

Fig. 4.13 The imaging echocardiographic techniques that identify latest activated LV area: A Global longitudinal strain; B circumferential strain, C radial strain, D 3D speckle tracking echocardiography

of relevant cardiac perforation (Domenichini et al. 2012; Biffi et al. 2018; Zhang et al. 2020; Cho et al. 2005). Other clinical risk factors are elderly and low body mass index. A septal position is to be preferable in such cases. The coronary sinus is to be used in the case of difficulties in deploying an RV lead, such as the tricuspid valve prosthesis (Glikson et al. 2021; Biffi et al. 2018; Ali et al. 2022; Zhang et al. 2020; Cho et al. 2005; Saito et al. 2015).

RVA pacing can induce interventricular and intraventricular dyssynchrony in patients with single- and dual-chamber pacemakers. It was also associated with reduced LV systolic dysfunction (Ali et al. 2022; Merchant and Mittal 2018; Schleifer et al. 2018; Burri et al. 2007). months after implantation. STE identified more radial dyssynchrony in patients with RVA pacing compared with those with non-apical lead position (Ali et al. 2022; Schleifer et al. 2018). Older age, higher percentage of pacing, and device type are prognostic factors for developing pacemaker-induced cardiomyopathy (Ali et al. 2022; Schleifer et al. 2018). Pacing-induced cardiomyopathy (PICM) is most commonly defined as the decrease in LVEF in patients with RVA pacing (Merchant and Mittal 2018). In the long-term, RV pacing influenced the time-to-peak radial strain of different LV segments, with 57% percent of patients developing LV dyssynchrony (Tops et al. 2007). The pacing percentage is the most sensitive prognostic factor for PICM. Other factors involved are device type and patient age (Zhang et al. 2020; Inoue et al. 2011). It has also been demonstrated that ventricular dyssynchrony induced by long-term RV apical pacing increases the risk of cardiac morbidity and mortality in heart failure patients. This pacing modality also reduces the LV systolic function (Ypenburg et al. 2009; Djavadzadehgan et al. 2013). RVA pacing can initiate asynchrony between LV interventricular septum (IVS) and free wall (Manolis 2006;

Baronaite et al. 2014) and between RV and LV (Tops et al. 2006; Teima et al. 2020). Patients with ventricular asynchrony have a high risk of cardiac morbidity and death (Cho et al. 2005; Choudhary et al. 2016).

The right ventricle septal (RVS) pacing is a more physiological alternative to the RVA to reduce the adverse effects of pacing-induced dyssynchrony (Shimony et al. 2012; Bongiorni et al. 2013; Ali et al. 2022; Manolis 2006). Right ventricular systolic function (Saito et al. 2015; Burri et al. 2012) and tricuspid regurgitation (Saito et al. 2015; Schleifer et al. 2018; Burri et al. 2012; Osmancik et al. 2013) are similar to apical pacing. The main advantage is less frequency of free wall peroration, with electrical parameters comparable to apical pacing (Burri et al. 2007; Kolb et al. 2014; Pang et al. 2014; Majauskiene et al. 2018).

In the acute setting, seven days after implantation, echocardiography parameters favor septal pacing (Inoue et al. 2011; Nishiyama et al. 2012). In short-term follow-up (3 months), RVS pacing is a better pacing alternative compared with RVA pacing. STE demonstrated less LV dysfunction and dyssynchrony in RV septal lead position patients (Djavadzadehgan et al. 2013; Pang et al. 2015). In the short-term (Baronaite et al. 2014; Sharma et al. 2016) and long-term follow-up (Teima et al. 2020; Choudhary et al. 2016; Chen et al. 2016; Wei et al. 2018) both dual-chamber and single-chamber pacemakers decreased LVEF and GLS at STE evaluation.

Studies have validated echocardiography in the final RV septum lead position established (Shimony et al. 2012; Ng et al. 2009; Merchant and Mittal 2018; Merchant and Mittal 2018; Tops et al. 2007; Burri et al. 2012; Osmancik et al. 2013; Pang et al. 2014; Zeitler et al. 1629; Kirkfeldt et al. 2014; Armaganijan et al. 2012) resulting in left ventricular dysfunction (Shimony et al. 2012; Ng et al. 2009; Merchant and Mittal 2018; Tops et al. 2007) perforation (Cho et al. 2005; Choudhary et al. 2016) and myocardial infarction, due to the left anterior descending artery damage (Majauskiene et al. 2018; Nishiyama et al. 2012; Pang et al. 2015; Dodson et al. 2014; Haines et al. 2011; Persson et al. 2014). Because of the funnel-shaped right ventricular outflow tract, pacing this small area may be challenging (Sharma et al. 2016; Chen et al. 2016; Wei et al. 2018; Poole et al. 2010; Hsu et al. 2013; Witt et al. 2016).

Right Atrial Lead

The atrial lead functions are:

- to maintain atrioventricular synchrony
- to confirm the atrial arrhythmias identification in patients without a VDD system and who do not require atrial pacing.
- follow-up of arrhythmic episodes with ICDs and decrease the number of inappropriate shocks without effects on mortality (Zeitler et al. 1629; Dilling-Boer et al. 2003)

Right atrial lead in patients with dual-chamber devices has been associated with an increased risk of complications compared to single-chamber VVI- pacemakers (Kirkfeldt et al. 2014; Armaganijan et al. 2012; Dodson et al. 2014; Haines et al. 2011; Persson et al. 2014; Poole et al. 2010; Hsu et al. 2013; Morales-Estrella et al. 2019; Sebastian et al. 2005; Srivathsan et al. 2003; Tanabe et al. 2019; Zoppo et al. 2015; Marco, et al. 2014; Kashani et al. 2004). The complications are lead dislodgement and perforation (Witt et al. 2016; Kaljusto and Tønnessen 2007) resulting in tamponade, pneumothorax or pneumopericardium.(Dilling-Boer et al. 2003; Morales-Estrella et al. 2019; Sebastian et al. 2005; Srivathsan et al. 2003; Sticco and Barrett 2006; Burri et al. 2021).

The preferred site for atrial pacing is the RA appendages, the lateral atrium lead placement increasing the risk of phrenic nerve capture. Tanabe et al. 2019. The tip of RAA should be avoided because this location may result in laceration of the aorta in patients with active fixation leads Zoppo et al. 2015; Marco, et al. 2014; Kashani et al. 2004; Kaljusto and Tønnessen 2007; Sticco and Barrett 2006. The

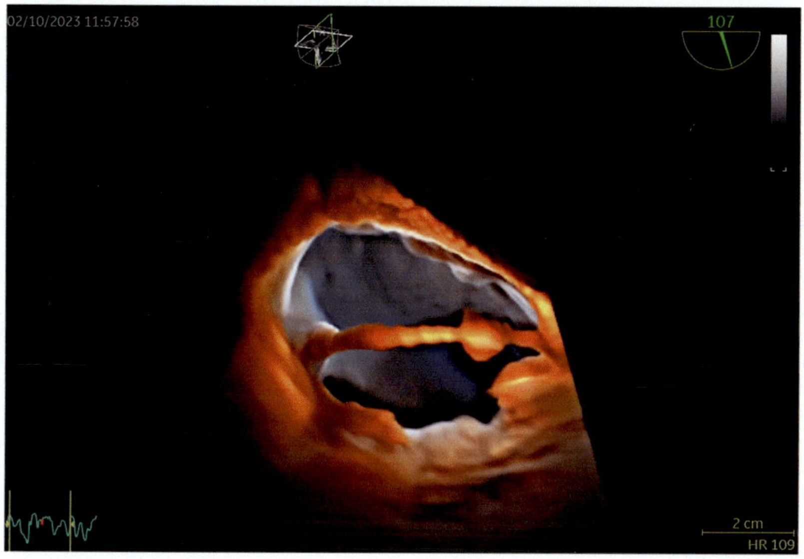

Fig. 4.14 Right atrial lead localization at the level of right atrial appendage evaluated by 3D transesophageal echocardiography

most appropriate site for the right atrial lead in the anterior RAA Burri et al. 2021 (Fig. 4.14, Suplementary material 4)

4.1 Conclusion

Echocardiography is valuable in identifying lead positions in patients with implanted devices. Conventional and advanced techniques help identify lead position before upgrading from a pacemaker with an apical right ventricle lead to CRT. In patients without reverse remodeling and LV function improvement after CRT, it is essential to identify the lead position from the fibrosis area. Transesophageal echocardiography is the most appropriate right atrial lead position evaluation technique.

References

Adelstein EC, Saba S. Scar burden by myocardial perfusion imaging predicts echocardiographic response to cardiac resynchronization therapy in ischemic cardiomyopathy. Am Heart J. 2007;153(1):105–12.

Adelstein E, Alam MB, Schwartzman D, et al. Effect of echocardiography-guided left ventricular lead placement for cardiac resynchronization therapy on mortality and risk of defibrillator therapy for ventricular arrhythmias in heart failure patients (from the Speckle tracking assisted resynchronization therapy for electrode region [STARTER] trial). Am J Cardiol. 2014;113:1518–22.

Aiba T, Hesketh GG, Barth AS, et al. Electrophysiological consequences of dyssynchronous heart failure and its restoration by resynchronization therapy. Circulation. 2009;119(9):1220–30.

Ali AN, Hawas AN, Ramadan AY. Impact of right ventricular lead position on left ventricular functions and early remodeling in permanent single- and dual chamber pacemakers. Herzschr Elektrophys. 2022;33:432–9.

Ansalone G, Giannantoni P, Ricci R, Trambaiolo P, Fedele F, Santini M. Doppler myocardial imaging to evaluate the effectiveness of pacing sites in patients receiving biventricular pacing. JACC. 2002;39:489–99.

Armaganijan LV, Toff WD, Nielsen JC, et al. Are elderly patients at increased risk of complications following pacemaker implantation? A meta-analysis of randomized trials. Pacing Clin Electrophysiol. 2012;35:131–4.

Bai R, Di Biase L, Mohanty P, et al. Positioning of left ventricular pacing lead guided by intracardiac echocardiography with vector velocity imaging during cardiac resynchronization therapy procedure. J Cardiovasc Electrophysiol. 2011;22:1034–41.

Bakos Z, Markstad H, Ostenfeld E, et al. Combined preoperative information using a bullseye plot from speckle tracking echocardiography, cardiac CT scan, and MRI scan: targeted left ventricular lead implantation in patients receiving cardiac resynchronization therapy. Eur Heart J Cardiovasc Imaging. 2014;15:523–31.

Baronaite DK, Vaškelyte J, Puodžiukynas A, et al. Evaluation of left ventricular longitudinal function and synchrony after dual chamber pacemaker implantation. Medicina. 2014;50(6):340–4.

Becker M, Hoffmann R, Kuhl HP, et al. Analysis of myocardial deformation based on ultrasonic pixel tracking to determine transmurality in chronic myocardial infarction. Eur Heart J. 2006;27:2560–6.

Becker M, Hoffmann R, Schmitz F, et al. Relation of optimal lead positioning as defined by three-dimensional echocardiography to long-term benefit of cardiac resynchronization. Am J Cardiol. 2007;100(11):1671–6.

Becker M, Ocklenburg C, Altiok E, et al. Impact of infarct transmurality on layer-specific impairment of myocardial function: a myocardial deformation imaging study. Eur Heart J. 2009;30(12):1467–76.

Becker M, Altiok E, Ocklenburg C, et al. Analysis of LV lead position in cardiac resynchronization therapy using different imaging modalities. JACC Cardiovasc Imaging. 2010;3:472–81.

Becker M, Zwicker C, Kaminski M, et al. Dependency of cardiac resynchronization therapy on myocardial viability at the LV lead position. JACC Cardiovasc Imaging. 2011;4:366–74.

Biffi M, de Zan G, Massaro G, et al. Is ventricular sensing always right, when it is left? Clin Cardiol. 2018;41:1238–45.

Bleeker GB, Kaandorp TA, Lamb HJ, et al. Effect of posterolateral scar tissue on clinical and echocardiographic improvement after cardiac resynchronization therapy. Circulation. 2006;113:969–76.

Bongiorni MG, Proclemer A, Dobreanu D, Marinskis G, Pison L, Blomstrom Lundqvist C et al.; conducted by the Scientific Initiative Committee, European Heart Rhythm Association. Preferred tools and techniques for implantation of cardiac electronic devices in Europe: results of the European Heart Rhythm Association survey. *Europace* 2013;15:1664–1668.

Boogers MJ, Chen J, van Bommel RJ, Borlefs CJ, Dibbets-Schneider P, van der Hiel B, et al. Optimal left ventricular lead position assessed with phase analysis on gated myocardial perfusion SPECT. Eur J Nucl Med Mol Imaging. 2011;38:230–8.

Bordachar P, Alonso C, Anselme F, et al. Addition of a second LV pacing site in CRT nonresponders rationale and design of the multicenter randomized V(3) trial. J Card Fail. 2010;16(9):709–13.

Burri H, Sunthorn H, Dorsaz PA, et al. Thresholds and complications with right ventricular septal pacing compared to apical pacing. Pacing Clin Electrophysiol. 2007;30:S75-78.

Burri H, Domenichini G, Sunthorn H, Ganiere V, Stettler C. Comparison of tools and techniques for implanting pacemaker leads on the ventricular midseptum. Europace. 2012;14:847–52.

Burri H, Starck C, Auricchio A, et al. EHRA expert consensus statement and practical guide on optimal implantation technique for conventional pacemakers and implantable cardioverter-defibrillators: endorsed by the Heart Rhythm Society (HRS), the Asia Pacific Heart Rhythm Society (APHRS), and the Latin-American Heart Rhythm Society (LAHRS). Europace. 2021;23:983–1008.

Cano O, Andres A, Alonso P, et al. Incidence and predictors of clinically relevant cardiac perforation associated with systematic implantation of active-fixation pacing and defibrillation leads: a single-centre experience with over 3800 implanted leads. EP Europace. 2017;19:96–102.

Chakir K, Daya SK, Tunin RS, et al. Reversal of global apoptosis and regional stress kinase activation by cardiac resynchronization. Circulation. 2008;117(11):1369–77.

Chan NY, Choy CC. Cheung KC et alal, Echocardiographic mapping of left ventricular resynchronization during cardiac resynchronization therapy procedures. Chin Med J. 2010;123:1645–51.

Chen D, Wei H, Tang J, Liu L, Wu S, Lin C, et al. A randomized comparison of fluoroscopic techniques for implanting pacemaker lead on the right ventricular outflow tract septum. Int J Cardiovasc Imaging. 2016;32:721–8.

Cho GY, Song JK, Park WJ. Mechanical dyssynchrony assessed by tissue Doppler imaging is a powerful predictor of mortality in congestive heart failure with normal QRS duration. J Am Coll Cardiol. 2005;46:2237–43.

Choudhary D, Chaurasia AK, Kumar SM, et al. Radial left ventricular dyssynchrony by speckle tracking in apical versus non apical right ventricular pacing-evidence of dyssynchrony on medium termfollow up. J Cardiovasc Thorac Res. 2016;8(1):20–5.

Daya HA, Alam MB, Adelstein E, et al. Echocardiographyguided left ventricular lead placement for cardiac resynchronization therapy in ischemic vs nonischemic cardiomyopathy patients. Heart Rhythm. 2014;11(4):614–9.

Delgado V, van Bommel RJ, Bertini M, et al. Relative merits of left ventricular dyssynchrony, left ventricular lead position, and myocardial scar to predict long-term survival of ischemic heart failure patients undergoing cardiac resynchronization therapy. Circulation. 2011;123(1):70–8.

Derval N, Steendijk P, Gula LJ, et al, Optimizing hemodynamics in heart failure patients by systematic screening of left ventricular pacing sites: the lateral left ventricular wall and the coronary sinus are rarely the best sites. *J Am Coll Cardiol*, 2010;55 566–575.

Dilling-Boer D, Ector H, Willems R, Heidbu¨chel H. Pericardial effusion and right-sided pneumothorax resulting from an atrial active-fixation lead. *Europace* 2003;5:419–423.

Djavadzadehgan H, Tabrizi MT, Mohammadi K. Comparison of left ventricle segments contraction pattern by 3dimentional speckle tracking echocardiography in right ventricular apical pacing with right ventricular septal pacing. JAmSci. 2013;9(11):34–7.

Dodson JA, Reynolds MR, Bao HK, et al. Developing a risk model for in-hospital adverse events following implantable cardioverter-defibrillator implantation. J Am Coll Cardiol. 2014;63:788–96.

Domenichini G, Sunthorn H, Fleury E, et al, Pacing of the interventricular septum versus the right ventricular apex: a prospective, randomized study Eur J InternMed 2012;23:621–627.

Duckett SG, Ginks M, Shetty A, et al. Adverse response to cardiac resynchronisation therapy in patients with septal scar on cardiac MRI preventing a septal right ventricular lead position. J Interv Card Electrophysiol. 2012;33(2):151–60.

Ghio S, Freemantle N, Scelsi L, et al. Long-term left ventricular reverse remodelling with cardiac resynchronization therapy: results from the CARE-HF trial. Eur J Heart Fail. 2009;11(5):480–8.

Gjesdal O, Hopp E, Vartdal T, et al. Global longitudinal strain measured by two-dimensional speckle tracking echocardiography is closely related to myocardial infarct size in chronic ischaemic heart disease. Clin Sci. 2007;113(6):287–96.

Glikson M, Nielsen JC, Kronborg MB, et al. 2021 ESC Guidelines on cardiac pacing and cardiac resynchronization therapy Developed by the Task Force on cardiac pacing and cardiac resynchronization therapy of the European Society of Cardiology (ESC). Eur Heart J. 2021;00:1–94.

Gorcsan J 3rd, Yu CM, Sanderson JE. Ventricular resynchronization is the principle mechanism of benefit with cardiac resynchronization therapy. Heart Fail. 2012;7(6):737–46.

Haines DE, Wang Y, Curtis J. Implantable cardioverter-defibrillator registry risk score models for acute procedural complications or death after implantable cardioverter-defibrillator implantation. Circulation. 2011;123:2069–76.

Hsu JC, Varosy PD, Bao H, Dewland TA, Curtis JP, Marcus GM. Cardiac perforation from implantable cardioverter-defibrillator lead placement: insights from the national cardiovascular data registry. Circ Cardiovasc Qual Outcomes. 2013;6:582–90.

Hussain MA, Furuya-Kanamori LUIS, Kaye G, et al. J, The effect of right ventricular apical and nonapical pacing on the short- and long-term changes in left ventricular ejection fraction: a systematic review and meta analysis of randomized-controlled trials. Pacing Clin Electrophysiol. 2015;38:1121–36.

Inoue K, Okayama H, Nishimura K, et al. Right ventricular septal pacing preserves global left ventricular longitudinal function in comparison with apical pacing. Circ J. 2011;75(7):1609–15.

Jacob S, Kondur A, Khetarpal V, Afonso L. Reversal of right ventricular apex pacing-induced left ventricular apical dyskinesis: utility of intraoperative 3D echocardiography in resynchronization therapy. Circ Arrhythm Electrophysiol. 2009;2:e21–3.

Kaljusto ML, Tønnessen T. Aortic perforation with cardiac tamponade two weeks after pacemaker implantation. J Thorac Cardiovasc Surg. 2007;134:502–3.

Kashani A, Mehdirad A, Fredman C, Barold SS. Aortic perforation by activefixation atrial pacing lead. Pacing Clin Electrophysiol. 2004;27:417–8.

Kass DA. Pathobiology of cardiac dyssynchrony and resynchronization. Heart Rhythm. 2009;6(11):1660–5.

Khan FZ, Virdee MS, Fynn SP, Dutka DP. Left ventricular lead placement in cardiac resynchronization therapy: where and how? Europace. 2009;11:554–61.

Khan FZ, Virdee MS, Read PA, et al. Effect of low-amplitude two-dimensional radial strain at left ventricular pacing sites on response to cardiac resynchronization therapy. J Am Soc Echocardiogr. 2010;23:1168–76.

Khan FZ, Virdee MS, Palmer CR et al, Targeted left ventricular lead placement to guide cardiac resynchronization therapy. The TARGET study: a randomized, controlled trial. *J Am Coll Cardiol,* 2012; 59:1509–1518.

Kirkfeldt RE, Johansen JB, Nohr EA, Jorgensen OD, Nielsen JC. Complications after cardiac implantable electronic device implantations: an analysis of a complete, nationwide cohort in Denmark. Eur Heart J. 2014;35:1186–94.

Kolb C, Solzbach U, Biermann, et al. Safety of mid-septal electrode placement in implantable cardioverter defibrillator recipients–results of the SPICE (Septal Positioning of ventricular ICD Electrodes) study. *Int J Cardiol* 2014;174:713–720.

Kydd AC, McCormick LM, Dutka DP. Optimizing benefit from CRT: role of speckle tracking echocardiography, the importance of LV lead position and scar. Expert Rev Med Devices. 2012;9(5):521–36.

Kydd AC, Khan FZ, Watson WD, et al. Prognostic benefit of optimum left ventricular lead position in cardiac resynchronization therapy: follow-up of the TARGET Study Cohort (Targeted Left Ventricular Lead Placement to guide Cardiac Resynchronization Therapy). JACC Heart Fail. 2014;2:205–12.

Lambiase PD, Rinaldi A, Hauck J, et al. Non-contact left ventricular endocardial mapping in cardiac resynchronisation therapy. Heart. 2004;90(1):44–51.

Lancellotti P, Senechal M, Moonen M, et al. Myocardial contractile reserve during exercise predicts left ventricular reverse remodelling after cardiac resynchronization. Eur J Echocardiogr. 2009;10(5):663–8.

Lim P, Bars C, Mitchell-Heggs L, et al. Importance of contractile reserve for CRT. Europace. 2007;9:739–43.

Lim P, Donal E, Lafitte S, et al. Multicentre study using strain delay index for predicting response to cardiac resynchronization therapy (MUSIC study). Eur J Heart Fail. 2011;13(9):984–91.

Majauskiene E, Aucina G, Semeniene P, et al. Myocardial in farction caused by active-fixation ventricular pacing lead screwed into the anterior descending coronary artery. Int Cardiovasc Res J. 2018;12:154–60.

Manolis AS. The deleterious consequences of right ventricular apical pacing: time to seek alternate site pacing. Pacing Clin Electrophysiol. 2006;29:298–315.

Di Marco A, Nu~nez E, Osorio K, et al. Aortic perforation by active-fixation atrial pacing lead: an unusual but serious complication. *Tex Heart Inst* J 2014;41:327–328.

Mele D, Agricola E, Monte AD, et al. Pacing transmural scar tissue reduces left ventricle reverse remodeling after cardiac resynchronization therapy. Int J Cardiol. 2013;167:94–101.

Mele D, Bertini M, Malagù M. Current role of echocardiography in cardiac resynchronization therapy. Heart Fail Rev. 2017;22:699–722.

Mele D, Nardozza M, Malagù M, et al, Left ventricle lead position guided by parametric strain echocardiography improves response to cardiac resynchronization therapy. J Am Soc Echocardiogr; in press, 2017;30(10):1001–1011.

Merchant FM, Mittal S. Pacing-induced cardiomyopathy. Card Electrophysiol Clin. 2018;10(3):437–45.

Molhoek SG, Bax JJ, Bleeker GB, et al. Comparison of response to cardiac resynchronization therapy in patients with sinus rhythm versus chronic atrial fibrillation. Am J Cardiol. 2004;94(12):1506–9.

Morales-Estrella J, Huded C, Bhargava M, Gildea T, Sampaio Rodrigues T, Almeida FA. Right-sided pneumothorax after cardioverter-defibrillator implantation. Heart Lung Circ. 2019;28:e137-138.

Morgan JM, Delgado V, Lead positioning for cardiac resynchronization therapy: techniques and priorities. *Europace* 11, 2009,(Suppl 5):v22–v28

Murphy RT, Sigurdsson G, Mulamalla S, et al. Tissue synchronization imaging and optimal left ventricular pacing site in cardiac resynchronization therapy. Am J Cardiol. 2006;97:1615–21.

Nesser HJ, Mor-Avi V, Gorissen W, et al. Quantification of left ventricular volumes using three-dimensional echocardiographic speckle tracking: comparison with MRI. Eur Heart J. 2009;30(13):1565–73.

Ng ACT, Allman C, Vidaic J, et al. Long-term impact of right ventricular septal versus apical pacing on left ventricular synchrony and function in patients with second- or third-degree heart block. Am J Cardiol. 2009;103:1096–101.

Nishiyama N, Takatsuki S, Kimura T, et al. Implantation of the right ventricular lead of an implantable cardioverter defibrillator complicated by apical myocardial infarction. Circulation. 2012;126:1314–5.

Norisada K, Kawai H, Tanaka H, et al. Myocardial contractile function in the region of the left ventricular pacing lead predicts the response to cardiac resynchronization therapy assessed by two-dimensional speckle tracking echocardiography. J Am Soc Echocardiogr. 2010;23:181–9.

Osmancik P, Stros P, Herman D, Curila K, Petr R. The insufficiency of left anterior oblique and the usefulness of right anterior oblique projection for correct localization of a computed tomography-verified right ventricular lead into the midseptum. Circ Arrhythm Electrophysiol. 2013;6:719–25.

Pang BJ, Joshi SB, Lui EH, et al. Validation of con ventional fluoroscopic and ECG criteria for right ventricular pacemaker lead position using cardiac computed tomography. Pacing Clin Electrophysiol. 2014;37:495–504.

Pang BJ, Barold SS, Mond HG. Injury to the coronary arteries and related structures by implantation of cardiac implantable electronic devices. Europace. 2015;17:524–9.

Persson R, Earley A, Garlitski AC, Balk EM, Uhlig K. Adverse events following implantable cardioverter defibrillator implantation: a systematic review. J Interv Card Electrophysiol. 2014;40:191–205.

Poole JE, Gleva MJ, Mela T, et al.; for the REPLACE Registry Investigators. Complication rates associated with pacemaker or implantable cardioverter-defibrillator generator replacements and upgrade procedures: results from the REPLACE registry. *Circulation* 2010;122:1553–1561.

Popovic ZB, Benejam C, Bian J, et al. Speckle-tracking echocardiography correctly identifies segmental left ventricular dysfunction induced by scarring in a rat model of myocardial infarction. Am J Physiol Heart Circ Physiol. 2007;292(6):H2809–16.

Saito M, Iannaccone A, Kaye G, et al. Effect of right ventricular pacing on right ventricular mechanics and tricuspid regurgitation in patients with high-grade atrioventricular block and sinus rhythm (from the protection of left ventricular function during right ventricular pacing study). Am J Cardiol. 2015;116:1875–82.

Schleifer JW, Pislaru SV, Lin G, et al. Effect of ventricular pacing lead position on tricuspid regurgitation: a randomized prospective trial. Heart Rhythm. 2018;15:1009–16.

Sebastian CC, Wu WC, Shafer M, Choudhary G, Patel PM. Pneumopericardium and pneumothorax after permanent pacemaker implantation. Pacing Clin Electrophysiol. 2005;28:466–8.

Sénéchal M, Lancellotti P, Magne J, et al. Contractile reserve assessed using dobutamine echocardiography predicts left ventricular reverse remodeling after cardiac resynchronization therapy: prospective validation in patients with left ventricular dyssynchrony. Echocardiography. 2010;27:668–667.

Shanks M, Delgado V, Ng AC, et al. Clinical and echocardiographic predictors of nonresponse to cardiac resynchronization therapy. Am Heart J. 2011;161(3):552–7.

Sharma G, Salahuddin S, Sanders P, et al. Inadequacy of fluoroscopy and electrocardiogram in predicting septal position in RVOT pacing - Validation with cardiac computed tomography. Indian Heart J. 2016;68:174–80.

Shimony A, Eisenberg MJ, Filion KB, Amit G. Beneficial effects of right ventricular non-apical vs. apical pacing: a systematic review and meta-analysis of randomized-controlled trials. Europace 2012;14:81–91.

Singh JP, Klein HU, Huang DT, et al. Left ventricular lead position and clinical outcome in the multicenter automatic defibrillator implantation trial-cardiac resynchronization therapy (MADIT-CRT) trial. Circulation. 2011;123(11):1159–66.

Smiseth OA, Russell K, Skulstad H. The role of echocardiography in quantification of left ventricular dyssynchrony: state of the art and future directions. Eur Heart J Cardiovasc Imaging. 2012;13(1):61–8.

Sogaard P, Egeblad H, Pedersen AK, et al. Sequential versus simultaneous biventricular resynchronization for severe heart failure: evaluation by tissue Doppler imaging. Circulation. 2002;106:2078–84.

Srivathsan K, Byrne RA, Appleton CP, Scott LRP. Pneumopericardium and pneumothorax contralateral to venous access site after permanent pacemaker implantation. Europace. 2003;5:361–3.

Sticco CC, Barrett LO. Delayed cardiac tamponade by iatrogenic aortic perforation with acemaker implantation. J Thorac Cardiovasc Surg. 2006;131:480–1.

Suffoletto MS, Dohi K, Cannesson M, Saba S, Gorcsan J 3rd. Novel speckletracking radial strain from routine black-and-white echocardiographic images to quantify dyssynchrony and predict response to cardiac resynchronization therapy. Circulation. 2006;113(7):960–8.

Tanabe K, Kotoda M, Nakashige D, et al, Sudden onset pacemaker-induced diaphragmatic twitching during general anesthesia. *JA ClinR* ep2019;5:36.678.

Tanaka H, Hara H, Saba S, et al. Usefulness of threedimensional speckle tracking strain to quantify dyssynchrony and the site of latest mechanical activation. Am J Cardiol. 2010;105:235–42.

Teima SM, Bedier AI, Eladawy AH, et al. Assessment of left ventricular dyssynchrony after permanent cardiac pacing by using two dimensional speckle tracking echocardiography. World Heart J. 2020;12(1):41–50.

Thebault C, Donal E, Meunier C, et al. Sites of left and right ventricular lead implantation and response to cardiac resynchronization therapy observations from the REVERSE trial. Eur Heart J. 2012;33:2662–71.

Tops LF, Schalij MJ, Holman ER, et al. Right ventricular pacing can induce ventricular dyssynchrony in patients with atrial fibrillation after atrioventricular node ablation. J Am Coll Cardiol. 2006;48:1642–8.

Tops LF, Suffoletto MS, Bleeker GB, Boersma E, van der Wall EE, Gorcsan J III. Schalij MJ & Bax JJ : Speckle-tracking radial strain reveals left ventricular dyssynchrony in patients with permanent right ventricular pacing. J Am Coll Cardiol. 2007;50(12):1180–8.

Uebleis C, Ulbrich M, Tegtmeyer R, et al. Electrocardiogram-gated 18F-FDG PET/ CT hybrid imaging in patients with unsatisfactory response to cardiac resynchronization therapy: initial clinical results. J Nucl Med. 2011;52(1):67–71.

van Bommel RJ, Ypenburg C, Mollema SA, et al. Site of latest activation in patients eligible for cardiac resynchronization therapy: patterns of dyssynchrony among different QRS configurations and impact of heart failure etiology. Am Heart J. 2011;161:1060–10660.

Van De Veire NR, Schuijf JD, De Sutter J, et al. Noninvasive visualization of the cardiac venous system in coronary artery disease patients using 64-slice computed tomography. J Am Coll Cardiol. 2006;48(9):1832–8.

Voight J-U, Pendrizzetti G, Lyssyansky P, et al. Definitions for a common standard for 2D speckle tracking echocardiography: consensus document of the EACVI/ASE/Industry Task Force to standardize deformation imaging. Eur Heart J - Cardiovasc Imaging. 2015;16:1–11.

Wei H, Tang J, Chen D, et al. Electrocardiographic predictors of validated right ventricular outflow tract septal pacing for correct localization of transthoracic echocardiography. Clin Cardiol. 2018;41:354–9.

Wikstrom G, Blomström-Lundqvist C, Andren B et al.; CARE-HF Study investigators. The effects of aetiology on outcome in patients treated with cardiac resynchronization therapy in the CARE-HF trial. *Eur. Heart J.*, 2009;30(7):782–788.

Witt CM, Lenz CJ, Shih HH, et al. Right atrial lead fixation type and lead position are associated with significant variation in complications. J Interv Card Electrophysiol. 2016;47:313–9.

Woo GW, Petersen-Stejskal S, Johnson JW, et al. Ventricular reverse remodeling and 6-month outcomes in patients receiving cardiac resynchronization therapy: analysis of the MIRACLE study. J Interv Card Electrophysiol. 2005;12(2):107–13.

Ypenburg C, Sieders A, Bleeker GB, et al. Myocardial contractile reserve predicts improvement in left ventricular function after cardiac resynchronization therapy. Am Heart J. 2007;154(6):1160–5.

Ypenburg C, van Bommel RJ, Delgado V, et al. Optimal left ventricular lead position predicts reverse remodeling and survival after cardiac resynchronization therapy. J Am Coll Cardiol. 2008;52(17):1402–9.

Ypenburg C, van Bommel RJ, Borleffs CJW. Longterm prognosis after cardiac resynchronization therapy is related to the extent of left ventricular reverse remodeling at midterm follow-up. J Am Coll Cardiol. 2009;53(6):483–90.

Yu CM, Zhang Q, Fung JW, et al. A novel tool to assess systolic asynchrony and identify responders of cardiac resynchronization therapy by tissue synchronization imaging. J Am Coll Cardiol. 2005;45:677–84.

Zeitler EP, Sanders GD, Singh K, et al. Single vs. dual chamber implantable cardioverter-defibrillators or programming of implantable cardioverter-defibrillators in patients without a bradycardia pacing indication: systematic review and meta-analysis. *Europace* 2018;20:1621– 1629.

Zhang H, Zhou Y-J, Zeng Y-J, Prognostic factors of pacing-induced cardiomyopathy. Chin Med J(Engl), 2020;133(13):1533–1539.

Zoppo F, Rizzo S, Corrado A, et al. Morphology of right atrial appendage for permanent atrial pacing and risk of iatrogenic perforation of the aorta by active fixation lead. Heart Rhythm. 2015;12:744–50.

Right Ventricle Function Evaluation in Patients with Implanted Devices

5

Abstract

Right ventricle dysfunction is a strong and independent predictor of mortality and morbidity in patients with implanted devices. It is critical to use adequate echocardiographic methods for right ventricle echocardiographic evaluation after device implantation. Clinical trials targeting the cardiac resynchronization therapy effect on heart failure have principally focused on left ventricle evaluation. Some studies revealed that this therapy might produce reverse remodelling of the right ventricle. Few data are available for right function evaluation in this group of patients. The right ventricle has a complex geometry, and evaluating cardiac resynchronization therapy effects on its performance may be challenging.

In patients with chronic left ventricular (LV) HF, right ventricle (RV) dysfunction is a strong and independent predictor of mortality and morbidity (Meyer et al. 2010; Field et al. 2006; Ghio et al. 2001; Haddad et al. 2008; Karatasakis et al. 1998; Rigolin et al. 1995; Ogunyankin and Puthumana 2010; Kaul et al. 1984).

Supplementary Information The online version contains supplementary material available at https://doi.org/10.1007/978-3-031-64079-7_5.

HF patients with left LV and RV systolic dysfunction have a worse prognosis whether or not they undergo CRT (Brignole et al. 2013). LV contraction significantly affects the RV systolic function. An LV function improvement after CRT might also act on the RV (Donal et al. 2017). Transthoracic echocardiography is the most widely used method for RV function evaluation (Ghio et al. 2000). It is critical to use adequate RV echocardiographic evaluation methods after device implantation. The clinical trials targeting the CRT effect on heart failure has focused on LV evaluation (Delgado and Bax 2010).

The RV has a complex geometry, and evaluating CRT effects on its performance may be challenging (Delgado and Bax 2010).

5.1 Mechanism of the Response of RV at CRT and RV Reverse Remodeling

Some analyses demonstrated a bidirectional relation between the CRT and the RV response. CRT acts on ventricular interdependence, inducing a more synchronous contraction. These actions reduce mitral regurgitation and pulmonary vein hypertension, leading to reverse remodeling in both LV and RV (Delgado and Bax 2010). Several studies also revealed reverse RV remodeling as a determinant of response to CRT (Fleming et al. 2011; Campbell et al. 2013; Donal et al. 2008).

D.-M. Toader, *Echocardiographic Evaluation of Patients with Implanted Devices*, https://doi.org/10.1007/978-3-031-64079-7_5

The response of RV at CRT has two phases:

- *Short-term response after first days.* Some studies demonstrated a CRT early improvement of the RV function and the tricuspid regurgitation (TR) before decreasing RV dimensions and pulmonary artery systolic pressure (PASP). The explanation for this effect might be better contractility coordination of the interventricular septum and the RV lateral wall, providing evidence of prompt hemodynamic relief obtained after device implantation (Fleming et al. 2011; Campbell et al. 2013; Donal et al. 2008)
- *Long-term response.* Long-term RV reverse remodeling refers to the six-month response after CRT implantation (Fleming et al. 2011; Campbell et al. 2013; Donal et al. 2008). The mechanisms involved are:
  (1) LV systolic function improvement
  (2) Decrease in mitral regurgitation and pulmonary vein hypertension
  (3) Reverse remodeling of the LV associated with the CRT effect on the interventricular septum CRT also acts on the neurohormonal status and may affect RV function and dimensions and PASP (Delgado and Bax 2010; Fleming et al. 2011).

The RV is a complex chamber, heavily influenced by pre-load and after-load (Haddad et al. 2008). Echocardiography is crucial for RV dimension and function assessment (Fiegenbaum 1994). The RV echocardiographic systolic function evaluation involves parameters such as RV index of myocardial performance (RIMP), tricuspid annular plane systolic excursion (TAPSE), 2D fractional area change (FAC), 3D EF, Doppler tissular imaging-derived (DTI) of the tricuspid lateral annular systolic velocity wave (S′), RV global longitudinal strain (RVGLS) by 2D DTI, and by speckle tracking echocardiography (STE) (Badano and Muraru 2011; Lang et al. 2015). Many studies used different methods to find the effect of CRT on the RV. Measurements used for RV function evaluation after CRT were RV long-axis and short-axis dimensions, TAPSE, RV strain, and RV fractional area change, (Sadeghian et al. 2022a) tissue Doppler imaging (D'Andrea et al. 2009).

The guidelines recommend multiple acoustic windows for evaluation (Fig. 5.1a–d) (Supplementary material 1–6). The final echocardiographic report should present the qualitative and quantitative parameters, including size and function (Lang et al. 2015).

Measurements of the RV dimensions by 2DE are challenging because of the complex geometry of the cavity and the absence of specific anatomic landmarks (Lang et al. 2015). RV linear dimensions should be measured from a four-chamber view from the apical window at end-diastole (Kusiak et al. 2012). RV basal diameter—is the maximal transversal dimension in the basal one-third of RV inflow (Lang et al. 2015; Rudski et al. 2010). *RV linear inflow measurements* must be obtained from the apical four-chamber (A4c)-focused on the RV (Langet al. 2015) (Fig. 5.2). RV linear dimensions should be measured from a four-chamber view from the apical window at end-diastole (Kusiak et al. 2012). RV basal diameter—is the maximal transversal dimension in the basal one-third of RV inflow (Lang et al. 2015) (Fig. 5.2a1). RV mid diameter—is the transversal RV diameter in the middle third of RV inflow, halfway between the maximal basal diameter and the apex, at the level of papillary muscles (Lang et al. 2015) (Fig. 5.2a2) RV longitudinal diameter (mm)—is the dimension from the middle of the tricuspid line to the apex (Lang et al. 2015) (Fig. 5.2a3)

RV linear outflow measurements are

- Right ventricle outflow tract proximal diameter (proximal RVOT) (mm)—measured from the anterior RV wall to the junctions between interventricular septum and aorta, in parasternal long-axis view) (Lang et al. 2015) (Fig. 5.2b) or the aortic valve (in parasternal short-axis) (Lang et al. 2015) (Fig. 5.2c1)
- RVOT distal diameter (distal RVOT) (mm)—measured proximal to the pulmonary valve in parasternal short-axis view (Lang et al. 2015) (Fig. 5.2c2)

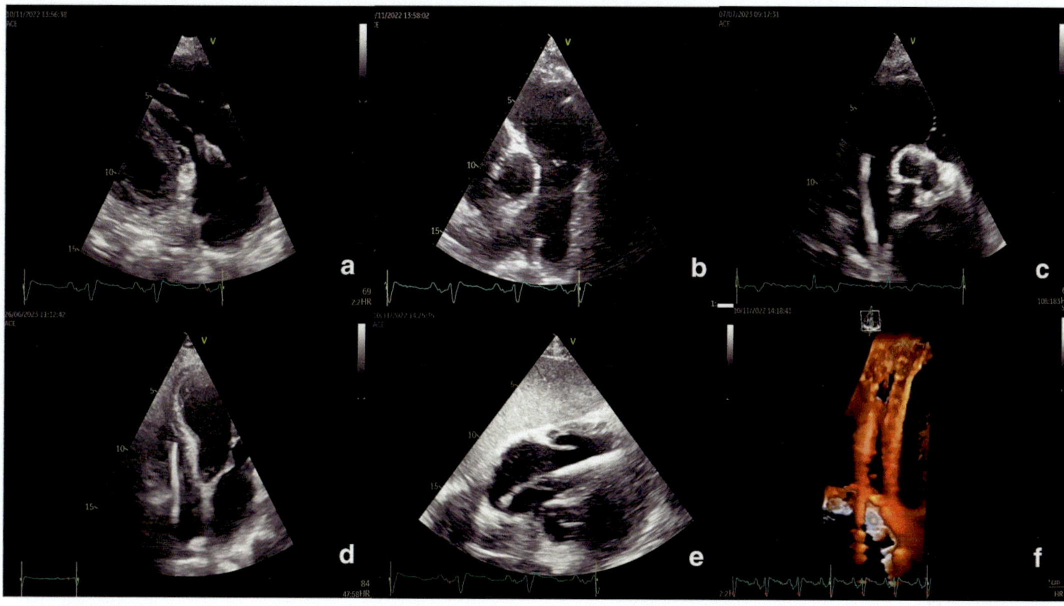

Fig. 5.1 Echocardiographic views for right ventricle evaluation. **a** Right ventricle inflow view, **b** right ventricle outflow view, **c** parasternal short axis view at the level of great arteries, **d** apical four-chamber view focused on the RV, **e** subcostal view, **f** three-dimensional reconstruction of the right ventricle in a patient with dilated cardiomyopathy and implanted cardio defibrillator

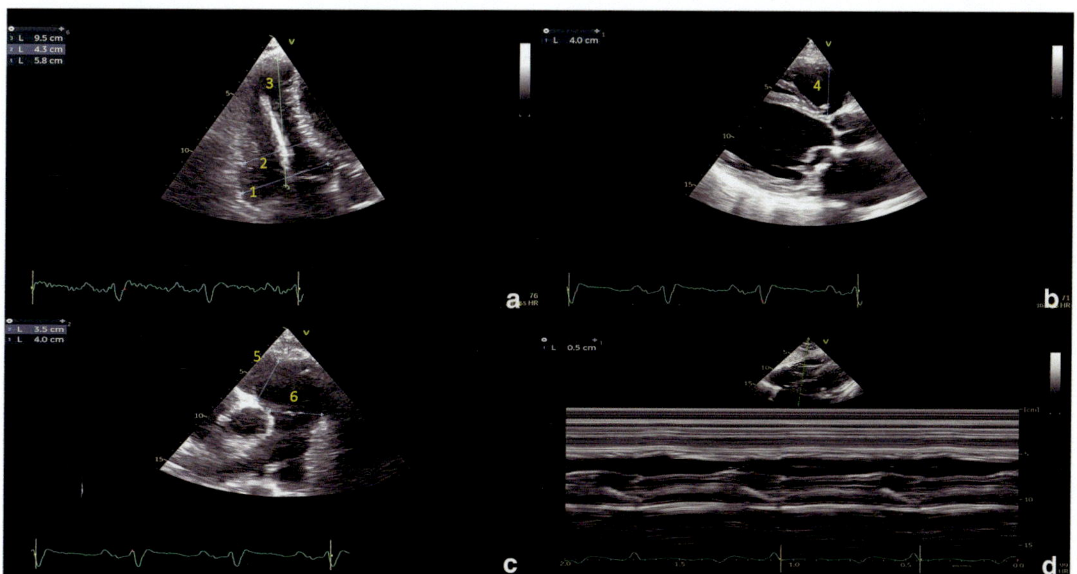

Fig. 5.2 Right ventricle linear measurements. **a** Apical four-chamber: **a1** basal diameter, **a2** mid diameter, **a3** longitudinal diameter; **b** outflow tract proximal diameter measured in parasternal long-axis view; **c** measurements in parasternal short-axis view: **c1** proximal outflow tract proximal diameter, **c2** distal outflow tract proximal diameter; **d** free wall thickness by M-mode from the subcostal window

All the linear measurements must be obtained at the end-diastole. These regional parameters may not reflect the global RV (Badano and Muraru 2011; Lang et al. 2015).

RV-free wall thickness should be measured at end-diastole by M-mode from the subcostal window (Kusiak et al. 2012) (Fig. 5.2d).

Because of the crescent RV shape, the report should inform the incidence approach. This data will avoid underestimation (Badano and Muraru 2011; Lang et al. 2015).

Tricuspid annular plane systolic excursion (TAPSE) reflects RV longitudinal function and has predictive value (Badano and Muraru 2011; Lang et al. 2015; Rudski et al. 2010). This parameter represents the distance of systolic excursion of the RV annulus along its longitudinal plane (Rajagopalan et al. 2007). The measurement uses M-mode echocardiography between end-diastole and peak systole, with the cursor aligned along with the direction movement of the lateral tricuspid annulus in the A4c view, averaging 3 cardiac cycles (Lang et al. 2015) (Fig. 5.3). TAPSE has correlated with other RV systolic function parameters, such as RV FAC and 2D echocardiographic EF in various studies. Guidelines validated this measurement against radionuclide RV EF. TAPSE is a one-dimensional measurement and may not offer an adequate RV function estimation because of overall heart motion (Lang et al. 2015; Rudski et al. 2010). The cutoff greater is 16 mm (Kaul et al. 1984; Tamborini et al. 2007).

RV fractional area change (RVFAC) evaluates global RV systolic function. This parameter has established predictive value and reflects longitudinal and radial RV contraction components (Badano and Muraru 2011; Lang et al. 2015).

The evaluation uses the A4c view focused on the RV:

$$\text{RV FAC (\%)} = 100 \times (\text{EDA}-\text{ESA})/\text{EDA}$$

EDA represents the end-diastolic area (Fig. 5.4a), and ESA represents the end-systolic area (Lang et al. 2015) (Fig. 5.4b). For RV fractional area change (RV FAC) evaluation, the RV endocardium will be measured in systole and diastole from the annulus to the apex along the free wall and from the apex to the annulus along the intraventricular septum. Tracing should avoid

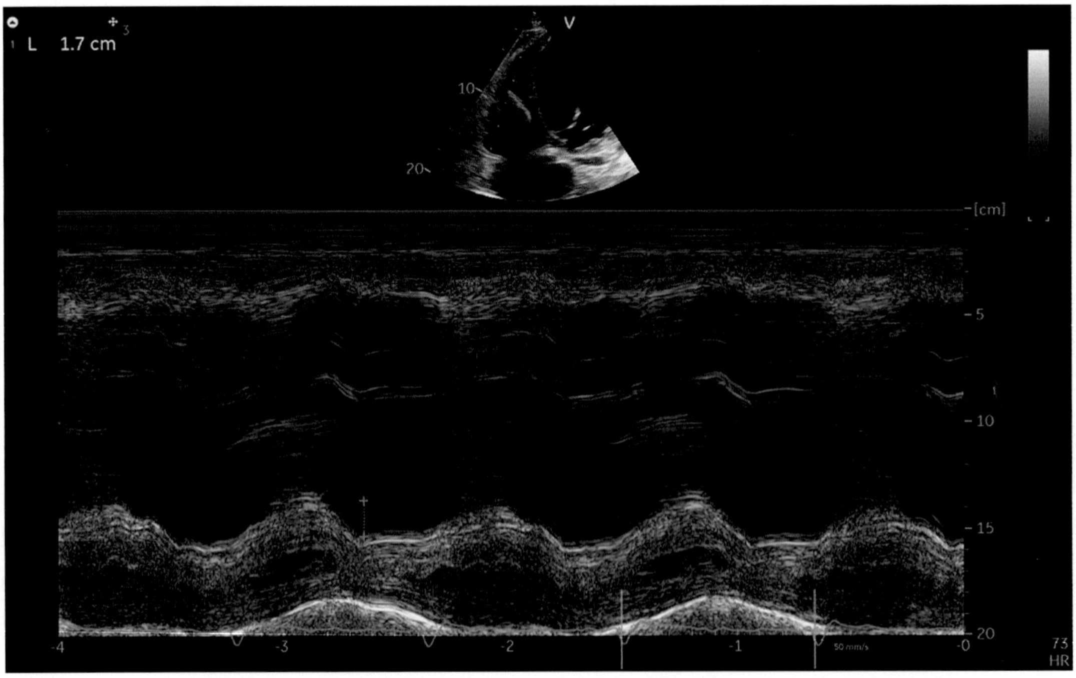

Fig. 5.3 Tricuspid annular plane systolic excursion

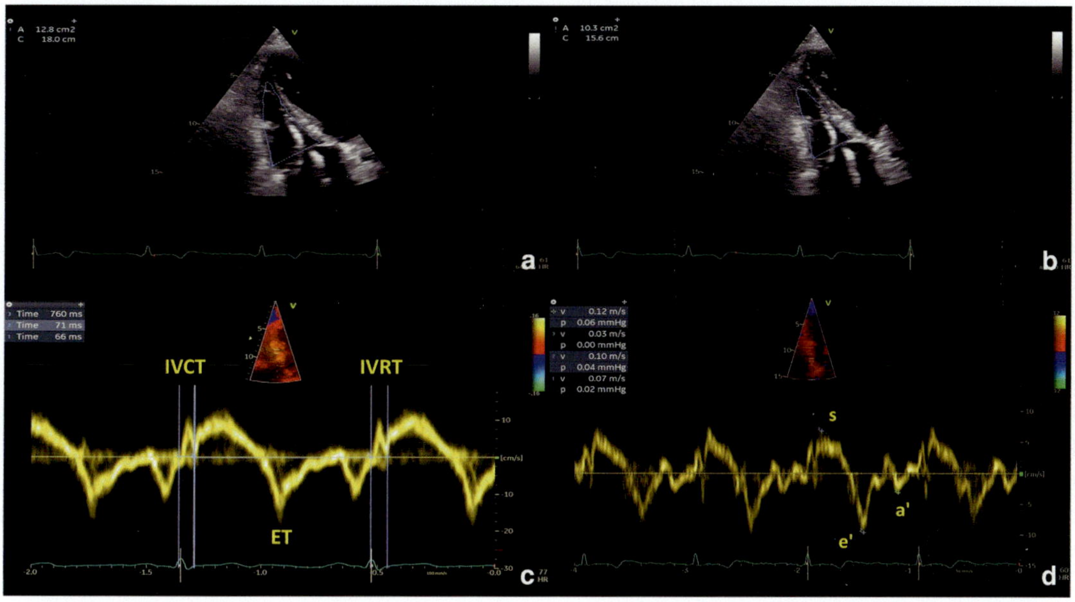

Fig. 5.4 RV FAC calculation. **a** End-diastolic area, **b** End-systolic area, **c** Right ventricular index of myocardial performance calculation by tissue Doppler echocardiography, **d** tissue Doppler-derived tricuspid lateral annular systolic velocity S' measurement

trabeculations (Lang et al. 2015; Kusiak et al. 2012; Rudski et al. 2010). RV FAC correlates with RV EF by cardiac magnetic resonance. A value < 35% indicates RV systolic dysfunction (Lang et al. 2015). The main limitation of this method is that it neglects the RV outflow tract contribution to systolic function (Badano and Muraru 2011; Lang et al. 2015).

Right Ventricular Index of Myocardial Performance (RIMP) reflects global RV function (Lang et al. 2015; Baumgartner et al. 2017; Lancellotti et al. 2013) measured by pulsed wave (PW) spectral Doppler or DTI at the lateral tricuspid annulus level. With PW spectral Doppler, the nonconsecutive beats must have similar RR intervals. This limitation does not apply to the DTI-based RIMP measurements (Badano and Muraru 2011; Lang et al. 2015; Rudski et al. 2010).

$$\text{RIMP} = (\text{IVRT} + \text{IVCT})/\text{ET}$$

IVRT represents the isovolumic relaxation time, ICVT represents the isovolumic contraction time and ET represents ejection time. Values of RIMP > 0.43 by PW Doppler or > 0.54 by DTI indicate an RV dysfunction (Lang et al. 2015) (Fig. 5.4c). This parameter has a prognostic value.

DTI-derived S′—tissue Doppler-derived tricuspid lateral annular systolic velocity (S′) represents the tricuspid annulus peak systolic velocity evaluated by PW DTI (cm/sec) (Badano and Muraru 2011; Lang et al. 2015) (Fig. 5.4d) For this parameter measurement, the ultrasound beam has to be parallel with RV free wall longitudinal displacement in an apical view. The studies revealed a good correlation with other parameters of global RV systolic function. An S′ wave velocity value < 9.5 cm/s at the free-wall level is a marker of RV systolic dysfunction (Lang et al. 2015).

For Tissue Doppler Echocardiography, gain and filters must be adjusted to remove background noise and generate a clear spectral display. Measurements are performed at a sweep speed of 100 mm/s, and digitally stored. Offline analysis consists of 3 successive beats of normal sinus rhythm and 10 cycles for patients with atrial fibrillation at end expiration, and the mean values will be calculated (Sadeghian et al. 2022a).

Tissue Doppler velocities of the tricuspid annulus are S′ in systole, E′, and A′ in diastole. The measurement is easy to perform and is reproducible. It has predictive value, validated against radionuclide EF, but is angle-dependent and influenced by heart motion (Rudski et al. 2010).

RV systolic dysfunction evaluated by **STE** is an independent prognostic marker (Giusca et al. 2010). The longitudinal **strain** represents the RV free wall percentage (%) of systolic shortening from the base to the apex. The longitudinal **strain rate** represents the shortening rate (Marwick et al. 2009). Compared to S′, RV longitudinal strain is less angle-dependent, but it depends on loading conditions (Marwick et al. 2009). 2D longitudinal strain uses an A-4c view focused on the RV (Lee and Park 2018). The reverberations and attenuation may influence the image quality. The region of interest should include the myocardium and exclude the pericardium (Marwick et al. 2009; Lee and Park 2018). **RV global longitudinal strain (RV GLS)** may refer to the averaging of tree segments of the RV free wall and tree septal segments or may include only the RV free wall segments (Lang et al. 2015) (Fig. 5.5a). The reference ranges were different because the studies involved multivendor equipment. According to the most recent chamber quantification guidelines, a value > −20% (< 20% in absolute value) of RV FWS is abnormal (Lang et al. 2015). The final echocardiographic report should also provide information about TR severity, PASP estimation, and RA dimensions (Lang et al. 2015; Rudski et al. 2010).

RV remodeling consists of volume increasing, tricuspid annular dilatation, papillary muscle displacing, leaflets tethering, and secondary **TR** (Fiegenbaum 1994; Rudski et al. 2010) (Fig. 5.5b). The final point is RV failure. **PASP** estimation uses CW Doppler imaging of the TR flow. Using the modified Bernoulli equation, the tricuspid valve gradient is measured from the peak velocity jet (Fig. 5.5c). Then, estimated right atrium (RA) pressure is added based on the inferior vena cava size and collapsibility (Fiegenbaum 1994).

Right ventricle systolic pressure (RVSP) is calculated from tricuspid regurgitation (TR) velocity and right atrium pressure, estimated

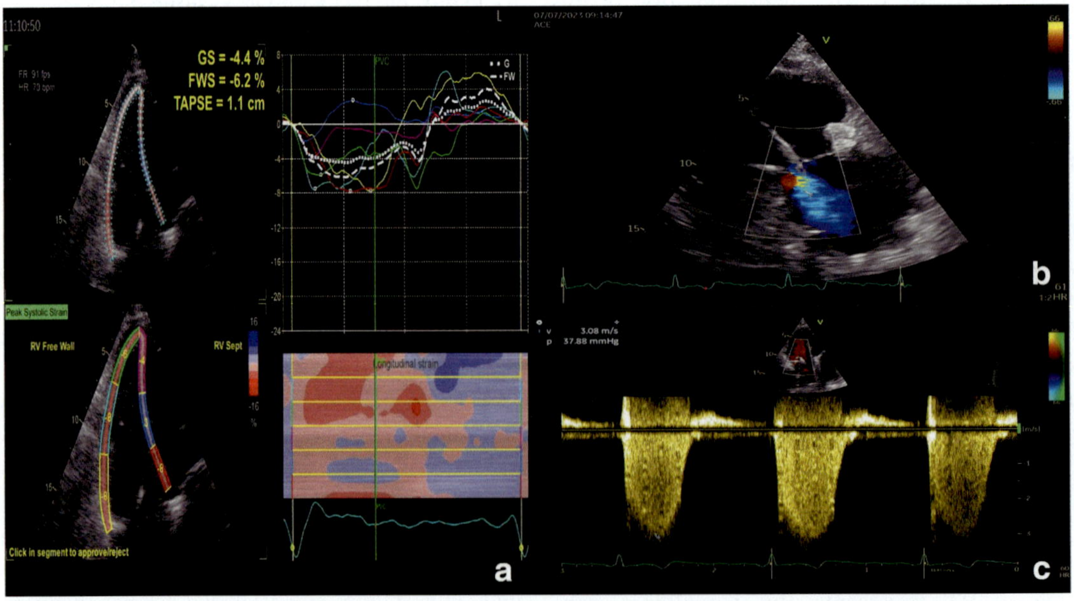

Fig. 5.5 **a** RV global longitudinal strain, **b** Tricuspid regurgitation, **c** Pulmonary systolic pressure calculation calculation from continuous Doppler envelope of tricuspid regurgitation

from the size and collapsibility of inferior vena cava (IVC) (Lang et al. 2015; Kusiak et al. 2012; Rudski et al. 2010).

RV volume measurement by **3D echocardiography** was validated against cardiac magnetic resonance (CMR). The technique is independent of geometric assumptions and includes the inflow, outflow, and apical regions. 3D RV volumes are usually lower compared to CMR (Lang et al. 2015).

3D RV EF assessment has some limitations linked to the loading conditions, septal motion, and imaging quality but correlates with RV EF by CMR. If available, guidelines consider it to be a method of quantifying RV systolic function (Fig. 5.4d). The RV systolic function is abnormal if the value is < 45% (Lang et al. 2015) (Fig. 5.6).

Doppler evaluation of RV diastolic function must be performed at end-expiration during quiet breathing. The parameters are peak early (E) and atrial (A) velocities of the tricuspid inflow. The pulse Doppler sample volume must be positioned in the apical four-chamber RV-focused view at the tip of the tricuspid valve (TV) leaflets. The measurements are the E/A ratio and the TV E-wave deceleration time (DT) (Singulane et al. 2016) (Fig. 5.7a). Tissue Doppler velocities are obtained by positioning the pulsed-wave tissue Doppler sample volume on the lateral tricuspid annulus. The measurements include the calculation of early (e′) and atrial (a′) diastolic velocities and the E/e′ ratio (Singulane et al. 2016) (Fig. 5.4d).

RA quantification size uses the A4-c view RA-focused view (Fig. 5.7b). RA linear dimensions should be measured from a four-chamber view from the apical window at end-systole.(Lang et al. 2015; Rudski et al. 2010) The minor-axis dimension is the plane perpendicular to the RA long-axis, extending from the RA lateral border to the interatrial septum (Fig. 5.7b). Guidelines indicate a single-view area-length and/or disk summation method for RA volume measurement using 2D echocardiography (Fig. 5.7c). 2D echocardiographic technique underestimates **RA volume** compared with 3D (Lang et al. 2015). 2D speckle tracking imaging can measure RA longitudinal strain in a

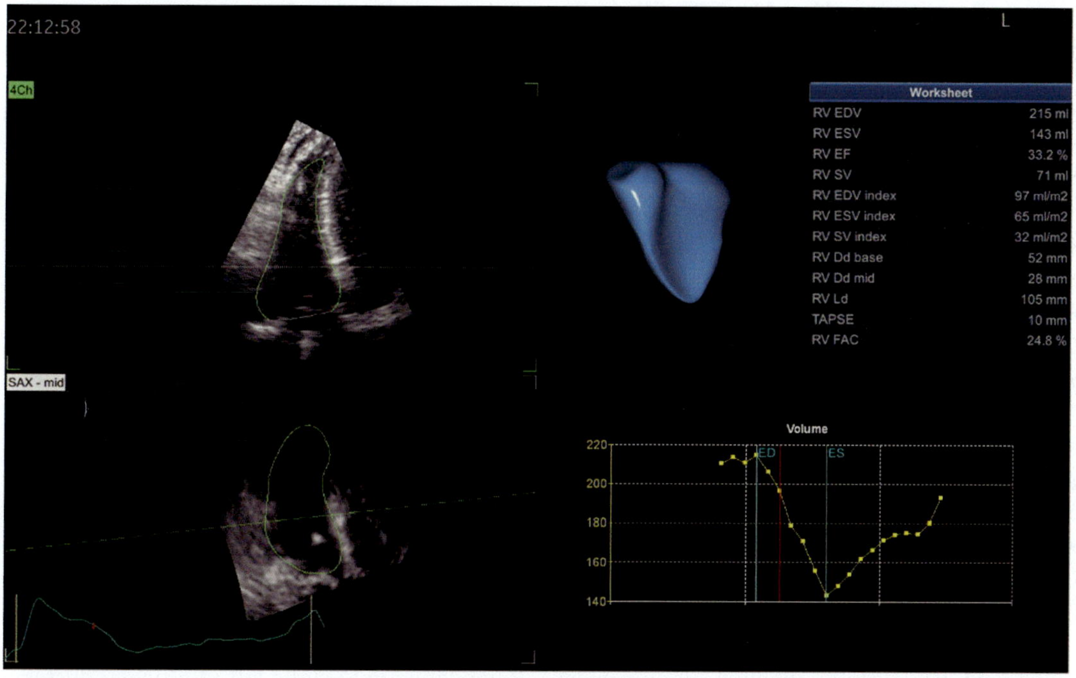

Fig. 5.6 Right ventricle quantification by three echocardiography using dedicated software

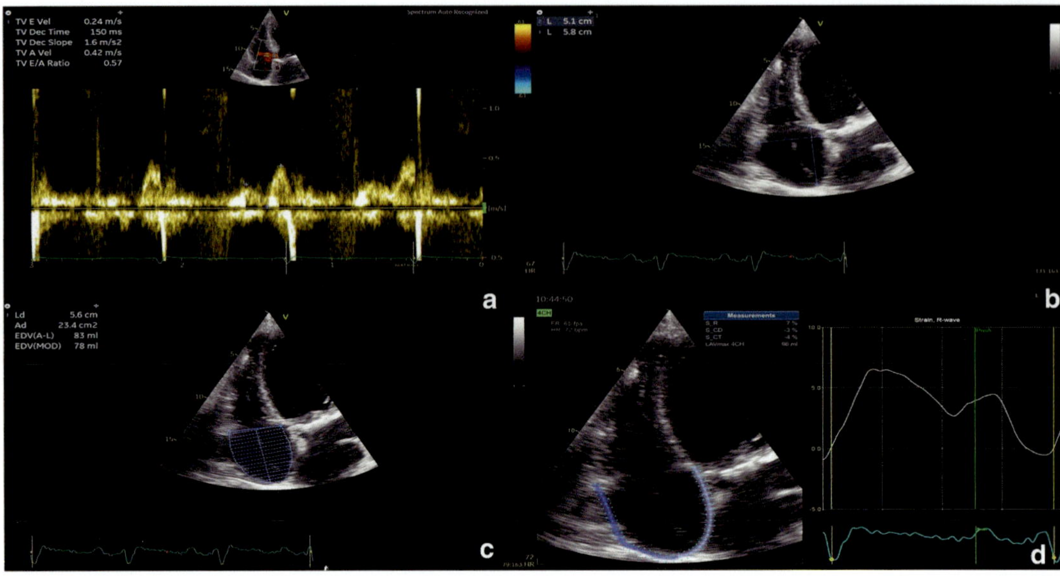

Fig. 5.7 **a** Right ventricle diastolic function evaluation form tricuspid inflow; **b** right atrium linear dimensions measurement; **c** right atrium volume measurement; **d** right atrium strain easurement by speckle tracking echocardiography

dedicated view for atrial analysis (Badano and Muraru 2011; Singulane et al. 2016) (Fig. 5.7d).

5.1.1 RV Echocardiographic Parameters Used in CRT Clinical Trials

Patients with nonischemic etiology of HF referred to CRT have a better improvement of RV dysfunction after CRT compared with those with an ischemic etiology of HF (Ghio et al. 2009; Sutton et al. 2006). Other studies did not find a link between the HF etiology and RV longitudinal axis function response to CRT (D'Andrea et al. 2009; Rajagopalan et al. 2007; Scuteri et al. 2009).

RV reverse remodeling is parallel to LV evolution in patients with CRT.

The effect of CRT on RV function is not clearly understood (Sadeghian et al. 2022b). RV systolic function improvement after CRT is linked to MR decrease and PASP reduction (Bleeker et al. 2005; Kanzaki et al. 2004) or to LV reverse remodeling, with better RV diastolic filling and RV systolic function improvement (Voelkel et al. 2006).

Some studies showed reverse remodeling of the RV concomitant with decreased PASP in patients with heart failure who received CRT. Other studies did not obtain any improvement of the RV function with CRT despite favorable changes to LV function. However, the evaluation methods had many limitations regarding the quantification methods (Cleland et al. 2005).

The Cardiac Resynchronization—Heart Failure (CARE-HF) trial used classical echocardiographic techniques for RV evaluation after CRT: TAPSE, RV EDA, RV ESA, RV FAC, TR, and the gradient pressure between RA and RV (Cleland et al. 2005). CRT increased LVEF, reduced LV volumes and MR at three months of implantation with benefit extension at nine and eighteen months, but did not improve RV structure and function (Cleland et al. 2005).

MADIT-CRT (the Multicenter Automatic Defibrillator Implantation with Cardiac Resynchronization Therapy) trial analysis identified an increase in RV FAC and a decrease in TR parallel with LV function improvement one year after implantation (Campbell et al. 2013).

In REVERSE (REsyncronization reVErses Remodeling in Systolic left vEntricular dysfunction) trial TAPSE was an independent predictor of LV reverse remodeling (Kjaergaard et al. 2011).

Echocardiographic parameters showing an RV function improvement *early* after CRT are RV FAC (Kusiak et al. 2012; Stolfo et al. 2016; Janousek et al. 2004). RV free wall tissue Doppler systolic velocity (Rajagopalan et al. 2007; Donal et al. 2007), and longitudinal strain (Donal et al. 2008). RV FAC increases in parallel with LV echocardiographic parameters changes such as severity of MR, restrictive filling pattern, E/E′ ratio, and PASP (Stolfo et al. 2016). S′ wave velocity and RV lateral wall basal and mid strain increased significantly three months after CRT (Donal et al. 2008). The effect on RV strain was evident in patients with septal RV lead position and correlated with the magnitude of RV dyssynchrony baseline evaluation. RV function improvement might precede RV reverse remodeling after CRT (Donal et al. 2008).

Some studies reported improvement in RV chamber size 6 months after CRT (Bleeker et al. 2005).

The parameters for RV evaluation *long-term* after CRT are RV dimensions at the level of the tricuspid annulus, RV short-axis, RV long-axis (Bleeker et al. 2005; Cappelli et al. 2010) TAPSE (Cappelli et al. 2010; Leong et al. 2013; Nagy et al. 2015) RVFAC (Nagy et al. 2015; Helsen et al. 2017) RV GLS, RV free wall strain (Helsen et al. 2017) the severity of TR, and PASP, (Bleeker et al. 2005) dyssynchrony at baseline (Bleeker et al. 2005).

RV function evaluation by TAPSE was significantly associated with LV diastolic function improvement 44 months after CRT (Leong et al. 2013). LV remodeling and MR correlated with RV FAC improvement (Helsen et al. 2017). RV systolic function evaluated by RV FAC was associated with clinical outcome at one year, independently of NYHA class and LV reverse remodeling (Helsen et al. 2017). RVGLS and RV-free wall strain improved six months after CRT implantation. These two parameters predicted survival at six months, independent of other parameters (Nagy et al. 2015).

Some studies showed RV tissue Doppler imaging velocity and RV lateral wall basal and mid-strain improvement after CRT (Donal et al. 2008).

5.2 Conclusions

RV evaluation plays an essential role in HF patients with CRT. Different studies studied different parameters at various times after CRT to evaluate the benefit on RV dimensions and function, and therefore, the results were discordant. The most appropriate approach is an integrative echocardiographic evaluation. CRT is associated with reverse remodeling of the RV. This action influences CRT's favorable effects. Future more extensive perspective studies help identify the most appropriate RV evaluation after CRT.

References

Badano LP, Muraru D. Assessment of right heart function and haemodynamics. In: Galiuto L, Badano L, Fox K, et al, editors. The EAE textbook of echocardiography. New York: Oxford University Press; 2011, p. 165–82.

Baumgartner H, Falk V, Bax JJ, et al. 2017 ESC/EACTS guidelines for the management of valvular heart disease The Task Force for the management of valvular heart disease of the European Society of Cardiology (ESC) and the European Association for Cardio-ThoracocSurgery (EACTS). Eur Heart J. 2017;38:2739–91.

Bleeker GB, Schalij MJ, Nihoyannopoulos P, et al. Left ventricular dyssynchrony predicts right ventricular remodeling after cardiac resynchronization therapy. J Am Coll Cardiol. 2005;46:2264–226910.

Brignole M, Auricchio A, Baron-Esquivias G, et al. 2013 ESC Guidelines on cardiac pacing and cardiac resynchronization therapy TheTask Force on cardiac pacing and resynchronization therapy of the European Society of Cardiology (ESC). Developed in collaboration with the European Heart Rhythm Association (EHRA). Eur Heart J. 2013;34:2281–2329.

Campbell P, Takeuchi M, Bourgoun M, et al. Right ventricular function, pulmonary pressure estimation, and clinical outcomes in cardiac resynchronization therapy. Circ Heart Fail. 2013;6:435–42.

Cappelli F, Porciani MC, Ricceri I, et al. Tricuspid annular plane systolic excursion evaluation improves selection of cardiac resynchronization therapy patients. Clin Cardiol. 2010;33(9):578–82.

Cleland GF, Daubert, Erdmann E, et al. The Effect of Cardiac Resynchronization on Morbidity and Mortality in Heart Failure, N Engl J Med. 2005;352:1539–49.

D'Andrea A, Salerno G, Scarafile R, et al. Right ventricular myocardial function in patients with either idiopathic or ischemic dilated cardiomyopathy without clinical sign of right heart failure: effects of cardiac resynchronization therapy. Pacing Clin Electrophysiol. 2009;32(8):1017–29.

Delgado V, Bax JJ. Cardiac resynchronization therapy: relevance of right ventricular function evaluation. Europace. 2010;12:311–2.

Donal E, Vignat N, De Place C, et al. Acute effects of biventricular pacing on right ventricular function assessed by tissue Doppler imaging. Europace. 2007;9(2):108–12.

Donal E, Thibault H, Bergerot C, et al. Right ventricular pump function after cardiac resynchronization therapy: a strain imaging study. Arch Cardiovasc Dis. 2008;101:475–84.

Donal E, Hernandez A, Hubert A, et al. Should the implantation of a CRT device in patients with a sick RV be discouraged? Acta Cardiol. 2017;3:237–9.

Fiegenbaum. Echocardiography, 5th ed. Baltimore: Lippincott Williams and Willis; 1994, p. 158–60.

Field ME, Solomon SD, Lewis EF, et al. Right ventricular dysfunction and adverse outcome in patients with advanced heart failure. J Card Fail. 2006;12(8):616–20.

Fleming LM, Haffajee C, Cang JD. Use of echocardiography to manage cardiac resynchronization therapy. J Innov Card Rhythm Manag. 2011;2:464–74.

Ghio S, Recusani F, Klersy C, et al. Prognostic usefulness of the tricuspid annular plane systolic excursion in patients with congestive heart failure secondary to idiopathic or ischemic dilated cardiomyopathy. Am J Cardiol. 2000;85(7):837–42.

Ghio S, Gavazzi A, Campana C, et al. Independent and additive prognostic value of right ventricular systolic function and pulmonary artery pressure in patients with chronic heart failure. J Am Coll Cardiol. 2001;37(1):183–8.

Ghio S, Freemantle N, Scelsi L, et al. Long-term left ventricular reverse remodelling with cardiac resynchronization therapy: results from the CARE-HF trial. Eur J Heart Fail. 2009;11(5):480–8.

Giusca S, Dambrauskaite V, Scheurwegs C, et al. Deformation imaging describes right ventricular function better than longitudinal displacement of the tricuspid ring. Heart. 2010;96:281–8.

Haddad F, Doyle R, Murphy DJ, Hunt SA. Right ventricular function in cardiovascular disease, part II: pathophysiology, clinical importance, and management of right ventricular failure. Circulation. 2008;117(13):1717–73.

Helsen F, Van De Bruaene A, Gabriels C. Prognostic significance of improvement in right ventricular systolic function during cardiac resynchronization therapy. Acta Cardiol. 2017;72(3):267–75.

Janousek J, Tomek V, Chaloupecky VA, et al. Cardiac resynchronization therapy: a novel adjunct to the treatment and prevention of systemic right ventricular failure. J Am Coll Cardiol. 2004;44:1927–31.

Kanzaki H, Bazaz R, Schwartzman D, et al. A mechanism for immediate reduction in mitral regurgitation after cardiac resynchronization therapy: insights from mechanical activation strain mapping. J Am Coll Cardiol. 2004;44:1619–25.

Karatasakis GT, Karagounis LA, Kalyvas PA, et al. Prognostic significance of echocardiographically estimated right ventricular shortening in advanced heart failure. Am J Cardiol. 1998;82(3):329–34.

Kaul S, Tei C, Hopkins JM, Shah PM. Assessment of right ventricular function using two-dimensional echocardiography. Am Heart J. 1984;107(3):526–31.

Kjaergaard J, Ghio S, Sutton MSJ, Hassager C. Tricuspid annular plane systolic excursion and response to cardiac resynchronization therapy: results from the REVERSE trial. J Card Fail. 2011;17(2):100–7.

Kusiak A, Wiliński J, Wojciechowska W, et al. Effects of biventricular pacing on right ventricular function assessed by standard echocardiography. Kardiol Pol. 2012;70(9):883–8.

Lancellotti P, Tribouilloy C, Hagendorff A, et al. Recommendations for the echocardiographic assessment of native valvular regurgitation: an executive summary from the European Association of Cardiovascular Imaging. Eur Heart J Cardiovasc Imag. 2013;14:611–44.

Lang RM, Badano LP, Mor-Avi V, et al. Recommendations for cardiac chamber quantification by echocardiography in adults: an update from the American Society of Echocardiography and the European Association of Cardiovascular Imaging. Eur Heart J Cardiovasc Imaging. 2015;16:233–71.

Lee J-H, Park J-H. Strain analysis of the right ventricle using two-dimensional echocardiography. J Cardiovasc Imaging. 2018;26(3):111–24.

Leong DP, Höke U, Delgado V. Right ventricular function and survival following cardiac resynchronisation therapy. Heart. 2013;99(10):722–8.

Marwick TH, Leano RL, Brown J, et al. Myocardial strain measurement with 2-dimensional speckle-tracking echocardiography: definition of normal range. JACC-Cardiovasc Imag. 2009;2(1):80–4.

Meyer P, Filippatos GS, Ahmed MI, et al. Effects of right ventricular ejection fractionon outcomes in chronic systolic heart failure. Circulation. 2010;121:252–8.

Nagy VK, Széplaki G, Apor A, et al. Role of right ventricular global longitudinal strain in predicting early and long-term mortality in cardiac resynchronization therapy patients. PLoS ONE. 2015;10(12):e0143907.

Ogunyankin KO, Puthumana JJ. Effect of cardiac resynchronization therapy on right ventricular function. Curr Opin Cardiol. 2010;25(5):464–8.

Rajagopalan N, Suffoletto MS, Tanabe M, et al. Right ventricular function following cardiac resynchronization therapy. Am J Cardiol. 2007;100(9):1434–6.

Rigolin VH, Robiolio PA, Wilson JS, Harrison JK, Bashore TM. The forgotten chamber: the importance of the right ventricle. Cathet Cardiovasc Diagn. 1995;35(1):18–28.

Rudski LG, Lai WW, Afilalo J, et al. Guidelines for the echocardiographic assessment of the right heart in adults: a report from the American Society of Echocardiography endorsed by the European Association of Echocardiography, a registered branch of the European Society of Cardiology, and the Canadian Society of Echocardiography. J Am Soc Echocardiogr. 2010;23:685–713.

Sadeghian H, Kazemisaied A, Rezvanfard M, et al. Improved right ventricular systolic function after cardiac resynchronization therapy in patients with heart failure. Tex Heart Inst J. 2022a;49(5):e207499.

Sadeghian H, Kazemisaied A, Rezvanfard M, et al. Improved right ventricular systolic function after cardiac resynchronization therapy in patients with heart failure, Sadeghian H, Kazemisaied A, Rezvanfard M, et al. Tex Heart Inst J. 2022;49(5):e207499.

Scuteri L, Rordorf R, Marsan NA, et al. Relevance of echocardiographic evaluation of right ventricular function in patients undergoing cardiac resynchronization therapy. Pacing Clin Electrophysiol. 2009;32(8):1040–9.

Singulane CC, Singh A, Miyoshi T, et al. Sex-, age-, and race-related normal values of right ventricular diastolic function parameters: data from the world alliance societies of echocardiography study, world alliance societies of echocardiography normal values study. J Am Soc Echocardiogr. 2016;35(4):426–34.

Stolfo D, Tonet E, Merlo M. Early right ventricular response to cardiac, resynchronization therapy: impact on clinical outcomes. Eur J Heart Fail. 2016;18:205–13.

Sutton MG, Plappert T, Hilpisch KE, Abraham WT, Hayes DL, Chinchoy E. Sustained reverse left ventricular structural remodeling with cardiac resynchronization at one year is a function of etiology: quantitative Doppler echocardiographic evidence from the Multicenter InSync Randomized Clinical Evaluation (MIRACLE). Circulation. 2006;113(2):266–72.

Tamborini G, Pepi M, Galli CA, et al. Feasibility and accuracy of a routine echocardiographic assessment of right ventricular function. Int J Cardiol. 2007;115(1):86–9.

Voelkel NF, Quaife RA, Leinwand LA et al. Right ventricular function and failure: report of a National Heart, Lung, and Blood Institute working group on cellular and molecular mechanisms of right heart failure. Circulation. 2006; 1141883–1891.

Mitral Regurgitation Echocardiographic Evaluation in Patients with Implanted Devices

6

Abstract

Patients with implanted devices and mitral regurgitation present a complex pathology, making accurately measuring the severity of the condition challenging. However, echocardiography remains essential for confirming the diagnosis, assessing the disease's severity, and predicting its prognosis. The decrease in mitral regurgitation parallels left ventricle reverse remodeling in CRT responders. Recent research showed a possible correlation between the right ventricle lead's position and mitral regurgitation severity in post-implantation patients. Updated guidelines recommend a comprehensive two-dimensional evaluation, including a detailed assessment of the mitral valve, the right ventricle, and the lead position. A systematic three-dimensional echocardiographic assessment of the mitral valve and surrounding structures should follow this approach. Three-dimensional echocardiographic software packages provide more detailed information about the etiology and severity of mitral regurgitation. Combining two-dimensional and three-dimensional echocardiographic evaluations will help better understand the condition, enabling treatment decisions. This promising development has the potential to improve patient outcomes significantly.

Supplementary Information The online version contains supplementary material available at https://doi.org/10.1007/978-3-031-64079-7_6.

Because of the right ventricle (RV) apical lead position, mitral regurgitation (MR) may persist after implantation or aggravate in cardiac resynchronization therapy (CRT) and pacemaker patients. In CRT responders, left ventricle (LV) reverse remodeling is linked to improvement in MR (Galiuto et al. 2011). Functional mitral regurgitation (FMR) is a complex cardiac pathology that affects the mitral valve (MV) in the absence of organic lesions. The primary determinant of FMR is the phenomenon of "systolic tenting," which occurs as a result of the displacement of the coaptation points of the valve leaflets away from the mitral annulus (MA) and towards the LV cavity. This displacement culminates with FMR (Galiuto et al. 2011). FMR can potentially exacerbate left ventricular remodeling, leading to a vicious cycle where the enlargement of the left ventricle and FMR worsen each other (Galiuto et al. 2011).

6.1 The Complexity of Functional Mitral Regurgitation in Patients with CRT

The studies revealed a robust correlation between moderate to severe FMR severity and all-cause mortality and hospitalization in

D.-M. Toader, *Echocardiographic Evaluation of Patients with Implanted Devices*, https://doi.org/10.1007/978-3-031-64079-7_6

patients diagnosed with dilated cardiomyopathy (DCM) and LV systolic dysfunction. This association was observed irrespective of the patient's implanted device status. The findings underscore the importance of identifying and managing FMR, particularly in patients with DCM and LV systolic dysfunction (Ponikowski et al. 2016). According to echocardiography studies, the estimated prevalence of FMR in DCM ranges from 8 to 74%. In ischemic cardiomyopathy, it is approximately 50%, while in nonischemic cardiomyopathy, it ranges from 56 to 65% (Ponikowski et al. 2016). FMR severity assessment has emerged as a critical determinant in the response to CRT, underscoring the significance of developing effective methods for FMR evaluation post-CRT (Brignole et al. 2013). An imbalance between the closing and tethering forces causes FMR in patients with DCM and CRT.

Understanding the mechanisms underlying FMR is critical for effective management and improved patient outcomes:

- LV contractile dysfunction and dilatation are the primary causes of decreased closing force (Enriquez-Sarano et al. 1999; Otsuji et al. 1997).
- Papillary muscle (PM) displacement is the leading cause of increased tethering force (Spartera et al. 2016).

Due to LV remodeling and dilation, PMs can be displaced away from the mitral annulus (MA) (You et al. 2000). PMs pull MV leaflets apically and/or posteriorly, increasing the tethering forces (Fig. 6.1a, Supplementary material 1). Posterior and lateral PM displacement also contribute to the lack of leaflets coaptation (Otsuji et al. 1997). (Fig. 6.1b, Supplementary material 2)

6.2 FMR Mechanisms in Patients with CRT and Heart Failure

FMR ensues from various underlying mechanisms such as decreased contractility, ventricular remodeling, impairment of MA function, and ventricular dyssynchrony (Enriquez-Sarano et al. 1999).

Other factors that contribute to FMR are:

1. The geometrical distortions of the **MA** caused by LV dilatation (Gorman et al. 2004; Watanabe et al. 2005). The annulus shape, dimension and function are impaired, and the annulus becomes flattened (Otsuji et al. 2002). (Fig. 6.2) The coaptation reserve decreases over time due to the increasing tethering forces. MA dilatation promoted by left atrial (LA) enlargement worsens FMR in patients with heart failure (HF) and atrial fibrillation

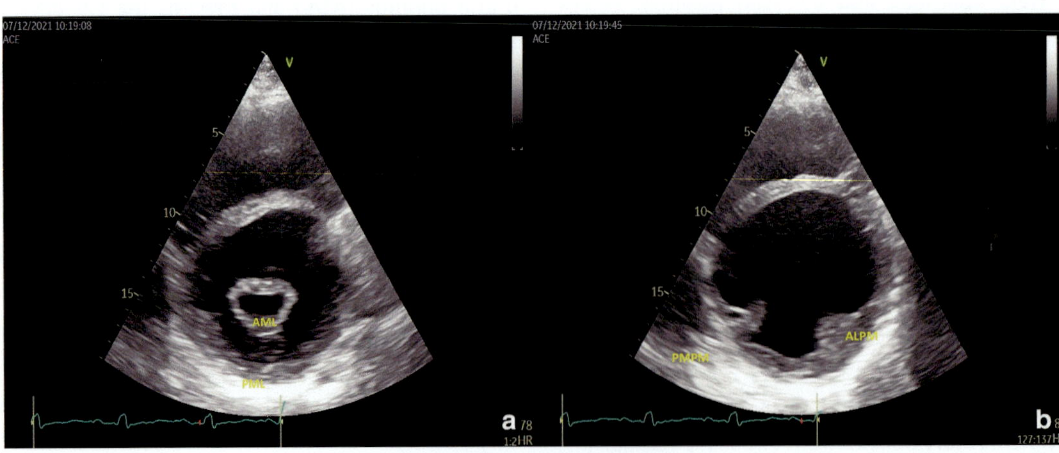

Fig. 6.1 A Mitral valve in a patient with dilated cardiomyopathy and CRT viewed from parasternal short axis view; B Posterior and lateral papillary muscles displacement in a patient with dilated cardiomyopathy and CRT viewed from parasternal short axis view

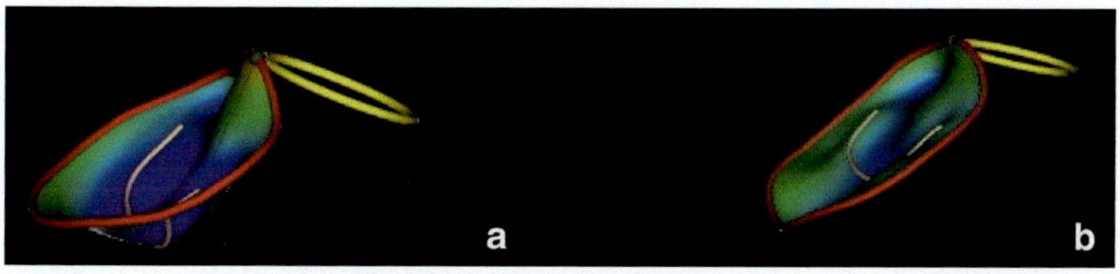

Fig. 6.2 A Normal shape of mitral mitral annulusş B Flattened shape of the mitral annulus in patients with dilated cardiomyopathy

(AF) (Ponikowski et al. 2016). MV leaflets are attached to the atrial wall in this setting, causing improper valve closure. This process is called "atriogenic leaflet tethering." The posterior MV leaflet is stretched across the LV wall by LA dilatation, tethering MV leaflets away from the PMs (Silbiger 2014).

2. The theory of **organic components** of FMR. HF has been shown to produce structural and biochemical alterations in MV leaflets, resulting in an increased concentration of cells and a decreased concentration of water—a vital component. This phenomenon subsequently leads to a reduction in the viscoelasticity of the tissue, rendering the leaflets stiffer. These findings underline the importance of understanding the impact of HF on MV leaflets (Grande-Allen et al. 2005a, 2005b; Stephens et al. 2009).
3. The **mechanical dyssynchrony** increases the tethering forces. Uncoordinated regional mechanical activation distorts MV apparatus geometry (He et al. 1997). The mechanical dyssynchrony decreases the closing forces and impairs MV tenting (Spartera et al. 2016).

The severity of FMR depends on:

1. *LV remodeling* can be either local, after an acute myocardial infarction, or global, caused by conditions like DCM, volume overload, or pressure overload (Spartera et al. 2016).
2. *The MA tenting* phenotypes based on LV remodeling:

- Symmetrical pattern in which both leaflets are equally affected owing to the apical displacement of both papillary muscles. As a result, the coaptation point is set apically, and the regurgitant jet is centralized. This group of patients is characterized by a more advanced stage of LV dilatation and dysfunction (Galiuto et al. 2011) (Fig. 6.3a).
- asymmetric pattern is characterized by posterior displacement of the posterior leaflet, PMs, and the coaptation point. It is more frequent in inferolateral myocardial infarctions, and the jet direction is opposite the affected leaflet. It is related to a lesser degree of LV dysfunction (Galiuto et al. 2011) (Fig. 6.3b).

MA dilation or dysfunction can lead to FMR by reducing MV coaptation. Research findings have indicated that isolated annulus dilation does not result in regurgitation without mitral leaflet tethering. This approach suggests that mitral leaflet tethering may be a necessary condition for FMR to occur (Donal et al. 2009). The enlargement or malfunction of the MA is considered a predisposing factor that can increase the MV tenting area (Donal et al. 2009).

3. *Cardiac dyssynchrony:*

- Atrioventricular dyssynchrony contributes to late diastolic regurgitation (Spartera et al. 2016) (Fig. 6.4).
- Interventricular dyssynchrony affects the synchrony between the left and right ventricles, decreasing cardiac output.(Spartera et al. 2016)
- Intraventricular dyssynchrony is characterized by different contraction times between myocardial segments of the LV, reducing systolic performance (Donal et al. 2009).

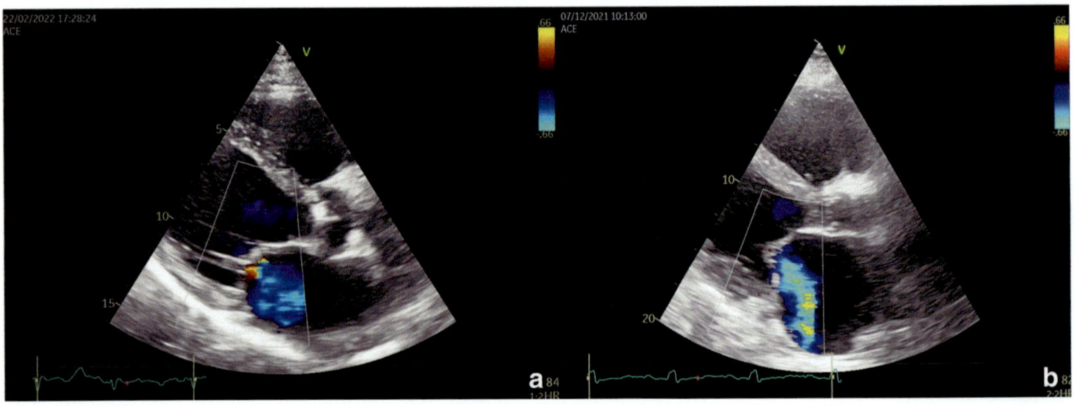

Fig. 6.3 A Central mitral regurgitation jet in a patient with symmetric mitral valve tethering; B: Posterior mitral regurgitation jet in a patient with asymmetric mitral valve tethering;

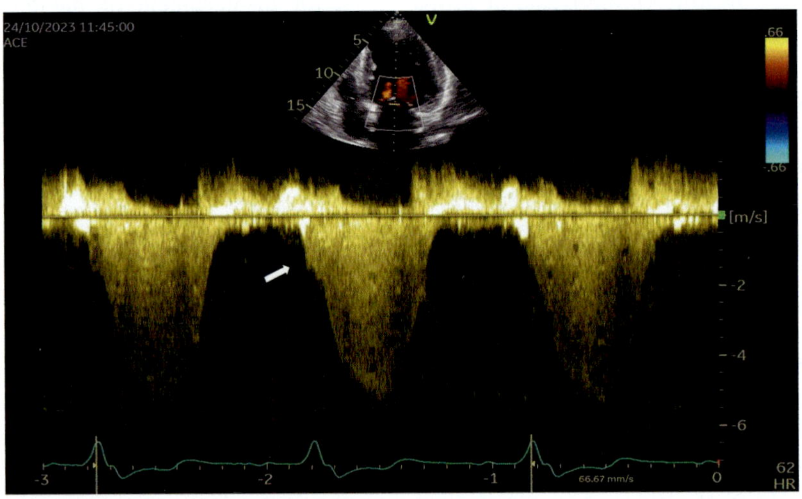

Fig. 6.4 Diastolic mitral regurgitation in a patient with VVI pacemaker

The studies have shown a link between the dyssynchrony of the myocardium surrounding the PMs and FMR (Donal et al. 2009; Kanzaki et al. 2004).

FMR is a dynamic lesion in patients with CRT and HF, with variation over time. It is essential to note that FMR is affected by the patient's condition and the loading conditions. Additionally, some patients may be taking medications that modify preload, which can lead to errors in color Doppler flow mapping of the LA and regurgitant jet width. Therefore, it is crucial to consider all relevant factors when evaluating FMR. Doppler measurement or proximal velocity surface area (PISA) method is more accurate. The regurgitant volume, specifically the (Effective Regurgitant Orifice Area) EROA, which is less load-dependent, is more reliable (McDonagh et al. 2012).

Intra-beat FMR variation is a medical condition caused by an imbalance between opposing forces. It is characterized by variation in the timing of the regurgitant orifice area, also known as the "loitering pattern." An increase in orifice area and regurgitation during early and late systole typically marks this condition. In contrast, regurgitation is lower during mid-systole when the LV pressure facilitates valve closure (Russo et al. 2022).

Beat-to-beat FMR variation depends on tethering and closing forces balance, which is influenced by physiological and pharmacological factors. Diuretics reduce preload, ventricular size, and tethering forces, decreasing MR. Inotropic agents also reduce MR severity by increasing contractility and closing forces. These interventions should be considered when managing MR (Russo et al. 2022; Baumgartner et al. 2017).

MR worsens over time due to chronic volume overload, creating a vicious circle where "MR begets MR" (Enriquez-Sarano et al. 1999).

Patients requiring CRT may experience LV reverse remodeling and decreased FMR. This could offer a multifaceted benefit in treating HF, including improved cardiac function, exercise capacity, and reduced risk of adverse events (Cazeau et al. 2001; Cleland et al. 2005). Multiple factors cause FMR in HF patients; LV dyssynchrony is not the only mechanism. Some patients do not respond to CRT and do not have an improvement in FMR (Russo et al. 2022).

FMR may predict mortality independently of LV volume and clinical CRT response (Brignole et al. 2013). Multiple studies have demonstrated that reducing the severity of FMR is critical in determining the response to CRT. Responders are less likely to experience a positive outcome if regurgitation persists (Brignole et al. 2013).

6.3 Effects of CRT on FMR

FMR is a condition that can exhibit varied outcomes following implantation, with the potential to improve, remain stable, or worsen. FMR has been identified as a prognostic factor in patients undergoing CRT, indicating its significance in patient outcomes (Brignole et al. 2013). It has been observed that a reduction in the severity of MR by at least one degree occurs in a significant proportion of patients, ranging from 30 to 40%, after the implant procedure. This improvement has been consistently demonstrated, irrespective of the etiology of the underlying cardiomyopathy (Kanzaki et al. 2004; Vinereanu 2008; Breithardt et al. 2003; Porciani et al. 2006).

CRT potentially addresses the underlying pathophysiologic determinants of FMR. This benefit stems from the correction of LV dyssynchrony and reverse remodeling. The efficacy of CRT in treating FMR lies in its ability to synchronize and optimize the contraction of the ventricles. This synchronization results in a reduction of MR and an improvement in LV function (Spartera et al. 2016).

It has been found that correcting apical rocking (AR) and septal flush (SF) can lead to a significant reduction in the severity of MR after CRT (Spartera et al. 2016). The short-term decrease in FMR severity in CRT patients is due to improved, coordinated timing of mechanical activation of PMs insertion sites and increased contraction efficiency. LV reverse remodeling causes changes in the geometry of the MV, leading to a decrease in FMR over time (You et al. 2000; Breithardt et al. 2003; Porciani et al. 2006; Karvounis et al. 2006; Naqvi et al. 2008; Ypenburg et al. 2008). CRT has been found to have positive long-term effects on FMR, including increased closing forces and global LV inverse remodeling after 3–6 months of therapy. The increase in closing forces reduces regurgitation volume and subsequently reduces the degree of FMR. LV remodeling resulting from CRT reduces LV volume and improves its function (Kanzaki et al. 2004).

CRT may alter annular geometry and function, decreasing sphericity indices and affecting FMR (Solis et al. 2009; Mihos et al. 2020). Studies suggest that CRT can induce LA reverse remodeling and reduce the burden of AF in patients with HF, which is essential as AF has been implicated in the development of MA dilatation (Lellouche et al. 2007). Optimizing atrioventricular delay can eliminate diastolic MR and improve outcomes in patients with cardiac disease (Spartera et al. 2016).

The patients presenting with persistent and significant mitral MR may exhibit a lower response to CRT than those with mild/absent or improved MR following electrical treatment. Moreover, the absence of improvement in MR after CRT serves as an independent predictor of all-cause and cardiovascular mortality, highlighting the importance of monitoring MR progression in patients undergoing CRT for HF (Cipriani et al. 2016). Persistent MR after biventricular stimulation may indicate poor long-term response to CRT (Cleland et al. 2005; Cipriani et al. 2016; Biase et al. 2011; Verhaert et al. 2012). Excessive ventricular dilatation is associated with reduced reverse remodeling and MR improvement after CRT. The ischemic etiology is more frequent in patients with worsening MR after CRT (Onishi et al. 2013; Bommel et al. 2011). The resynchronization effect may be constrained by a scar at the PM site or by the gradual loss of viable myocardium due to ischemia. These factors merit consideration when assessing the effectiveness of the resynchronization treatment (Vinereanu 2008; St John Sutton et al. 2006).

The optimal impact of CRT on FMR and LV remodeling may be most beneficial in patients with mild MR rather than those with severe MR and irreversible LV dysfunction and dilatation. Patients with mild MR may benefit from CRT through improved FMR and LV remodeling. However, patients with severe MR and irreversible LV dysfunction and dilatation may not experience the same degree of benefit (Cipriani et al. 2016).

The specific mechanisms of CRT on FMR involve two main aspects. Firstly, CRT restores the synchronous contraction of the LV and PMs, improving spatial relations and function of the sub-valvular apparatus and the mitral valve. This subsequently reduces the tethering force. Secondly, CRT improves the coordination of the left ventricular wall contraction, contributing to an increase in the transmitral pressure gradient, thereby increasing the closing force. These two mechanisms work cohesively to improve the function of the MV and reduce FMR (Spartera et al. 2016).

Two phases can characterize the response of FMR following CRT

1. The initial, short-term reduction in FMR occurs immediately after the CRT implantation and is considered the primary determinant of a favorable response. This reduction in FMR is attributed to better left ventricular contraction, including PM-bearing segments, and an improvement in the transmitral pressure gradient, which results in increased closing forces. Additionally, due to the correction of the atrioventricular delay, diastolic or presystolic MR is eliminated (Spartera et al. 2016).
2. The long-term reduction in FMR occurs over weeks to months following CRT and is attributed to reverse remodeling. This reduction in FMR is due to decreased LV volume and sphericity, which leads to reduced tethering forces. Furthermore, the improved LV systolic function with increased closing forces characterizes this phase (Spartera et al. 2016).

6.4 FMR in Patients with Pacemaker

The pacing of the RVA results in ventricular dyssynchrony, causing consequential systolic and diastolic ventricular function impairment, LV remodeling, and MR. These adverse effects of RVA pacing have been documented in numerous studies and are of significant concern in the clinical management of patients with HF or other cardiac conditions (Tops et al. 2007) (Fig. 6.5). Hiss bundle pacing (HBP) is a recommended intervention for patients with moderate LV dysfunction who exhibit an LV ejection fraction (LVEF) of 36–50%. This treatment option is classified as a class IIa indication. It is especially suitable for individuals expected to require 40% ventricular pacing (Kusumoto et al. 2018). In patients with LV systolic dysfunction, HBP reduces functional MR through favorable ventricular remodeling. Physiological pacing via HBP is associated with improved LV remodeling (Upadhyay et al. 2021). The mechanisms

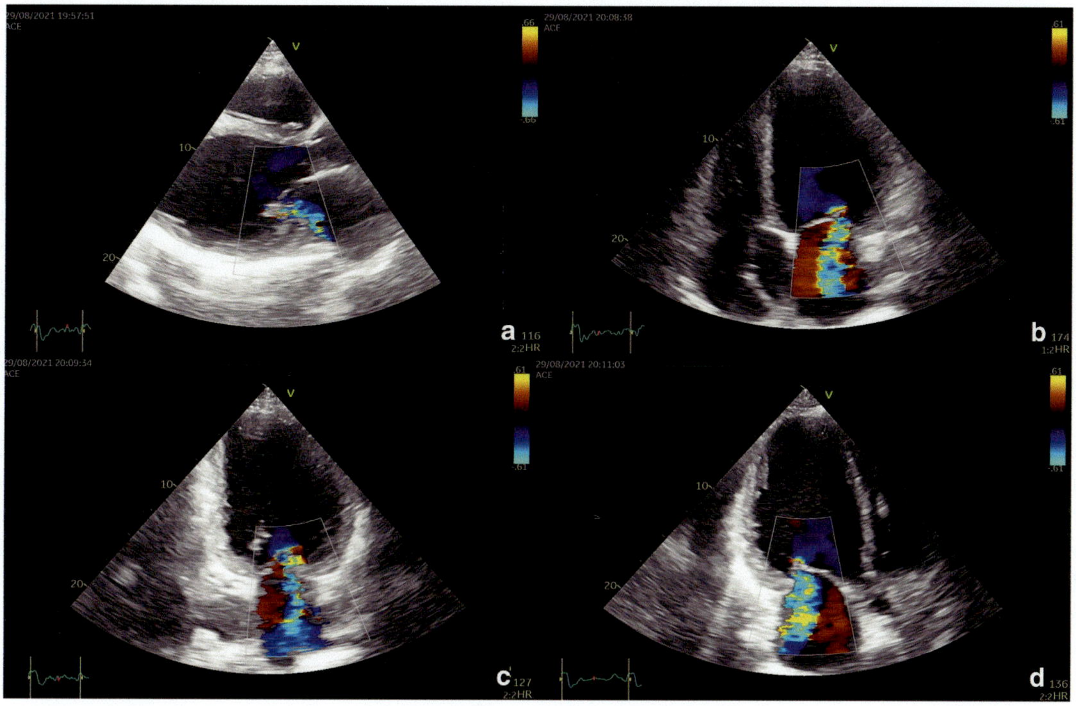

Fig. 6.5 Mitral regurgitation in a patient with VVI pacemaker; lead at the right ventricle apex: A parasternal long axis view; B Apical four-chamber view; C Apical two-chamber view; D Apical three-chamber view

for this improvement include enhancement of LV contractility and reduction in LV volume, which subsequently lead to improvements in MV and LV chamber geometry (Upadhyay et al. 2021). CRT may lead to a potential improvement in the severity of MR, LV hemodynamic parameters, and mechanical function (Eldadah et al. 2006; Marai et al. 2006). RVA-paced subjects receiving CRT exhibit similar short-term benefits as those with newly implanted CRTs (Lipar et al. 2016). CRT has also led to improvement in FMR in this group (Bommel et al. 2011). Irrespective of CRT response, moderate to severe FMR persistence after resynchronization is an essential indicator of bad prognosis (Trepa et al. 2020), underlying the importance of an adequate evaluation of severity and the most appropriate moment for intervention.

Echocardiography is a fundamental technique to confirm the FMR diagnosis and assess its severity and prognosis (Vahanian et al. 2022). A comprehensive approach considering various criteria is highly recommended to evaluate FMR effectively (Galiuto et al. 2011; Lee and Naqvi 2022). This approach is also applied in cases of FMR after CRT or pacemaker implantation (Lancellotti et al. 2013). As per current guidelines, it is also important to note that two-dimensional transthoracic echocardiography is typically regarded as the primary imaging method for valvular regurgitation (Vahanian et al. 2022).

Two-dimensional transthoracic echocardiography (2D TTE) is the first imaging technique used to assess valve leaflet anatomy, motion, and regurgitation severity evaluation (Lee and Naqvi 2022). In situations where transthoracic evaluation falls short or when dealing with intricate valve lesions, two-dimensional transesophageal (2D TEE) and three-dimensional echocardiography (3DE) can be highly beneficial. Among these diagnostic tools, TEE stands out for its ability to provide high-resolution images of valve leaflets and supporting structures, which can be instrumental in determining the mechanism of valve regurgitation (Lee and Naqvi 2022).

TEE is a diagnostic modality that enables the acquisition of detailed anatomical and functional information related to MR. This technique allows clinicians to evaluate the morphology and function of the MV and associated cardiac structures by providing high-resolution images of the heart. As a result, it serves as a valuable tool for identifying the underlying pathophysiology of FMR and guiding appropriate treatment strategies. The changes in LV loading conditions during the transesophageal evaluation might underestimate regurgitation severity (Lang et al. 2011).

Using three-dimensional transesophageal echocardiography (3DTEE) has enabled the quantification of valve regurgitation severity through direct 3D planimetry of valve area. This method has demonstrated an ability to identify the location and degree of valve regurgitation, irrespective of ventricular loading conditions. Such methodology effectively evaluates the severity of valve regurgitation (Lee and Naqvi 2022).

6.4.1 2D TTE FMR Quantification

Qualitative evaluation:—The **mitral valve morphology** has to be visually assessed in multiple views: parasternal long (PS LAX) (Fig. 6.6a) and short axis (PS SAX) view (Fig. 6.6b), apical four (A4ch)(Fig. 6.6c), two (A 2ch) (Fig. 6.6d), and three (A3ch) (Fig. 6.6e) chamber view (Baumgartner et al. 2017). From the 2D PS LAX view, the anterior MV leaflet is in continuity with the non-coronary cusp, and the scallops are A2 and P2 (Fig. 6.6a) as in A3ch-view. (Fig. 6.6d). The A4ch-view enables the evaluation of the MA, tenting area (TA), and tenting height (TH) (Baumgartner et al. 2017). From left to right, the scallops identified from this view are A3, A2, and P1 (Fig. 6.6b). A2ch-view visualizes P3, A2, and P1 (Fig. 6.6c). The PS SAX view at the MV level presents the anterior MV in the upper position and the posterior MV in the lower position, with scallops visible from left to right A3, A2, and A1 and P3, P2, and P1, respectively. (Fig. 6.6e) The PS SAX view at the PMs level reveals the anterolateral PM at the 3 o'clock position and the posterolateral PM at the 8 o'clock position. The MV and PM are posteriorly displaced in patients with DCM, leading to restricted leaflet movement (Baumgartner et al. 2017) (Fig. 6.7c, d).

The preferred MA dilatation assessment method is the 2D PS LAX view. This view also allows the TA and TH measurement (Lancellotti et al. 2013) (Fig. 6.8) Annulus/anterior leaflet ratio exceeds 1.3 in diastole, or the annulus diameter exceeds 35 mm typically diagnoses MA dilatation. The muscular posterior annulus is more involved in dilatation. The mitral annulus natural systolic contraction reduces its area by around 25%. These diagnostic criteria should be considered when assessing suspected MA dilatation patients. The interpapillary muscle distance is obtained from the end-systole parasternal PS SAX view (Lancellotti et al. 2013) (Fig. 6.7d). Normal leaflets with severe tenting or poor leaflet coaptation characterizes a severe FMR (Vahanian et al. 2022).

The CW Doppler of the MR jet is a valuable parameter for assessing the severity of mitral regurgitation (Vahanian et al. 2022). A dense holosystolic signal, as seen in Fig. 6.9a, may indicate severe MR. Other indicators of severe MR include a notched envelope with a triangular contour or a blunt early peak velocity. The CW Doppler can also identify and evaluate diastolic FMR (Lancellotti et al. 2013). Reducing CW Doppler signal intensity suggests improved regurgitation severity after CRT (Spartera et al. 2016). The presystolic component disappears early in all patients after the device implantation (Spartera et al. 2016).

Color M-mode is an imaging technique utilized to identify the dynamic variation of the regurgitant orifice area during different stages of the cardiac cycle. As illustrated in Fig. 6.9b, this technique can help detect early and late systolic peaks and a mid-systolic decrease of MR flow in patients with DCM (Lancellotti et al. 2013). These changes reflect the phasic variation in transmitral pressure that acts to close the mitral leaflets.

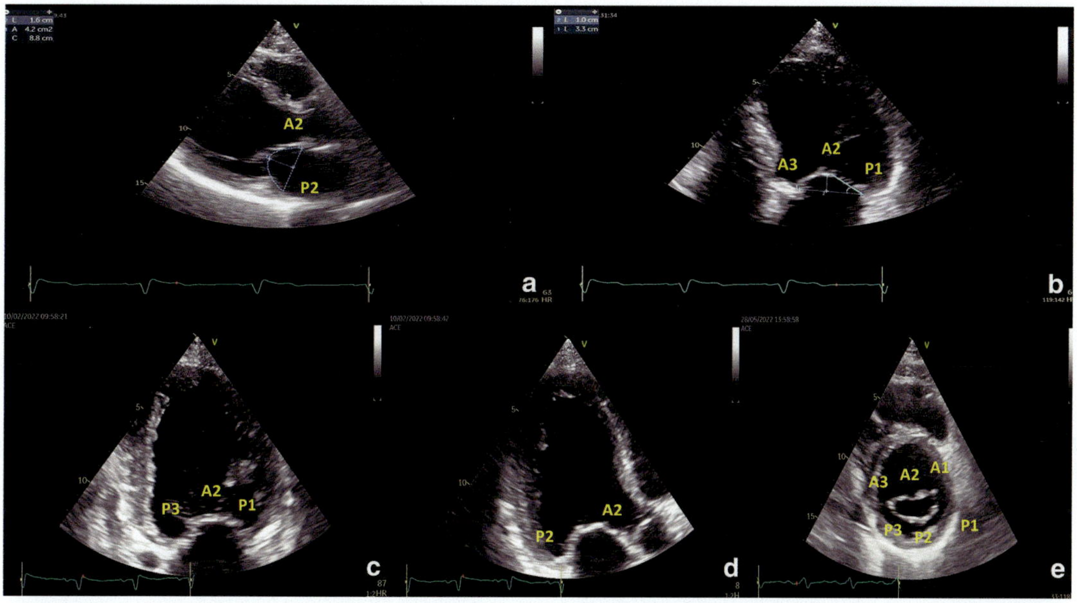

Fig. 6.6 Mitral valve visualization: **a** parasternal long axis view; **b** apical four-chamber view; **c** apical two-chamber view; **d** apical three-chamber view; **d** parasternal short axis view

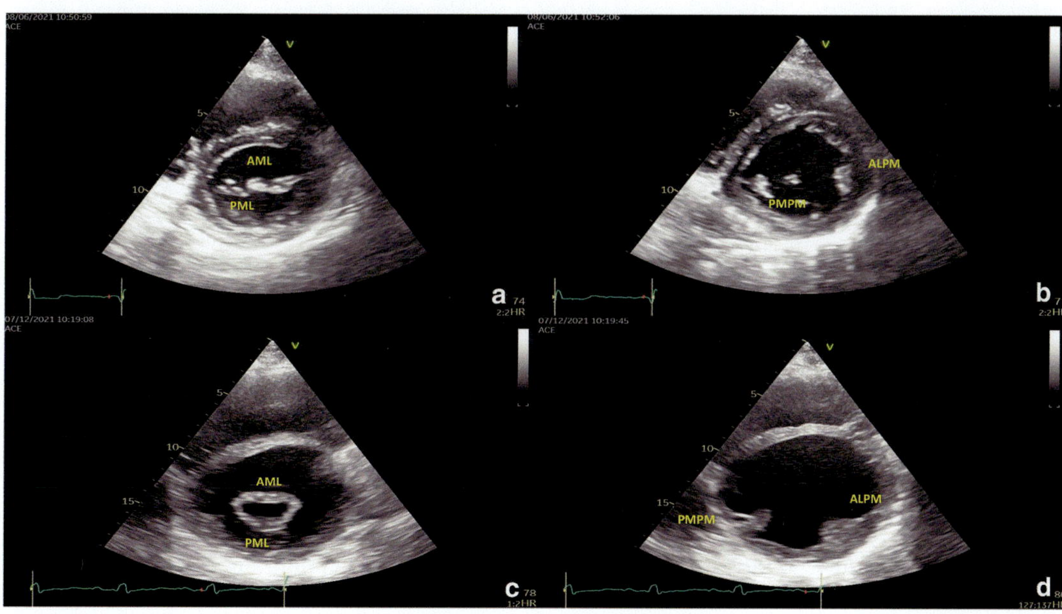

Fig. 6.7 **a** Normal position of the mitral valve; **b** The parasternal short-axis view at the papillary muscle level: anterolateral papillary muscle at the 3 o'clock position and the posterolateral PM at the 8 o'clock position of the image; **c** Posterior displaced mitral valve in a patient with dilated cardiomyopathy; **d** Posteriorly displaced papillary muscles in a patient with dilated cardiomyopathy

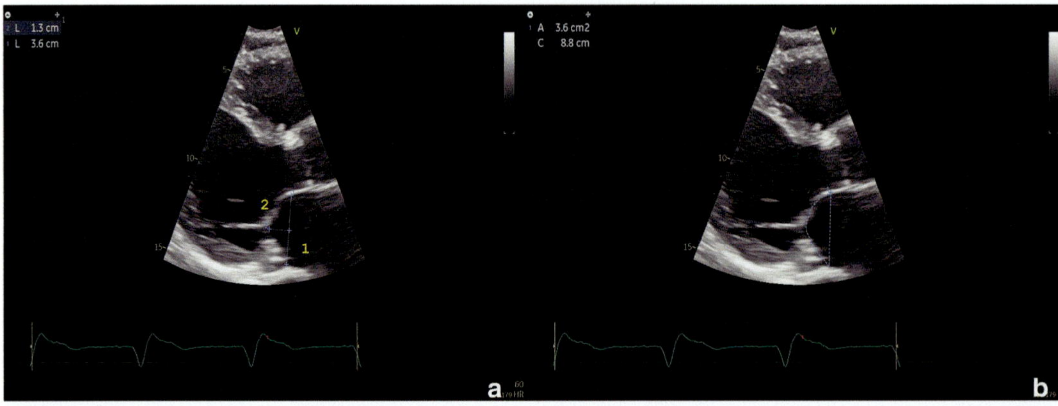

Fig. 6.8 Mitral annulus measurements from parasternal long axis view: A 1 mitral annulus dimension, 2 tenting height, B tenting area

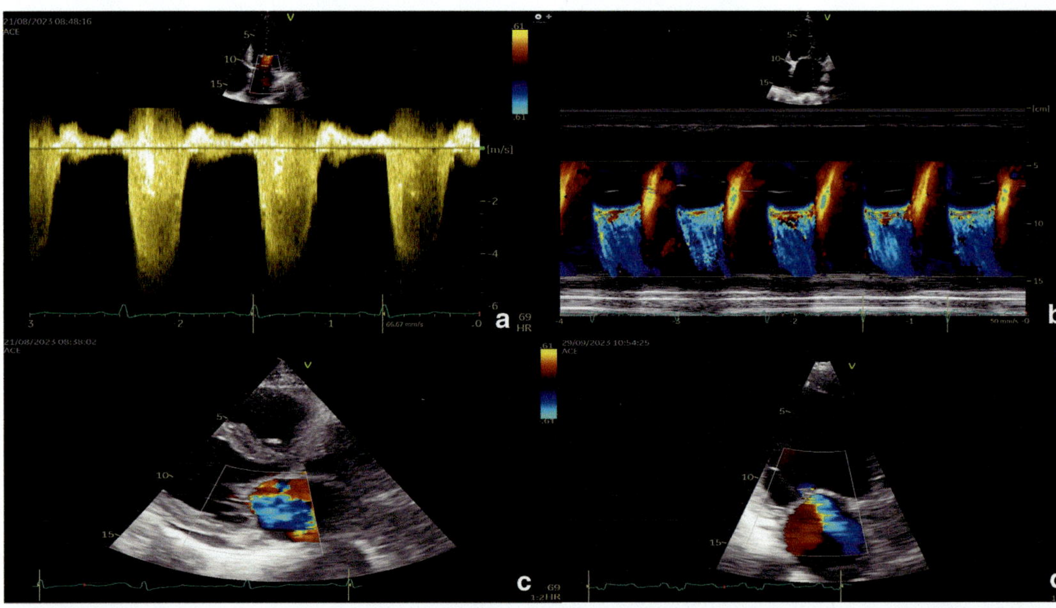

Fig. 6.9 Qualitative evaluation of mitral regurgitation **a** Continuous wave Doppler, **b** Color Mmode; **c**, **d** Color Doppler

Color flow Doppler regurgitant jet is a widely used method for assessing the presence of MR. This technique evaluates the jet's spatial orientation, differentiates between mild and severe regurgitation, and localizes the origin of the regurgitant jet. In qualitative terms, flow convergence at a Nyquist limit of 50–60 cm/s indicates severe MR (Baumgartner et al. 2017; Vahanian et al. 2022) (Fig. 6.9c, d). Large color jets extending deep into the LA are theoretically more severe than smaller ones. According to the guidelines, a large central jet (>50% of LA) or eccentric wall-impinging jet of variable size is a marker of severe MR (Baumgartner et al. 2017; Vahanian et al. 2022). However, it is essential to recognize that the relationship between jet size and MR severity is influenced by various technical factors such as transducer frequency, gain, Nyquist limit, frame rate, and hemodynamic factors such as the eccentricity of the jet and flow momentum (Lancellotti et al. 2013). It should be noted that this method may underestimate eccentric jets due to the Coanda effect (Fig. 6.9c, d). The current guidelines advocate using color flow imaging exclusively for MR detection. However, a more quantitative approach is imperative for cases where the MR jet is more substantial than a small central jet Zoghbi et al. (2017). Clinical trials used olor jet area to evaluate CRT effect in DCM and HF patients (Cleland et al. 2005; St John Sutton et al. 2006; Linde et al. 2002). Many studies used both the color jet area (Biase et al. 2011) and jet area/LA area ratio (Porciani et al. 2006; Ypenburg et al. 2008; Onishi et al. 2013; Brzezińska et al 2016) to evaluate the long-term effect of CRT on FMR in patients with CRT.

Semiquantitative parameters

- **Vena contracta (VC) width** is an essential parameter for quantifying MR. VC width is defined as the minimum thickness of the jet immediately distal to the regurgitant orifice, perpendicular to the jet's direction and reflecting the regurgitant orifice area (Baumgartner et al. 2017; Vahanian et al. 2022). VC width accurate measurement involves using a view perpendicular to the commissural line and average measurements over a minimum of two to three beats using two orthogonal planes (Lancellotti et al. 2013). Its accurate measurement can provide valuable insights into the severity of the condition (Lancellotti et al. 2013).
- In the context of secondary MR, the regurgitant orifice may be elongated along the mitral coaptation line results in a narrow VC in the A4ch view (Fig. 6.10a) and a broad VC in the A2ch view (Fig. 6.10b). By averaging the VC widths obtained from the A4ch and A2ch views, a better correlation with the 3D VC area can be achieved. A value exceeding 8 mm on 2D TTE indicates severe FMR and this method is relatively independent of hemodynamic and instrumentation factors and not influenced by other valve leaks (Vahanian et al. 2022). It can differentiate between mild and severe regurgitation. It has also been used for eccentric jet evaluation, but systolic changes in regurgitant flow may affect its accuracy (Vahanian et al. 2022). 2D TTE values of the VC width are not additive in the case of multiple jets. Many studies focused on LV and MR after CRT implantation and used VC for FMR quantification in the short-term (Onishi et al. 2013; Brzezińska et al. 2016) and long-term follow-up (Biase et al. 2011; Verhaert et al. 2012; Bommel et al. 2011).
- **A dominant E-wave** (>1.2 m/s) of the *pulsed wave of mitral inflow* (Fig. 6.11a) and a TVI mitral/TVI aortic ratio>1.4 also indicates a severe MR (Vahanian et al. 2022).
- Pulsed wave Doppler flow in pulmonary veins is best evaluated by interrogation of the left superior pulmonary vein from 2D TEE (Galiuto et al. 2011) (Fig. 6.11b). Doppler sample volume is placed within the left upper pulmonary vein with color Doppler guidance. The measured parameters are peak systolic (S) velocity, peak diastolic (D) velocity, and peak atrial reversal (AR) velocity (Vahanian et al. 2022; Camaj et al. 2023). **Systolic flow reversal in pulmonary veins** suggests a severe MR (Vahanian et al. 2022).

Quantitative parameters are obtained from the flow convergence method (Proximal isovelocity surface area—PISA method), which estimates EROA and RV (Galiuto et al. 2011; Vahanian et al. 2022).

- **EROA)**>40 mm2 (>30mm2 for elliptical orifices), **RV**>60 mL (> 45 in low flow conditions), or **regurgitant fraction (RF)**>50% reveals severe FMR. This group of patients has an increased risk of cardiovascular events (Baumgartner et al. 2017) (Fig. 6.12). The PISA method, which assumes hemispheric symmetry of the velocity distribution proximal to the circular regurgitant lesion, may be subject to several confounding factors affecting its accuracy (Lancellotti et al. 2013).

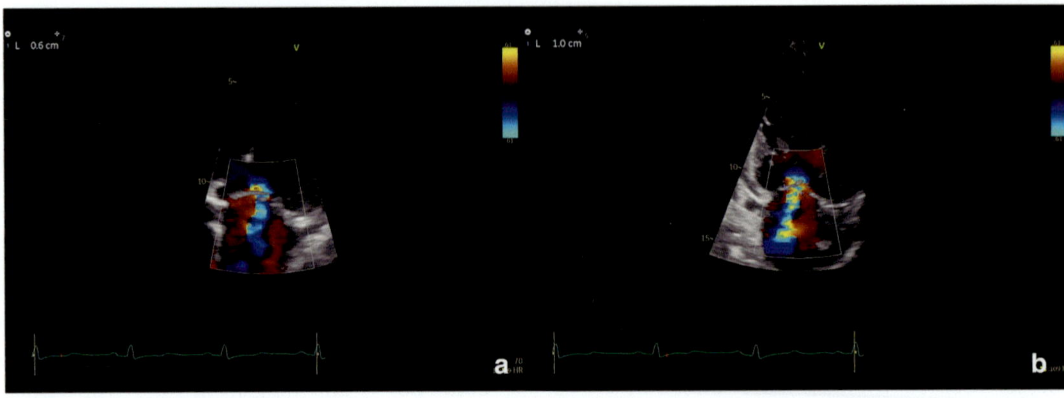

Fig. 6.10 Vena contracta measurement: **a**Apical four-chamber view; **b** Apical two-chamber view

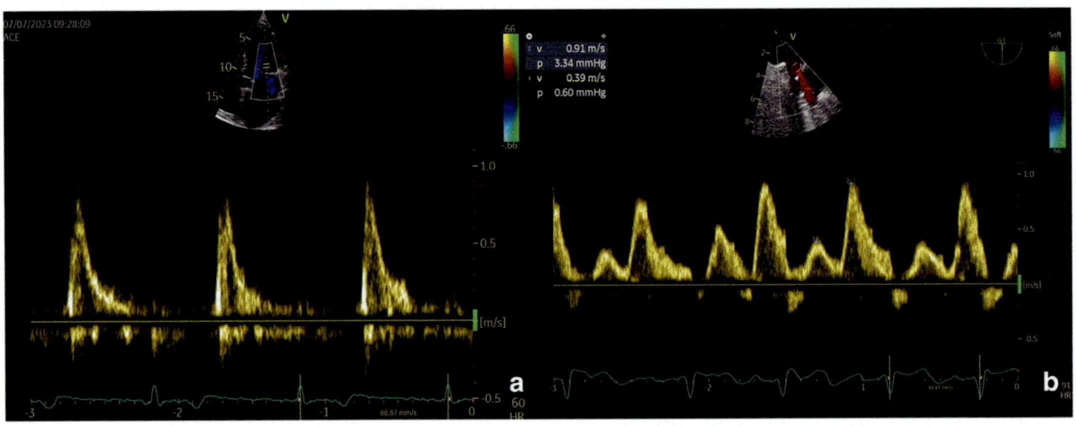

Fig. 6.11 Semiquantitative measurements: **a** Pulsed wave mitral inflow **b Pulsed wave Doppler flow in pulmonary veins**

These include the aliasing velocity, non-circular orifice, systolic changes in regurgitant flow, and adjacent structures. In cases of FMR, the PISA has an ellipsoidal shape and may manifest as two separate regurgitant jets originating from the medial and lateral sides of the coaptation line (Lancellotti et al. 2013). When the shape of the flow convergence zone deviates from a hemisphere and/or the ratio of the long-axis length to the short-axis length of the regurgitant orifice is more significant than 1,5, the PISA method may underestimate the degree of FMR and therefore not be valid (Lancellotti et al. 2013). Additionally, the PISA method is not suitable for use in cases of multiple jets. These factors should be considered when considering the accuracy and applicability of the PISA method in the assessment of mitral regurgitation (Lancellotti et al. 2013).

When assessing FMR severity, the recommended approach is to evaluate the jets using 3D TEE via multiplanar reconstruction and 3D planimetry. However, it is essential to consider the risk of TEE underestimating its severity (Zoghbi et al. 2017; Lang et al. 2015; Hahn et al. 2013). The guidelines highly recommend the PISA method for the severity of regurgitation evaluation whenever feasible (Vahanian et al. 2022). This method measures the EROA, RV, and RF (Camaj et al. 2023).

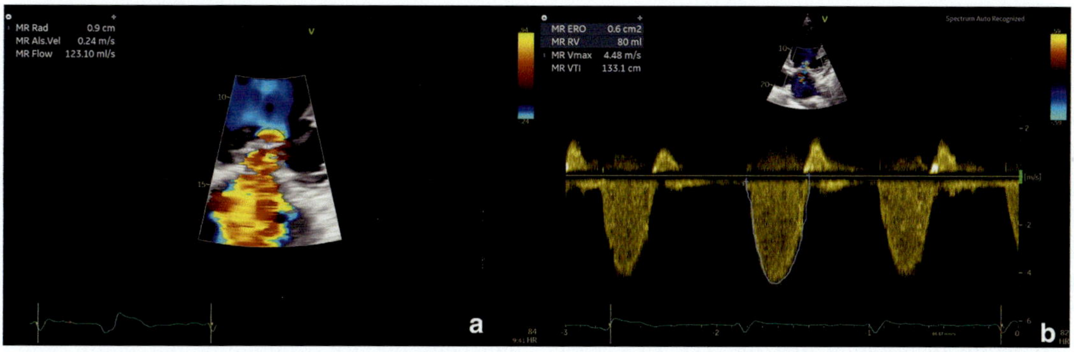

Fig. 6.12 Parameters resulted from Proximal Isovelocity Surface Area method calculation by Two-dimensional transthoracic echocardiography in a patient with severe mitral regurgitation after CRT: **a** Proximal Isovelocity Surface Area radius, **b** Effective Regurgitant Orifice Area, and regurgitant volume

Studies evaluating MR response to CRT in the short-term (Kanzaki et al. 2004) and the long-term conditions used EROA (Biase et al. 2011; Verhaert et al. 2012; Hahn et al. 2013).

In conclusion, the accuracy of FMR severity evaluation can be affected by the method used. Relying solely on color jet size or other traditional measures such as PISA and VC width may result in overestimating or underestimating FMR severity. It is essential to consider all available measures for a more accurate assessment (Vahanian et al. 2022).

Supplementary data provided by the 2D transthoracic echocardiography report of FMR evaluation after CRT are:

- **Ventricular and atrial size** (assessed by the Simpson method) LVEF should be carefully evaluated in patients with implanted devices and MR because this parameter is essential for the timing of intervention (Russo et al. 2022).
- **The right atrium and right ventricle dimensions and functions** (Baumgartner et al. 2017; Vahanian et al. 2022).
- Estimated **pulmonary artery systolic pressure**, considering the interference of the implanted device with tricuspid valve closure (Baumgartner et al. 2017; Vahanian et al. 2022).

6.5 2D TEE FMR Quantification

The evaluation of the MV apparatus using TEE involves rotating the probe through a range of 0 to 180 degrees to visualize various segments of leaflets. The mid-esophageal (ME) four-chamber view (0 degrees) visualizes the anterior and posterior mitral leaflets on the image's left and right sides, respectively (Galiuto et al. 2011; Hahn et al. 2013). The visualized leaflet segments in this view include A3A2 and P2P1 (Galiuto et al. 2011; Hahn et al. 2013) (Fig. 6.13a). The ME commissural view (50–70 degrees) displays the MV scallops from left to right as P3-A2-P1 and adjacent A3 and A1. (P3-A3A2A1- P1) This view also provides visibility of the anterolateral and posteromedial PMs and their corresponding chordae (Galiuto et al. 2011; Hahn et al. 2013) (Fig. 6.13b). Additionally, the ME two-chamber view (80–100 degrees) identifies the posterior mitral leaflet on the left side, the anterior leaflet on the right side of the image, and the MV leaflet segments P3-A3A2A1 (Galiuto et al. 2011; Hahn et al. 2013) (Fig. 6.13c). The ME LAX view (120–150 degrees) displays the P2-A2 scallops (Galiuto et al. 2011; Hahn et al. 2013) (Fig. 6.14d). The transgastric (TG) MV short-axis (SAX) views provide a unique perspective of the MV and PM. The TG MV SAX view (0–20 degrees at the MV level), in particular, reveals the anterior leaflet on the left and the posterior leaflet on the right, with the medial commissure situated in the near field and the lateral commissure in the far field (Hahn et al. 2013) (Fig. 6.13e). The TG mid-papillary SAX view (0–20 degrees at the MV level), on the other hand, shows the anterolateral PM at the 5-o'clock position and the posteromedial PM located approximately between 11- and 2-o'clock positions (Hahn et al. 2013). It is worth mentioning that the TG SAX view is highly effective in detecting MV and PM displacement in patients with DCM (Hahn et al. 2013) (Fig. 6.13f).

3D echocardiography has emerged as a valuable technique in providing additional information regarding the severity of mitral valve pathology. This is because orifice geometry in FMR can be noncircular or have multiple jets, which can be better evaluated using 3D imaging in contrast to 2D imaging (Galiuto et al. 2011) (Fig. 6.14, Supplementary material 3) 3D echocardiography is crucial in demonstrating the spatial interactions between different MV components (Robinson et al. 2021). The technique provides a unique perspective of the valve from both the LV and LA, known as the "en face view" or "surgical view" due to its similarity to the view seen during surgery (Robinson et al. 2021) (Fig. 6.15a, Supplementary material 4, 5).

Guidelines recommend acquiring narrow-angle and zoomed images from the PS LAXview and A4ch view for 3D TTE evaluation of the MV (Lang et al. 2012). The zoomed acquisition is recommended for a comprehensive evaluation of leaflet anatomy and motion due to its superior temporal and spatial resolution. Conversely, the full-volume acquisition is indispensable for examining the entire mitral valve apparatus (Lang et al. 2012). The posterior MV leaflet is optimally visualized from the parasternal window, while the anterior leaflet is adequately viewed from both the apical and parasternal windows (Lang et al. 2012). Long-axis views provide critical information regarding the sub-valvular apparatus. Moreover, the 3D surgical view of the MV is an excellent method for appreciating the MA (Lang et al. 2012).

The MV competence during systole depends on the normal motion and contraction of both the ventricles and the MA. Any alterations in the geometry of the LV, which affect the position of the PMs, can result in poor leaflet coaptation. Dynamic 3D rendering of the MV has the potential to differentiate between normal leaflet mobility and tethered leaflets caused by

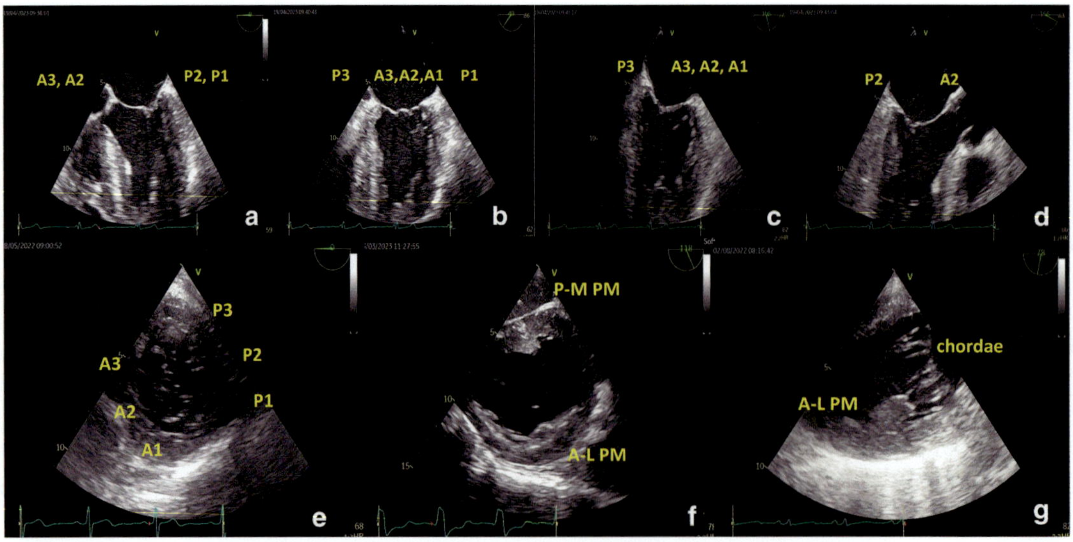

Fig. 6.13 Mitral valve evaluation by two-dimensional transesophageal echocardiography

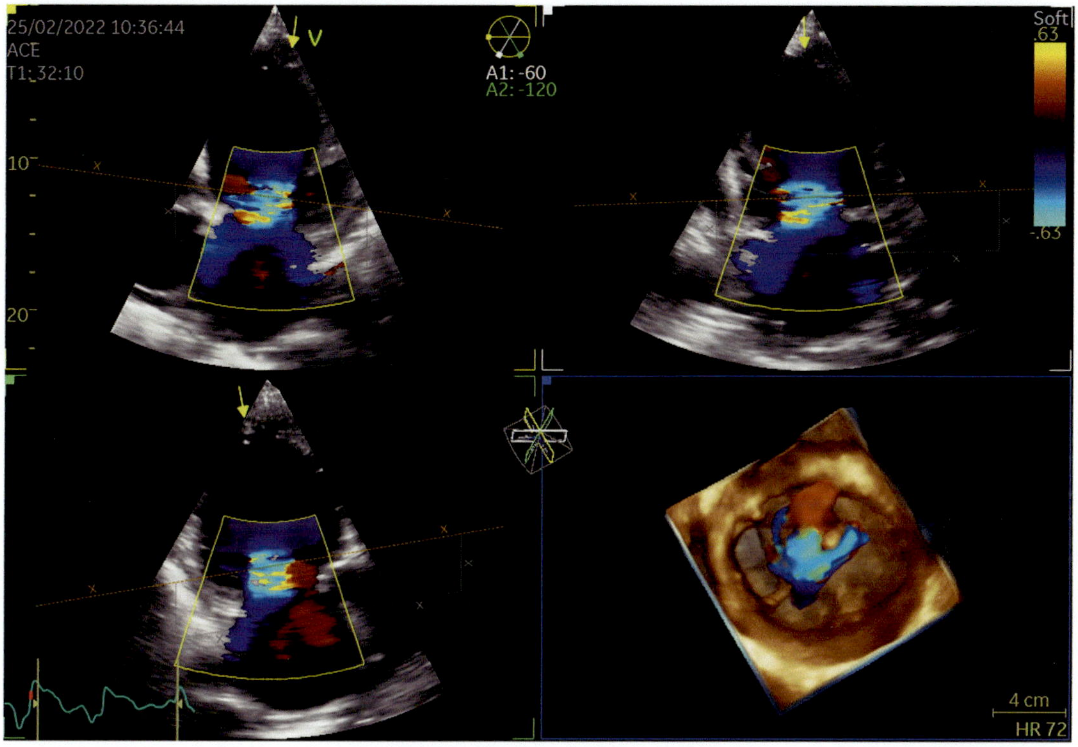

Fig. 6.14 Noncircular aspect of mitral regurgitation jet visualized from three-dimensional echocardiography

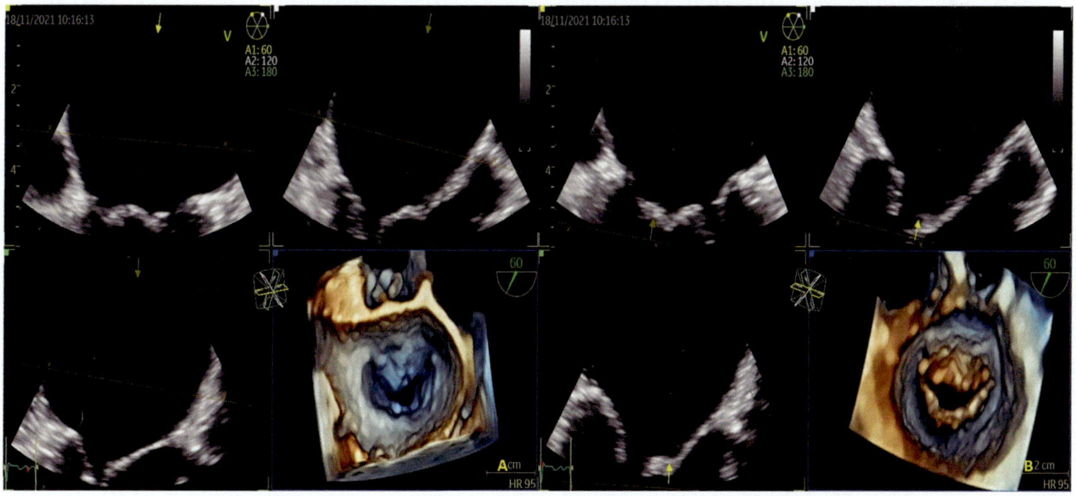

Fig. 6.15 3D perspectives of the mitral valve in a patient with dilated cardiomyopathy, **a** atrial perspective, **b** ventricular perspective

regional wall motion abnormalities or global LV enlargement (Lang et al. 2012). 3DE allows for a comprehensive evaluation of the MV apparatus. (Fig. 6.16, Supplementary material 6). Additionally, 3D TEE MV quantification (3D MVQ) provides valuable information regarding

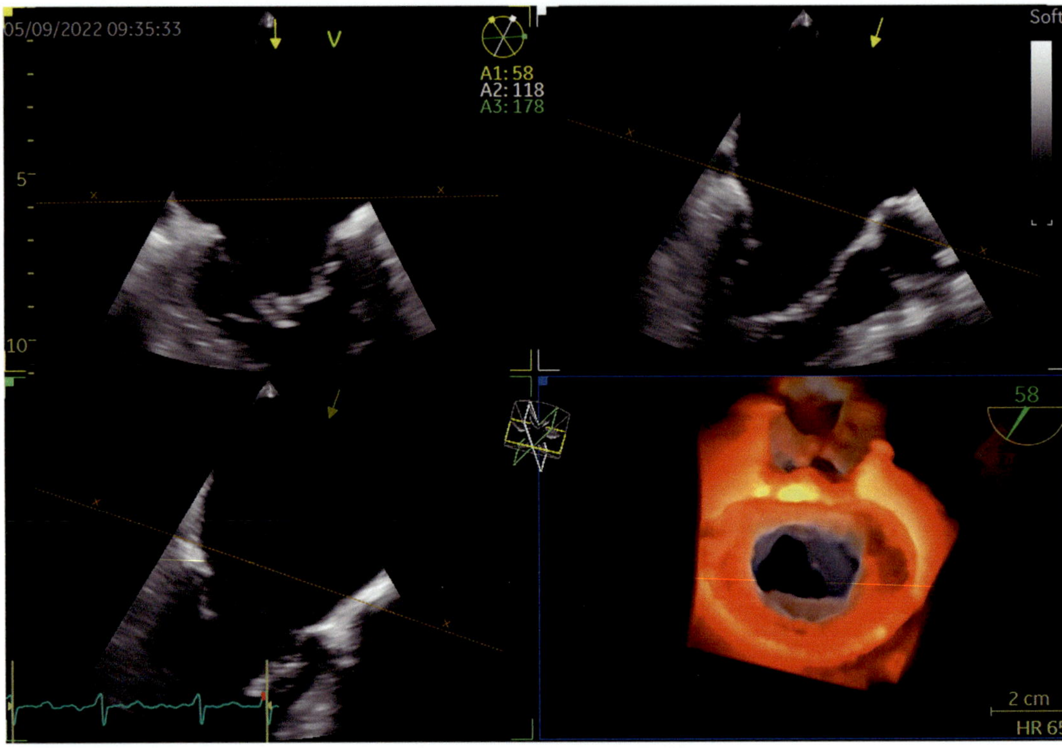

Fig. 6.16 3DTEE

the MA size, shape, and function (Grayburn et al. 2014; Faletra et al. 2019). Annular dilation, flattening, and reduced contractility are commonly associated with FMR (Cabrera-Bueno et al. 2010; Kovalova and Necas 2011). 3D MVQ in patients with ventricular FMR (VFMR) has shown that the condition is typically characterized by anteroposterior annular dilatation, loss of the typical saddle shape of the MA, a longer distance between the MA and inter-trigonal zone, a more significant annular nonplanarity scalar angle, and increased anteroposterior and anterolateral-posteromedial diameters (Levack et al. 2012) (Fig. 6.17).

Validation of 3DE for MV assessment has proven to be a valuable tool in several aspects, including defining the location and extent of pathology, identifying the severity and mechanism of valvular dysfunction, and enabling effective communication of results to interventional cardiologists or cardiac surgeons before intervention (Lang et al. 2012; Faletra et al. 2019; Zamorano et al. 2011). Two major advantages of 3DE in this regard are its capacity to delineate the effective regurgitant orifice area and the VC (Lang et al. 2012; Faletra et al. 2019; Zamorano et al. 2011).

The 3D-derived VC area closely correlates with the Doppler-derived effective regurgitant orifice area. It measures the cross-sectional area of the VC, which appears narrow in the A4ch view, broad in the A2ch view, and asymmetric along the commissural line in an "en face" view. (Fig. 6.18). The planar area measured from the "en face" view corresponds directly to the effective regurgitant orifice area (Lang RM et al. 2012; Zamorano et al. 2011). 3DE and color flow imaging can also quantify MR jet volumes, providing a comprehensive understanding of MV pathology beyond what is possible with 2D imaging methods. Current guidelines recommend using 3DE to assess MR, especially in complex cases where 2D imaging methods may underestimate regurgitation (Baumgartner

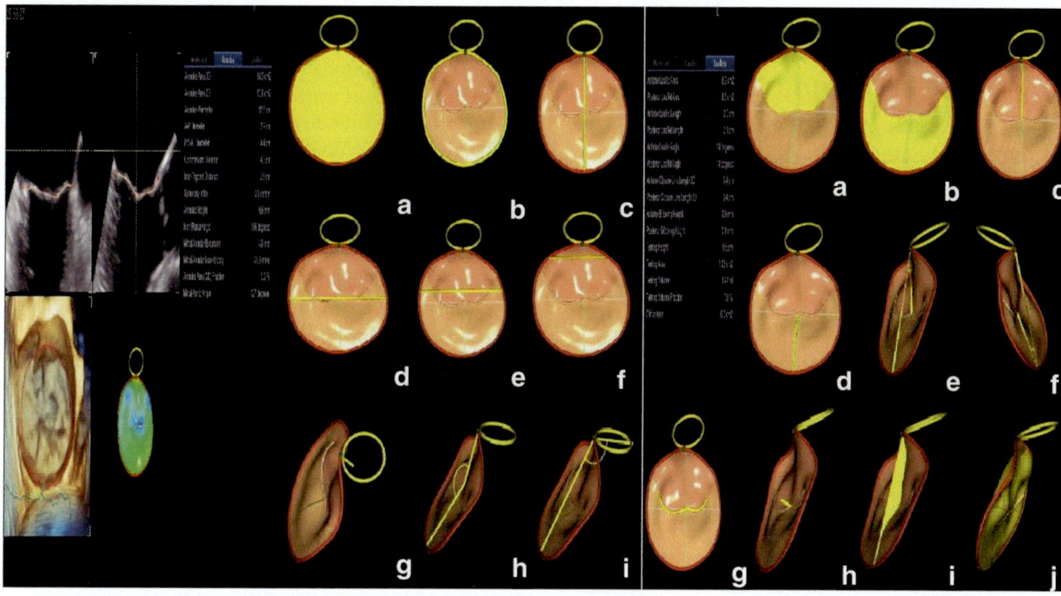

Fig. 6.17 Mitral valve quantification by three-dimensional echocardiography using dedicated software

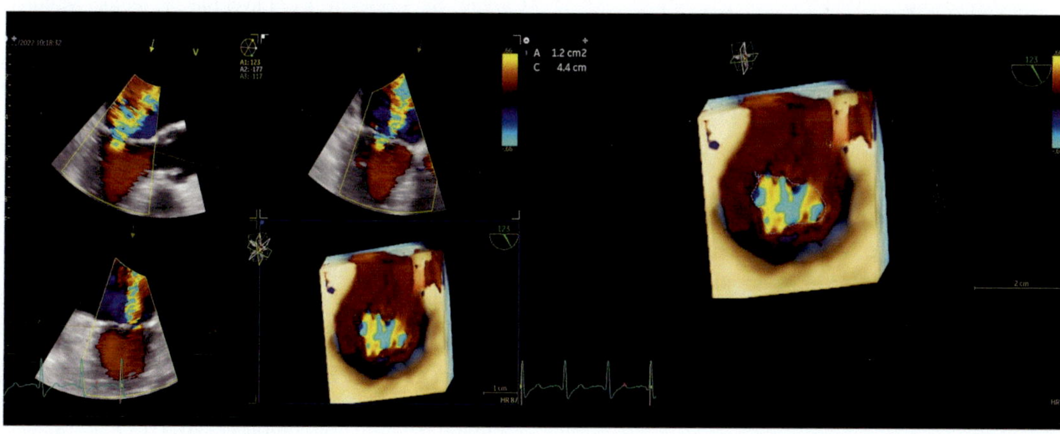

Fig. 6.18 Vena contracta area area measurement from three-dimensional echocardiography

et al. 2017; Vahanian et al. 2022). Incorporating 3D assessments of MV pathology into routine clinical practice provides the most comprehensive physiologic and morphologic information regarding this valve (Baumgartner et al. 2017; Vahanian et al. 2022).

The geometric features of the MV apparatus are critical factors in determining the response of MR to CRT implantation. Specifically, the MA area, mitral annular contraction, leaflet closing area, and tenting volume, as measured by 3D echocardiography, are considered essential parameters for assessing MR response (Solis et al. 2009). However, accurately evaluating secondary MR can be challenging, requiring multiple parameters. Thus, a multimodality assessment employing both 2DE and 3DE is optimal (Asgar et al. 2015). It should be noted that the persistence of FMR is associated with adverse outcomes (Cabrera-Bueno et al. 2010), and it is imperative to establish the optimal timing for FMR correction in non-responders (Biase et al. 2011).

6.6 Right Time of Intervention for MR in Patients with Implanted Devices

Research indicates that the optimal time for MV intervention is three months after CRT implantation. During this period, CRT may offer enhanced FMR for certain patients (Russo et al. 2022). Observations suggest that patients with at least mild MR experience the most significant benefits of CRT for FMR and LV remodeling. However, individuals with irreversible stages of LV dysfunction and dilatation who are unresponsive to electrical therapy have a low probability of MR improvement (Russo et al. 2022).

6.7 Conclusions

FMR in patients with implanted devices is a complex syndrome that requires a multilevel approach to address the underlying mechanisms. Clinical studies and trials suggest that MR improvement is achievable early after CRT implantation, but typically after three or six months, and more frequently in patients with sinus rhythm. Sometimes, CRT or pacemakers may neither modify nor improve MR, which has been linked to unfavorable long-term survival. The findings from clinical studies underscore the need for continued research efforts to optimize treatment strategies for patients with implanted devices.

References

Asgar AW, Mack MJ, Stone GW, et al. State-of-Art-Reiew, Secondary mitral regurgitation in heart failure pathophysiology Prognosis, and therapeutic considerations. J Am College Cardiol. 2015;65:1231–48.

Barold SS, Ovsyshcher IE. Pacemaker-induced mitral regurgitation. Pacing Clin Electrophysiol. 2005;28:357–60.

Baumgartner H, Falk V, Bax JJ, et al. 2017 ESC/EACTS Guidelines for the management of valvular heart disease The Task Force for the management of valvular heart disease of the European Society of Cardiology (ESC) and the European Association for Cardio-Thoracic Surgery (EACTS). Eur Heart J. 2017;38:2739–91.

Breithardt OA, Sinha AM, Schwammenthal E, et al. Acute effects of cardiac resynchronization therapy on functional mitral regurgitation in advanced systolic heart failure. J Am Coll Cardiol. 2003;41:765–70.

Brignole M, Auricchio A, Baron-Esquivias, et al. 2013 ESC Guidelines on cardiac pacing and cardiac resynchronization therapy TheTask Force on cardiac pacing and resynchronization therapy of the European Society of Cardiology (ESC). Developed in collaboration with the European Heart Rhythm Association (EHRA). European Heart J. 2013;34:2281–2329.

Brzezińska B, Łoboz-Grudzień K, Wita K, et al. Predictors of functional mitral regurgitation improvement during a short-term follow-up after cardiac resynchronisation therapy. Kardiol Pol. 2016;74:665–73.

Cabrera-Bueno F, Molina-Mora MJ, Alzueta J, et al. Persistence of secondary mitral regurgitation and response to cardiac resynchronization therapy. Eur J Echocardiogr. 2010;11:131–7.

Camaj A, Thourani VH, Gillam LD. Heart failure and secondary mitral regurgitation: a contemporary review. J Soc Cardiovascular Angiography Intervent. 2023;2: 101195.

Cazeau S, Leclercq C, Lavergne T, et al. Multisite Stimulation in Cardiomyopathies (MUSTIC) Study Investigators. Effect of multisite biventricular pacing in patients with heart failure and intraventricular conduction delay. N Engl J Med. 2001;344:873–880.

Cipriani M, Lunati M, Landolina M, et al. Prognostic implications of mitral regurgitation in patients after cardiac resynchronization therapy. Eur J Heart Fail. 2016;18:1060–8.

Cleland JG, Daubert JC, Erdmann E, et al. Cardiac Resynchronization-Heart Failure (CARE-HF) Study Investigators. The effect of cardiac resynchronization on morbidity and mortality in heart failure. N Engl J Med. 2005;352:1539–1549.

Di Biase L, Auricchio A, Mohanty P, et al. Impact of cardiac resynchronization therapy on the severity of mitral regurgitation. Europace. 2011;13:829–38.

Donal E, De Place C, Kervio G, et al. Mitral regurgitation in dilated cardiomyopathy: value of both regional left ventricular contractility and dyssynchrony. Eur J Echocardiography. 2009;10:133–8.

Eldadah ZA, Rosen B, Hay I, et al. The benefit of upgrading chronically right ventricle-paced heart failure patients to resynchronization therapy demonstrated by strain rate imaging. Heart Rhythm. 2006;3:435–42.

Enriquez-Sarano M, Basmadjian AJ, Rossi A, et al. Progression of mitral regurgitation: a prospective Doppler echocardiographic study. J Am Coll Cardiol. 1999;34:1137–44.

Faletra FF, Leo LA, Paiocchi VP, et al. Anatomy of mitral annulus insights from non-invasive imaging techniques. EHJ-CV Imaging. 2019;20:843–57.

Galiuto L, Badano L, Fox K, Sicari R, Zamorano JL et al. The EAE textbook of echocardiography. Oxford University Press New York; 2011

Gorman JH, Jackson BM, Enomoto Y. Gorman RC The effect of regional ischemia on mitral valve annular saddle shape. Ann Thorac Surg. 2004;77:544–8.

Grande-Allen KJ, Barber JE, Klatka KH, et al. Mitral valve stiffening in end-stage heart failure: Evidence of an organic contribution to functional mitral regurgitation. J Thorac Cardiovasc Surg. 2005a;130:783–90.

Grande-Allen KJ, Borowski AG, Troughton RW, et al. Apparently normal mitral valves in patients with heart failure demonstrate biochemical and structural derangements: an extracellular matrix and echocardiographic study. J Am Coll Cardiol. 2005b;45:54–61.

Grayburn PA, Carabello B, Hung J, et al. Defining "severe" secondary mitral regurgitation: emphasizing an integrated approach. J Am Coll Cardiol. 2014;64(25):2792–801.

Hahn RT, Abraham T, Adams MT, et al. Guidelines for performing a comprehensive transesophageal echocardiographic examination: recommendations from the American society of echocardiography and the society of cardiovascular anesthesiologists. J Am Soc Echocardiogr. 2013;26:921–64.

He S, Fontaine AA, Schwammenthal E, Yoganathan AP, Levine RA. Integrated mechanism for functional mitral regurgitation: leaflet restriction versus coapting force: In vitro studies. Circulation. 1997;96(6):1826–34.

Kanzaki H, Bazaz R, Schwartzman D, Dohi K, Sade LE, Gorcsan J. A mechanism for immediate reduction in mitral regurgitation after cardiac resynchronization therapy insights from mechanical activation strain mapping. J Am Coll Cardiol. 2004;8:1619–25.

Karvounis HI, Dalamaga EG, Papadopoulos CE, et al. Improved papillary muscle function attenuates functional mitral regurgitation in patients with dilated cardiomyopathy after cardiac resynchronization therapy. J Am Soc Echocardiogr. 2006;19:1150–7.

Kovalova S, Necas J. RT-3D TEE: characteristics of mitral annulus using mitral valve quantification (MVQ) program. Echocardiography. 2011;8:461–7.

Kusumoto FM, Schoenfeld MH, Barrett C, et al. 2018 ACC/AHA/HRS guideline on the evaluation and management of patients with bradycardia and cardiac conduction delay. Circulation 2018;:CIR000000000000

Lancellotti P, Tribouilloy C, Hagendorff A et al. Recommendations for the echocardiographic assessment of native valvular regurgitation: an executive summary from the European Association of Cardiovascular Imaging. Eur Heart J. Cardiovascular Imaging. 2013;14:611–44.

Lang RM, Badano LP, Tsang W, et al. EAE/ASE recommendations for image acquisition and display using three-dimensional echocardiography. Eur Heart J Cardiovasc Imaging. 2012;13:1–46.

Lang RM, Tsang W, Weinert L, et al. Valvular heart disease. The value of 3-dimensional echocardiography. J Am Coll Cardiol. 2011;58:1933–44.

Lang RM, Badano LP, Mor-Avi V, et al. Recommendations for cardiac chamber quantification by echocardiography in adults: an update from the american society of echocardiography and the european association of cardiovascular imaging, European Heart J Cardiovasc Imag. 2015;16:233–71.

Lee H, Naqvi TZ, Echocardiography in the assessment of valve regurgitation–incremental role of three dimensional echocardiography. Rev Cardiovasc Med. 2022;23(12):407.

Lellouche N, De Diego C, Vaseghi M, et al. Cardiac resynchronization therapy response is associated with shorter duration of atrial fibrillation. Pacing Clin Electrophysiol. 2007;30:1363–8.

Levack MM, Jassar AS, Shang EK, et al. Three-dimensional echocardiographic analysis of mitral annular dynamics: implication for annuloplasty selection. Circulation. 2012;126:S183–8.

Linde C, Leclercq C, Rex S, et al. Long-term benefits of biventricular pacing in congestive heart failure: Results From the Multisite STimulation In Cardiomyopathy (MUSTIC) Study. J Am Coll Cardiol. 2002;40:111–8.

Lipar L, Srivathsan K, Scott LR. Short-term outcome of cardiac resynchronization therapy—a omparison between newly implanted and chronically right ventricle-paced patients. Int J Cardiol. 2016;219:195–9.

Marai I, Gurevitz O, Carasso S, et al. Improvement of congestive heart failure by upgrading of conventional to resynchronization pacemakers. Pacing Clin Electrophysiol. 2006;29:880–4.

McDonagh TA, Metra M, Adamo M, et al. 2021 ESC Guidelines for the diagnosis and treatment of acute and chronic heart failure: Developed by the Task Force for the diagnosis and treatment of acute and chronic heart failure of the European Society of Cardiology (ESC) with the special contribution of the Heart Failure Association (HFA) of the ESC. Eur Heart J. 2012;42:3599–726.

Mihos CG, Yucel E, Upadhyay GA et al. Left ventricle and mitral valve reverse remodeling in response to cardiac resynchronization therapy in nonischemic cardiomyopathy. Echocardiography 2020;37:1557–1565

Naqvi TZ, Rafique AM, Swerdlow C, et al. Predictors of reduction in mitral regurgitation in patients undergoing cardiac resynchronisation treatment. Heart 2008;94:1580–158.8

Onishi T, Onishi T, Marek JJ, et al. Mechanistic features associated with improvement in mitral regurgitation after cardiac resynchronization therapy and their relation to long-term patient outcome. Circ Hear Fail. 2013;6:685–93.

Otsuji Y, Handschumacher MD, Schwammenthal E, et al. Insights from three-dimensional echocardiography into the mechanism of functional mitral regurgitation: direct in vivo demonstration of altered leaflet tethering geometry. Circulation. 1997;96:1999–2008.

Otsuji Y, Kumanohoso T, Yoshifuku S, et al. Isolated annular dilation does not usually cause important functional mitral regurgitation: comparison between patients with lone atrial fibrillation and those with idiopathic or ischemic cardiomyopathy. J Am Coll Cardiol. 2002;39:1651–6.

Ponikowski P, Voors AA, Anker SD, et al. 2016 ESC Guidelines for the diagnosis and Treatment of acute and chronic heart failure The Task Force for the diagnosis and treatment of acute and chronic heart failure of the European Society of Cardiology (ESC) Developed with the special contribution of the Heart Failure Association (HFA) of the ESC. Eur Heart J. 2016;37:2129–200.

Porciani MC, Macioce R, Demarchi G, et al. Effects of cardiac resynchronization therapy on the mechanisms underlying functional mitral regurgitation in congestive heart failure. Eur J Echocardiogr. 2006;7:31–3917.

Robinson S, Ring L, Augustine DX, et al. The assessment of mitral valve disease: a guideline from the British Society of Echocardiography. Echo Res Pract. 2021;8:G87–136.

Russo RE, Russo G, Cassese M, et al. The role of cardiac resynchronization therapy for the management of functional mitral. Cells. 2022;11:2407.

Silbiger JJ. Does left atrial enlargement contribute to mitral leaflet tethering in patients with functional mitral regurgitation? Proposed role of atriogenic leaflet tethering. J Heart Valve Dis. 2014;23:385–6.

Solis J, McCarty D, Levine RA, et al. Mechanism of decrease in mitral regurgitation after cardiac resynchronization therapy: optimization of the force-balance relationship. Circ Cardiovasc Imaging. 2009;2:444–50.

Solis J, McCarty D, Levine RA, et al. Mechanism of decrease in mitral regurgitation after cardiac resynchronization therapy optimization of the force–balance relationship. Circulation Cardiovascular Imag. 2009;2:444–450.

Spartera M, Galderisi M, Mele D, et al. On behalf of the Echocardiographic Study Group of the Italian Society of Cardiology (SIC), Role of cardiac dyssynchrony and resynchronization therapy in functional mitral regurgitation. Eur Heart J - Cardiovasc Imaging. 2016;17:271–80.

St John Sutton MG, Plappert T, Hilpisch KE, Abraham WT, Hayes DL, Chinchoy E. Sustained reverse left ventricular structural remodeling with cardiac resynchronization at one year is a function of etiology: quantitative Doppler echocardiographic evidence from the Multicenter InSync Randomized Clinical Evaluation (MIRACLE). Circulation 2006;113:266–272.

Stephens EJ, Timek TA, Daughters GT, et al. Significant changes in mitral valve leaflet matrix composition and turnover with tachycardia-induced cardiomyopathy. Circulation. 2009;120:S112–9.

Tops LF, Suffoletto MS, Bleeker GB, et al. Speckle-tracking radial strain reveals leftventricular dyssynchrony in patients with permanent right ventricular pacing. J Am Coll Cardiol. 2007;50(12):1180–8.

Trepa M, Baggen-Santos R, Fontes-Oliveira M, et al. Determinants and clinical outcomes of functional mitral regurgitation improvement following cardiac resynchronization therapy. Int Cardiovasc Res J. 2020;14(1):7–11.

Upadhyay GA, Henry M, Genovese D. Impact of physiological pacing on functional mitral regurgitation in systolic dysfunction: initial echocardiographic remodeling findings after His bundle pacing. Heart Rhythm. 2021;2(5):446–54.

Vahanian A, Beyersdorf F, Praz F, et al. 2021 ESC/EACTS Guidelines for the management of valvular heart disease Developed by the Task Force for the management of valvular heart disease of the European Society of Cardiology (ESC) and the European Association for Cardio-Thoracic Surgery (EACTS). Eur Heart J. 2022;43:561–632.

Van Bommel RJ, Marsan NA, Delgado V, et al. Cardiac resynchronization therapy as a therapeutic option in patients with moderate–severe functional mitral regurgitation and high operative risk. Circulation. 2011;124:912–9.

Verhaert D, Popovic ZB, De S, et al. Impact of mitral regurgitation on reverse remodeling and outcome in patients undergoing cardiac resynchronization therapy. Circ Cardiovasc Imaging. 2012;5:21–6.

Vinereanu D. Mitral regurgitation and cardiac resynchronization therapy. Echocardiography. 2008;25:1155–2116.

Watanabe N, Ogasawara Y, Yamaura Y, et al. Quantitation of mitral valve tenting in ischemic mitral regurgitation by transthoracic real-time three-dimensional echocardiography. J Am Coll Cardiol. 2005;45:763–769.

You SF, Enriquez-Sarano M, Tribouilloy C, et al. Determinants of the degree of functional mitral regurgitation in patients with systolic left ventricular dysfunction: a quantitative clinical study. Circulation. 2000;102(12):1400–6.

Ypenburg C, Lancellotti P, Tops LF, et al. Mechanism of improvement in mitral regurgitation after cardiac resynchronization therapy. Eur Heart J. 2008;29:757–65.

Zamorano JL, Alberto de Augustín J. Three-dimensional Echocardiographic Evaluation of the Mitral Valve. In: Badano L, Lang RM, Zamorano JL, Textbook of Real-Time Three Dimensional Echocardiography, London, UK: Springer, 2011;55–8.

Zoghbi WA, Adams D, Bonow RO, et al. Recommendations for noninvasive evaluation of native valvular regurgitation: a report from the American Society of Echocardiography developed in collaboration with the Society for Cardiovascular Magnetic Resonance. J Am Soc Echocardiogr. 2017;30(4):303–71.

Tricuspid Valve Evaluation in Patients with Implanted Devices

7

Abstract

The presence of cardiac implantable electronic devices is linked to the occurrence of tricuspid regurgitation. Understanding the structural mechanisms behind tricuspid regurgitation paramount in this group of patients as it facilitates establishing monitoring strategies through noninvasive imaging and refines implantation techniques. Echocardiography is the primary imaging technique for identifying tricuspid regurgitation's structural mechanisms and severity in patients with implanted devices. The guidelines indicate a multimodality approach using two-dimensional and three-dimensional echocardiography for this complex pathology evaluation.

Implantable cardioverter defibrillators (ICDs) and permanent pacemakers (PPMs) are employed for managing cardiac conduction disorders and life-threatening arrhythmias in contemporary medical practice. The presence of cardiac implantable electronic devices (CIEDs) is being linked (Arabi et al. 2015; Mediratta et al. 2014) to the occurrence of tricuspid regurgitation (TR), a condition not to be underestimated. CIED-lead implantation leads to progressive TR in 20–30% of cases (Vahanian et al. 2021; Kim et al. 2008; Hoke et al. 2014; Anvardeen et al. 2019) and progresses over time (Benfari et al. 2019). Understanding the structural mechanisms behind CIED-associated TR is paramount as it facilitates establishing monitoring strategies through noninvasive imaging and refines implantation techniques (Seo et al. 2008). Echocardiography and its associated imaging modalities remain the standard method for assessing TR and determining its severity. However, two-dimensional transthoracic echocardiography (2DTTE) has limitations (Hoke et al. 2014), as it can only visualize device leads traversing the tricuspid valve in a small percentage of patients (12–17%) (Mediratta et al. 2014).

In contrast, the utilization of three-dimensional imaging aids in identifying whether the device lead disrupts normal leaflet coaptation. Early detection of lead-related tricuspid regurgitation is crucial for selecting the most appropriate treatment approach, which may involve lead extraction or, in severe cases, tricuspid valve repair or replacement.

Tricuspid valve anatomy and physiology

The intricate TV system depends on multiple structures working harmoniously within a low-pressure environment. These structures play a vital role in maintaining valve integrity and are closely linked to the geometry and function of the right atrium (RA) and right ventricle (RV)

Supplementary Information The online version contains supplementary material available at https://doi.org/10.1007/978-3-031-64079-7_7.

D.-M. Toader, *Echocardiographic Evaluation of Patients with Implanted Devices*, https://doi.org/10.1007/978-3-031-64079-7_7

(Hoke et al. 2014). The tricuspid valve consists of three leaflets: septal, anterior, and posterior, positioned slightly more apical compared to the mitral valve. TV leaflets are thinner than the mitral ones, and calcification rarely occurs. The three commissures, antero-septal, antero-posterior, and postero-septal are defined by the free edges of each leaflet and a fan-like chorda is usually present.

Recently, a new classification for TV morphology using transesophageal echocardiography (TEE) (Volpato et al. 2021; Hołda et al. 2019; Hahn et al. 2021) has been proposed:

- Type I: typical three-leaflet valve
- Type II: 2 leaflet valves with the anterior and posterior leaflets not clearly separated and forming a single large leaflet
- Type III: 4 leaflet valve—(a) additional anterior leaflet, (b) additional posterior leaflet, (c) additional septal leaflet
- Type IV: more than four leaflet valve.

The tricuspid annulus (TA) is a complex, elliptical three-dimensional structure that differs from the more symmetric "saddle-shaped" mitral annulus (Fig. 7.1). In the TA, the posteroseptal part is situated more apically than the anteroseptal section (Smolarek and Gruchala, 2013; Spinner et al. 2011). Due to its significant size, even a 40% increase in the TA area can result in significant TR (Spinner et al. 2011). The TA is dynamic, changing in size throughout different phases of the cardiac cycle and under varying right ventricular load conditions (Smolarek and Gruchala, 2013; Spinner et al. 2011). 3D Echocardiography observed that the TA exhibited a biphasic pattern with two peaks during early and late diastole in healthy subjects (Spinner et al. 2011). In patients with functional TR (FTR), the early-diastolic peak was absent in 75% of cases (Fig. 7.2). Healthy subjects had a non-planar TA shape with consistent contraction. At the same time, FTR patients displayed TA dilation in the septal to lateral and posteroseptal to anterolateral directions, resulting in a more circular TA shape with asymmetrically reduced contraction (Spinner et al. 2011).

The sub-valvular apparatus consists of chordae and papillary muscles (PMs), with the anterior PM being the largest and the most apically displaced. The moderator band and the trabecula septo-marginalis divide the RV inflow from the outflow tract (Spinner et al. 2011).

The RV has a crescent-shaped configuration with three regions: the inlet, apical, and outflow portions. This intricate morphology renders two-dimensional echocardiography (2DE) inadequate for RV imaging (Fukuda et al. 2006). Conversely, three-dimensional transthoracic echocardiography (3D TTE) demonstrates promising results in measuring volumes and function, showing a strong correlation with cardiac magnetic resonance (CMR) (Fukuda et al. 2006; Shimada et al. 2010) which remains the gold standard for RV volume measurement and provides insights into tissue characterization.

The right atrium (RA) features anterior trabeculated and posterior smooth segments, which interface with the septum and the venae cavae. The RV and the RA are pivotal in developing functional tricuspid regurgitation (FTR). Dilatation of the RA and/or RV cavity can lead to tricuspid annulus enlargement, while conical remodeling of the RV can cause tenting of the TV (Fukuda et al. 2006).

Tricuspid regurgitation

Any disease affecting the intricate components of the TV apparatus can induce TR, with FTR being the predominant cause. The TV operates within a low-pressure system, making the severity of TR contingent upon loading conditions and respiratory fluctuations. Device-related dysfunction of the TV can manifest as either regurgitation or, less commonly, stenosis. Both forms of dysfunction are considered primary (organic) causes of TV dysfunction. The reported incidence of significant TR development following implantation of CIEDs varies widely, ranging from 7 to 45% (Hoke et al. 2014; Sugeng et al. 2010; Addetia et al. 2019).

Current guidelines advocate for a comprehensive assessment of TR using multiple parameters despite limitations associated with specific

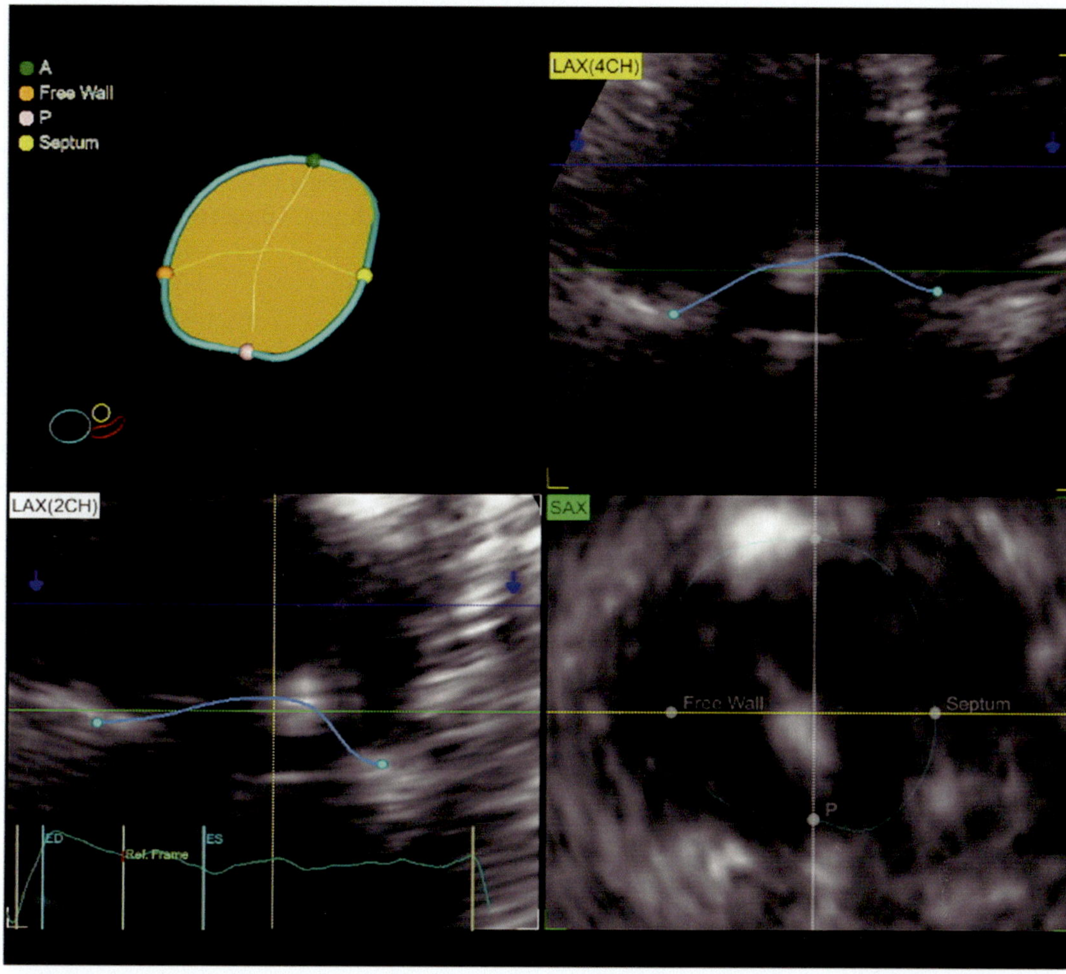

Fig. 7.1 Tricuspid annulus shape

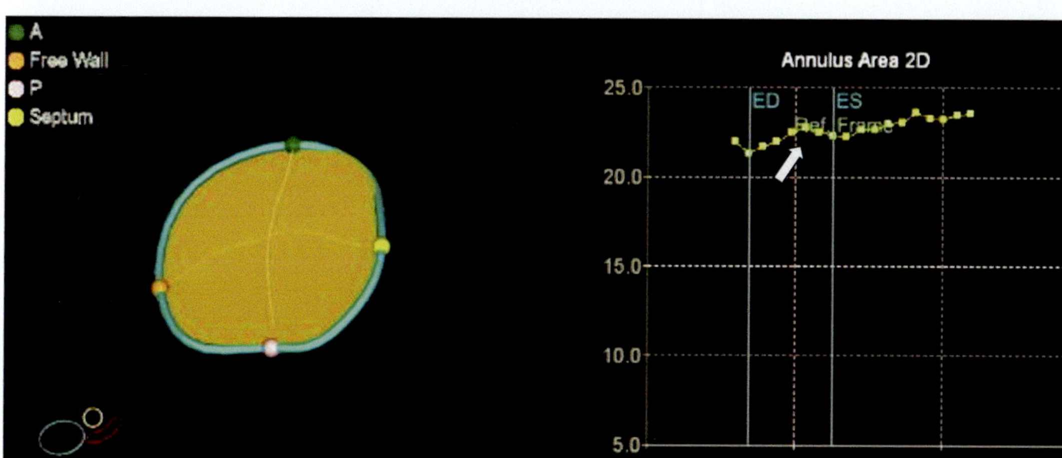

Fig. 7.2 Diastolic tricuspid annulus peak in patients with functional tricuspid regurgitation

metrics like vena contracta (VC) and effective regurgitant orifice area (EROA), measured via the proximal isovelocity surface area (PISA) method (Gelves-Meza et al. 2022; Hua et al. 2010). These measurements often rely on geometric assumptions that may not consistently apply to TR.

Echocardiography remains the primary imaging method for diagnosing the cause and severity of the TR. A VC of more than 0.7 cm (Fig. 7.3a), an EROA exceeding 0.40 cm^2 (Fig. 7.3b), and a regurgitant volume of more than 45 ml, define severe TR (Zoghbi et al. 2017; Hahn and Zamorano 2017; Muraru et al. 2022) (Fig. 7.3c). Notably, the SCOUT trial revealed that the conventional PISA method tends to underestimate the quantitative assessment of EROA in FTR (Hua et al. 2010). Some studies have proposed expanding the grading system to include categories like "massive" (VC measuring 1.4–2.0 cm, EROA ranging from 60 to 79 mm^2) and "torrential" (VC greater than 2.1 mm, EROA exceeding 80 mm^2) (Hahn and Zamorano 2017). Additionally, they aim to address the issue of PISA underestimation by introducing a new quantitative parameter, the VC 3D EROA (Addetia et al. 2019), with the following cutoff values for FTR severity: severe FTR (75–94 mm^2), massive FTR (95–114 mm^2), and torrential FTR (equal to or greater than 115 mm^2) (Fig. 7.3d).

In recent times, three-dimensional echocardiography (3DE) has become increasingly crucial for assessing both the anatomy and function of the TV as it is visualized from both atrial (Fig. 7.4a) and ventricular views (Hahn et al. 2017) (Fig. 7.4b). It offers valuable insights into the causes of TR (Supplementary material 1) and aids in comprehending the intricate valve structure. Moreover, 3DE is paramount for understanding pathophysiologic mechanisms resulting in lead-associated TR. The so-called "en face" view of the TV (Fig. 7.4a), made possible through 3DE, allows for a quantitative assessment of TR by calculating the three-dimensional VC area (Fig. 7.3d). Additionally, multiplying the velocity time integral of the TR jet by the VC size makes it possible to determine the regurgitation volume (Hahn and Zamorano 2017;

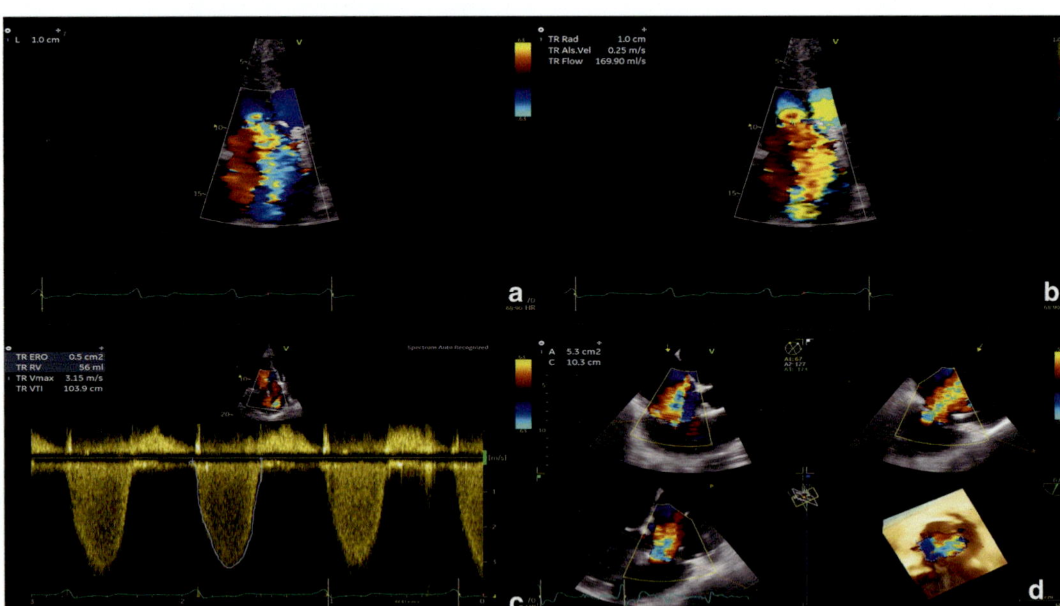

Fig. 7.3 Parameters of tricuspid regurgitation evaluation: **a** vena contracta; **b** PISA radius; **c** effective regurgitant orifice area and regurgitant volume; **d** three-dimensional vena contracta area

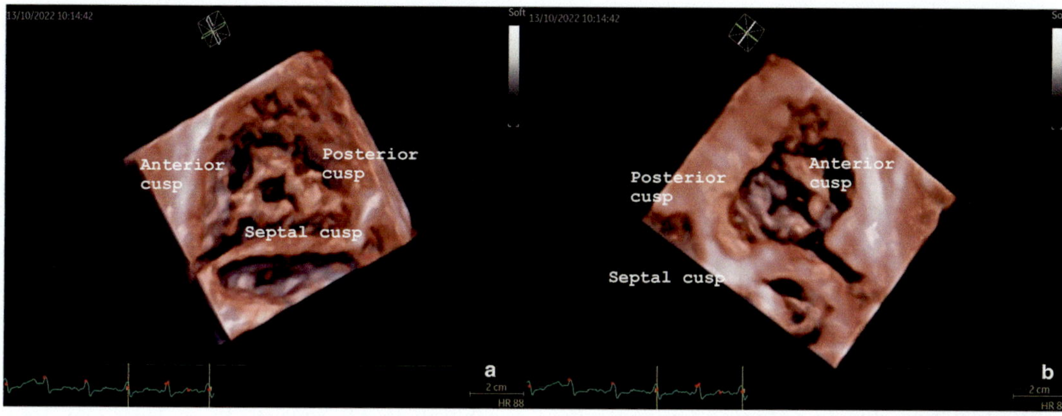

Fig. 7.4 Three-dimensional representation of the tricuspid valve: **a** right atrial view (surgical view); **b** right ventricle view

Muraru et al. 2022). Notably, 3D VC area correlates most closely with EROA, exhibits a moderate correlation with VC diameter, and shows a weaker correlation with the jet area/right atrial area ratio (Muraru et al. 2022).

Mechanisms of CIED-induced tricuspid regurgitation

A series of studies (Arabi et al. 2015; Mediratta et al. 2014; Muraru et al. 2019) have indicated that positioning device leads as they pass through the TV is a significant factor contributing to TR. Previously, diagnosis of device lead-related interference with the TV was typically made during autopsy or surgery. However, with the advent of three-dimensional echocardiography, it is now possible to diagnose this condition non-invasively. This advancement is particularly valuable as two-dimensional transthoracic imaging has been found inadequate for fully visualizing right ventricular (RV) leads (Arabi et al. 2015; Mediratta et al. 2014).

Placing implantable cardioverter defibrillators (ICDs), permanent pacemakers, and biventricular devices involves fluoroscopic guidance, aiming to position the lead tip at the apex, septum, or RV outflow tract (Mediratta et al. 2014; Addetia et al. 2019). Chronic RV apical pacing is often avoided due to its association with increased risks such as atrial fibrillation, heart failure hospitalization, pacing-induced cardiomyopathy, and mortality (Addetia et al. 2019). However, fluoroscopy cannot visualize TV leaflets or ascertain the final lead position within the tricuspid annulus once it is placed in the RV. Device leads can induce complications, including interference with TV function due to mechanical effects on leaflet mobility or coaptation. Techniques for right ventricle lead placement vary among operators and centers. Typically, one of three approaches is utilized (Arabi et al. 2015; Addetia et al. 2019; Muraru et al. 2019).

1. Prolapsing the lead across the tricuspid valve by forming a loop in the right atrium and then advancing it forward until it traverses the valve.
2. Directly crossing the valve toward the intended target location using a shaped stylet.
3. Directly crossing the valve toward the RV outflow tract with a curved stylet, then retracting the lead until it aligns with the target location.

Procedural variables can increase the risk of TV damage during lead placement (Arabi et al. 2015; Muraru et al. 2019). Among the three primary methods for positioning an RV lead, the "prolapsing technique" may reduce the likelihood of perforation and laceration because it involves less direct trauma to the leaflets or sub-valvular tissue.

CIED-induced TR can be categorized into primary and secondary forms. Up to 60% of cases of TR worsening after CIED implantation are due to secondary causes (Hołda et al. 2019; Addetia et al. 2014). Primary CIED-induced TR results from direct interaction between the lead and the tricuspid valve. In contrast, secondary CIED-induced TR stems from RV dilatation caused by pacing or heart failure. If primary CIED-induced TR is left untreated, it can lead to RV dilatation due to volume overload, ultimately resulting in secondary TR. Once this critical point is reached, it may not be possible to reverse TR through lead extraction (Hołda et al. 2019; Addetia et al. 2014).

CIED-associated TR can be classified into three main types: lead-related mechanical interference on TV coaptation, pacing-induced TR, or TV dysfunction following lead extraction (Sugeng et al. 2010; Addetia et al. 2019). Leads causing TR can be categorized either as interfering or non-interfering. The interfering leads are those that adhere to or impinge upon a leaflet, potentially impairing leaflet coaptation, which results in worsened TR severity compared to non-impinging leads (such as leads located in a commissural position or the middle of the valve).

Other mechanisms of lead-related interference on TV leaflets motion include (Addetia et al. 2019; Riesenhuber et al. 2021).

- lead adherence to valve leaflets or sub-valvular apparatus
- lead entrapment or entanglement within the sub-valvular apparatus
- valve perforation or laceration during RV lead placement
- valve avulsion, mainly during lead extraction in CIED implantation for > 1 year
- transection of papillary muscles or chordae tendineae.

The mechanism in severe CIED-associated TR was 39% mechanical interference (impingement) on leaflet mobility caused by the lead, 34% lead adherence, 17% leaflet perforation (with the septal leaflet being the most frequently affected), and 10% lead entanglement of the sub valvular apparatus (Riesenhuber et al. 2021).

Pacing-induced TR is based on RV electrical stimulation (Addetia et al. 2019). Dyssynchrony caused by high RV-pacing burden (>90%) (Addetia et al. 2019; Lin et al. 2005) induces RV geometric changes that result in inadequate mitral and tricuspid valve coaptation, even without mechanical leaflet interference.

RV apical (RVA) pacing correlates with an escalation in TR severity by at least one grade and, in some cases, two grades, compared to non-apical pacing. Additionally, lead impingement on the posterior leaflet is more prevalent among patients with RVA pacing. In contrast, placement of the lead in the middle position of the TV was more common in non-RVA pacing. A TV lead passage angle within the range of 15° to 15°, determined by the attachment site of the lead, is linked to minimal TR risk. This variation in lead-leaflet interaction might elucidate the higher incidence of TR with RVA pacing in contrast to non-RVA pacing (Lin et al. 2005).

Lead extraction may also cause harm to the tricuspid valve apparatus, potentially serving as an additional factor contributing to lead-induced dysfunction of the tricuspid valve.

Transvenous lead extraction (TLE) represents a complex therapeutic approach for managing lead-related infections or CIED-associated TR. The primary concern with TLE procedures is the potential for the avulsion of tricuspid valve tissue during the manual traction required for lead removal, leading to a subsequent exacerbation of TR severity (Addetia et al. 2019). Adherence of the leads typically begins within 4–5 days post-implantation. However, over time, fibrosis and adhesion between the lead and tricuspid valve tissue can escalate, accompanied by severe inflammation and calcification, increasing the risk of tissue avulsion during challenging TLE scenarios.

Furthermore, lead infections affecting the tricuspid valve apparatus pose a considerable mortality risk (Yu et al. 2020; Park et al. 2018) mainly as lead vegetation forms close to the valve. Distinguishing the direct involvement of the valve leaflets in these cases can be difficult, often necessitating TLE for treatment, which further elevates the potential for harm to the TV (Park et al. 2018).

Recent advancements in lead extraction techniques, such as laser-assisted dissection of the lead from adherent material, have reduced complications such as exacerbation of TR (ranging from 0 to 6%) (Yu et al. 2020; Park et al. 2018). Additionally, in cases where a lead proves resistant to extraction, it may either remain in the chest cavity or, if deemed necessary, be surgically extracted. Research indicates that older leads are more prone to encapsulation and thus may necessitate laser extraction tools compared to newer leads.

Diagnosis of tricuspid valve damage or dysfunction associated with CIED leads.

Achieving an accurate diagnosis of CIED-related TR necessitates the comprehensive integration of all available echocardiographic techniques because distinguishing between lead-induced TR, functional TR, and the presence of both can pose a significant diagnostic challenge (Vahanian et al. 2021; Addetia et al. 2019). The limitations inherent in 2DE have been surpassed by the introduction of 3DE imaging, particularly in evaluating lead-related TR. 3DE (Seo et al. 2008; Addetia et al. 2019) enables simultaneous visualization of the TV leaflets and their commissures, documentation of the relationship between the lead and leaflet mobility, assessment of valve coaptation, identification of lead impingement, and visualization of the lead course within the tricuspid annulus (Faletra et al. 2019).

Lead-related TR diagnosis involves multiple steps (Seo et al. 2008; Sugeng et al. 2010; Addetia et al. 2019).

1. Assessing the development of new-onset or aggravated TR by comparing transthoracic echocardiographic studies before and after implantation.
2. Evaluating TR severity using multimodality imaging techniques under updated guidelines.
3. Illustrating through both 2DE and 3DE imaging the mechanical obstruction or harm inflicted upon the TV leaflets or apparatus by the CIED lead.
4. Evaluating the hemodynamic impact on the right heart chambers in cases where moderate or greater TR is identified
5. Assessing the necessity and feasibility of early TLE or surgical intervention.

Transesophageal echocardiography (TEE) employing three-dimensional (3D) imaging is the following step when uncertainty persists regarding the mechanism of CIED-associated TR after suboptimal transthoracic echocardiography. (TTE) (Addetia et al. 2019) (Fig. 7.5a TEE 2D, supplementary material 2) Utilizing the trans-gastric short-axis view and obtaining optimal 3D volume-rendered TV images typically enhances the diagnostic precision for identifying lead-related TR (Mediratta et al. 2014; Vahanian et al. 2021) (Fig. 7.5b TEE 3D, supplementary material 3, 4).

TTE and TEE with 3D imaging make it possible to visualize all three TV leaflets simultaneously through "en face" visualization from both ventricular and atrial viewpoints (Seo et al. 2008; Hahn et al. 2017). Additionally, the positioning of the device lead can often be observed in relation to the TV leaflets and annulus. Previous investigations have indicated that the relationship between the lead and the TV leaflets could be delineated in approximately 12% to 17.2% of cases using 2DE (Spinner et al. 2011). In contrast, 3D imaging offers a significantly higher level of precision, enabling the determination of the route and position of the lead within the tricuspid apparatus in approximately 90–94% of cases (Mediratta et al. 2014; Seo et al. 2008).

2D TTE standard views of the tricuspid valve, including the apical four-chamber (A4ch) view, the A4ch view focused on the RV, and the parasternal short-axis view at the level of the great arteries, are commonly utilized (Seo et al. 2008; Hua et al. 2010; Muraru et al. 2022; Hahn et al. 2017) (Fig. 7.6a, b, c). The essential

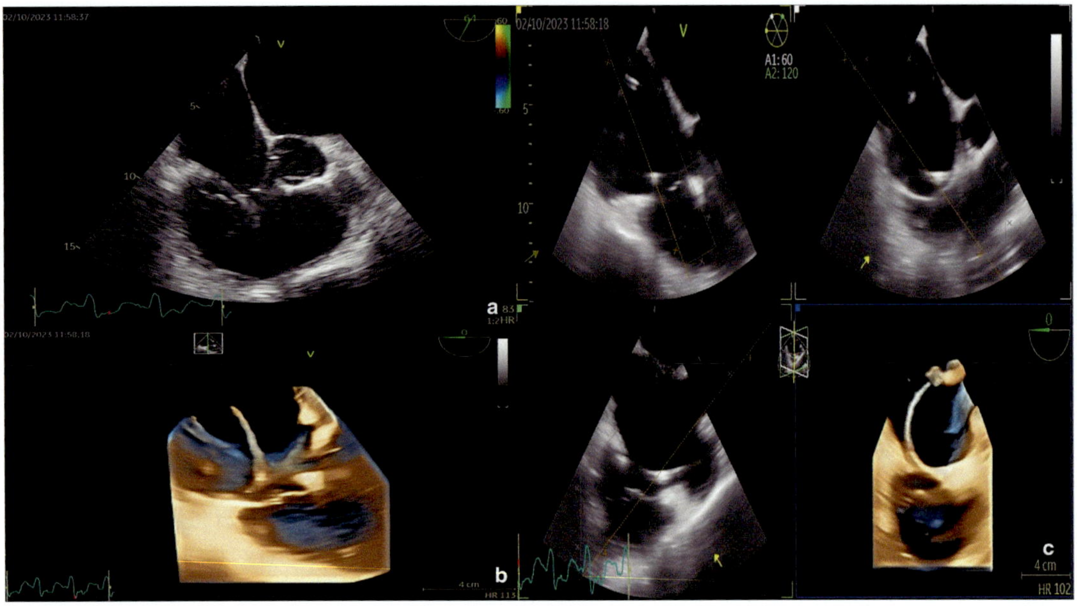

Fig. 7.5 Transesophageal evaluation of the tricuspid valve: **a** two-dimensional echocardiography; **b**, **c** three-dimensional echocardiography

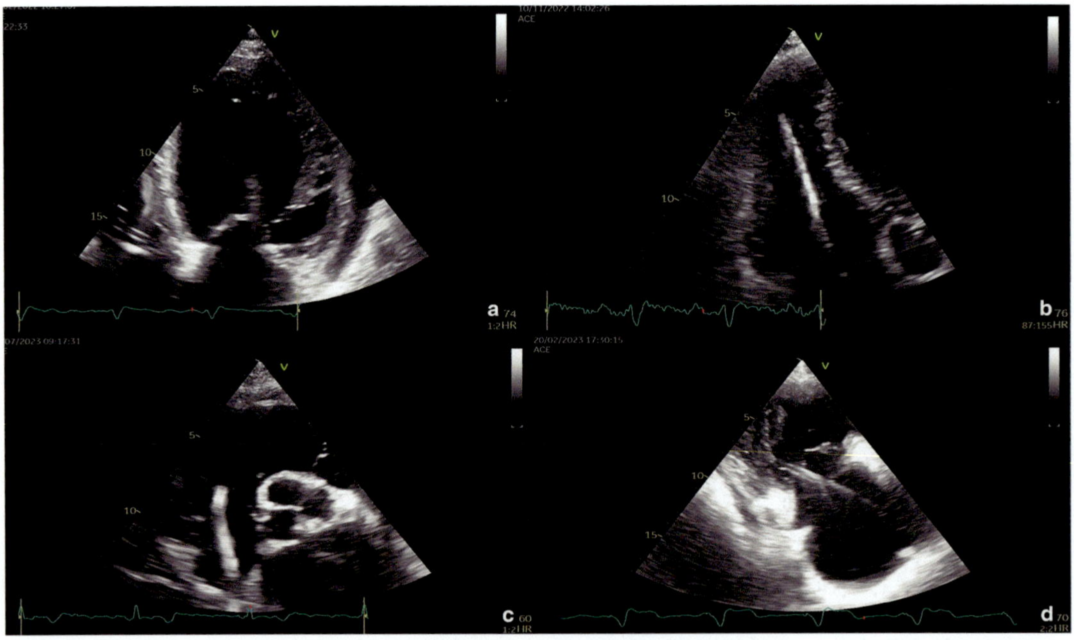

Fig. 7.6 Two-dimensional transthoracic echocardiography standard views of the tricuspid valve; **a** the apical four-chamber view; **b** the apical four-chamber view focused on the right ventricle; **c** and the parasternal short-axis view at the level of the great arteries; **d** the right ventricle inflow view

set of two-dimensional views for TV pathology comprises the standard views mentioned earlier, complemented by the RV-focused view with color Doppler interrogation, the RV inflow view encompassing the septum and coronary sinus, (Fig. 7.6 D) Focused examination of the TV leaflets is crucial for pinpointing the origin of TR (Muraru et al. 2022; Hahn et al. 2017) thereby facilitating the identification of TV pathology to a particular leaflet. This approach is particularly essential for understanding the mechanism of TR in patients with cardiac implantable electronic devices (CIEDs).

- RV inflow view: both the septal and anterior TV leaflets are visualized. Moreover, when the septum is seen, the septal leaflet is imaged in the far field, with the anterior leaflet imaged in the near field (Fig. 7.7a) (Supplementary material 5).
- A4ch view: the septal and anterior leaflets can be visualized. When the aortic valve is brought into view, the anterior and septal tricuspid leaflets are imaged. However, when the coronary sinus is seen, the septal and posterior leaflets are being imaged (Fig. 7.7b, c) (Supplementary material 6)
- In the parasternal short-axis view, if a single leaflet is visualized, this is always the anterior leaflet. (Fig. 7.7d) (Supplementary material 7)

According to the last guidelines, 2D TTE parameters indicating severe TR severity are:

Qualitative

Color flow regurgitant jet—a very large central jet or eccentric wall impinging jet (Fig. 7.8a)

CW signal of regurgitant jet—a dense/triangular with early peaking (Fig. 7.8b)

Semiquantitative

VC width (mm) > 7 (measured with a Nyquist limit of 50–60 cm/s, and preferably biplane) (Fig. 7.3a)

PISA radius (mm) > 9 (Baseline Nyquist limit shift of 28 cm/s) (Fig. 7.3b)

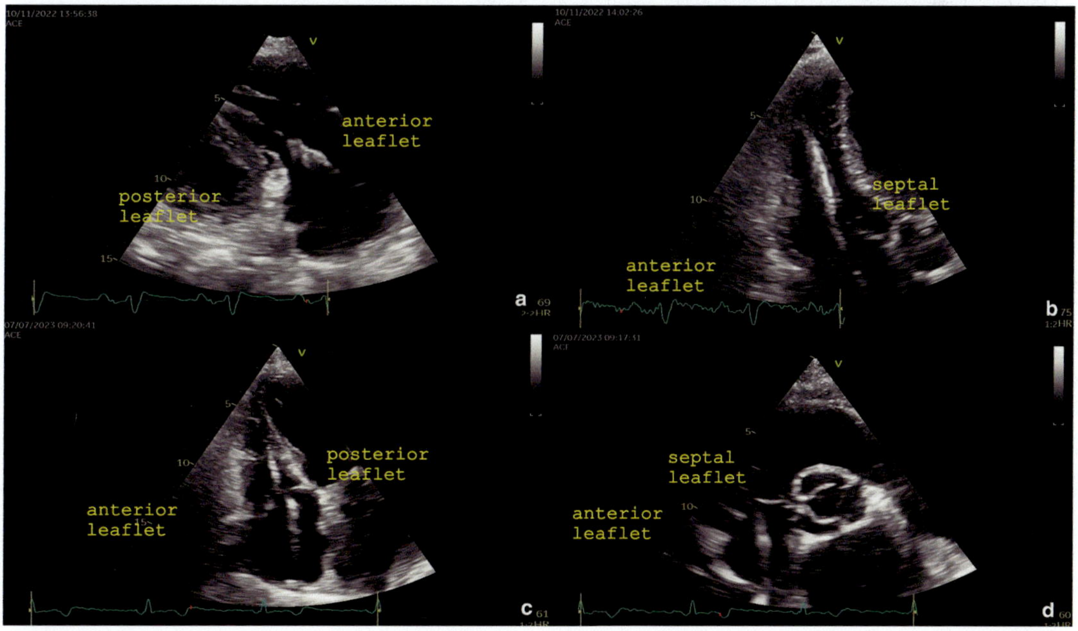

Fig. 7.7 Tricuspid leaflets imaging by two-dimensional transthoracic echocardiography: **a** from right ventricle inflow view; **b** from apical four-chamber view anterior angulated; **c** from apical four-chamber view posterior angulated; **c** parasternal short-axis view at the level of the great arteries

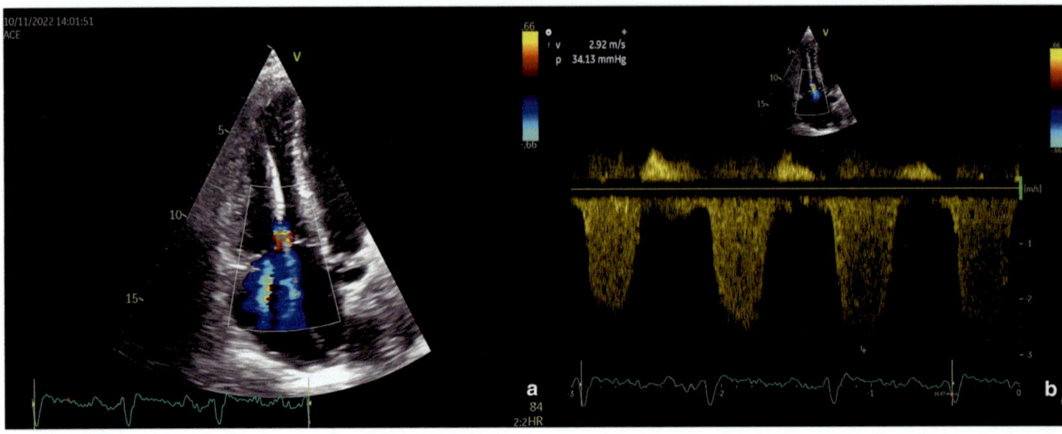

Fig. 7.8 Qualitative parameters for tricuspid regurgitation evaluation: **a** Color flow regurgitant jet; **b** CW signal of regurgitant jet

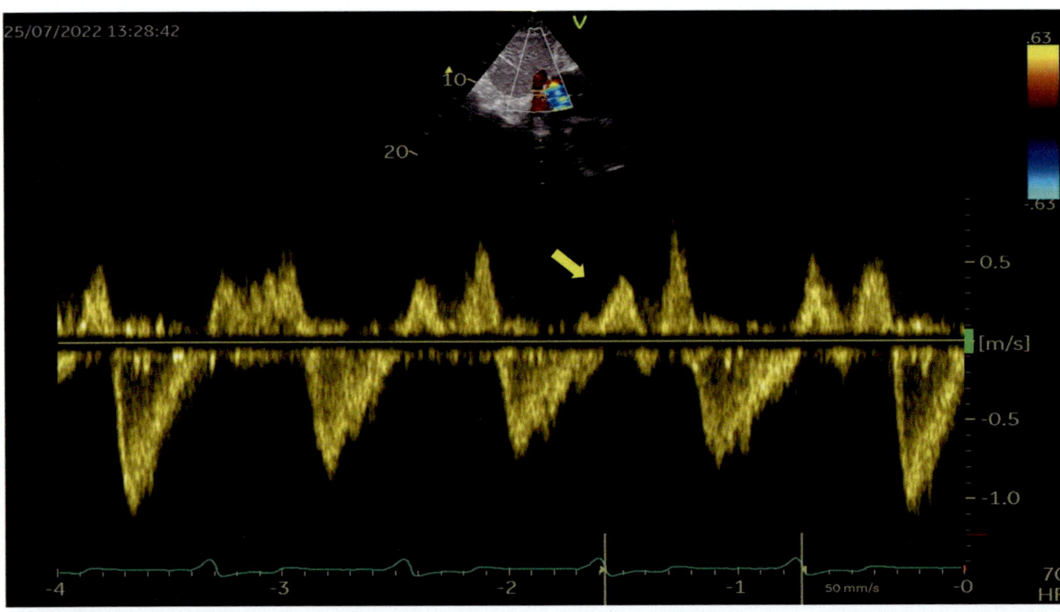

Fig. 7.9 Semiquantitative parameters for tricuspid regurgitation evaluation: Hepatic vein flow—Systolic flow reversal (arrow)

Hepatic vein flow—Systolic flow reversal (Fig. 7.9).

Tricuspid inflow E-wave dominant ≥ 1 m/s (in a patient without other causes of elevated RA pressure)

Quantitative

EROA ≥ 40 mm^2 (Fig. 7.3c)

Regurgitant volume ≥ 45 mL/beat (Fig. 7.3c)

Enlargement of cardiac chambers/vessels RV, RA, and inferior vena cava, Vahanian et al. 2021.

3DTTE examination can identify the lead position in 90% of the patients, with the interference of one leaflet in 47% of patients: the septal leaflet in 23% of patients, the posterior leaflet in 20% of patients, and the anterior leaflet in only 4% of patients (Mediratta et al. 2014)

(Fig. 7.4). When the lead is positioned near the postero-septal commissure or in the central portion of the tricuspid valve orifice, the lead does not interfere with leaflet motion in most cases (Mediratta et al. 2014). It is important to emphasize that patients with "impinging" leads on the body of the TV leaflets exhibited greater severity of TR compared to leads situated at the commissures or in the middle of the valve (non-impinging positions) (Mediratta et al. 2014).

Given these results, the 3D TTE guidance could be considered for placement in a commissural position, as 3D TTE-assisted device placement might reduce lead-associated TR. 3D TEE-guided lead placement in a commissure, predominantly in the postero-septal position, can be achieved in 95.2% of cases without exacerbating TR upon discharge (Patel et al. 2014).

Tricuspid annulus, RV, and RA dimensions (Fig. 7.10a–c), and RV function should also be measured because these parameters have prognostic value (Dietz et al. 2019). RV strain (Prihadi et al. 2019; Park et al. 2016) (Fig. 7.10c) and/or 3D measurements of RV volumes and EF measurement are indicated to overcome the limitations of 2D RV function evaluation (Lang et al. 2015) (Fig. 7.11). Advanced software allows tricuspid complex evaluation (tricuspid valve quantification—TVQ), providing information about its parameters structure function, and timing. (Fig. 7.12a–c). Tricuspid annulus parameters measured by TVQ are annulus area 3D and 2D (Fig. 7.13a), annulus area change, annulus perimeter (Fig. 7.13b), 4Ch diameter (Fig. 7.13c), 4Ch diastolic diameter (Fig. 7.13d), 2Ch diameter (Fig. 7.13e) major axis (Fig. 7.13f), major diastolic axis (Fig. 7.13g), minor axis (Fig. 7.13h), annulus sphericity index, annulus excursion. TV leaflets parameters (Fig. 7.14a) measured by TVQ are coaptation point height (Fig. 7.14b), maxim tenting height (Fig. 7.14c), and tenting volume (Fig. 7.14d) (Lang et al. 2015).

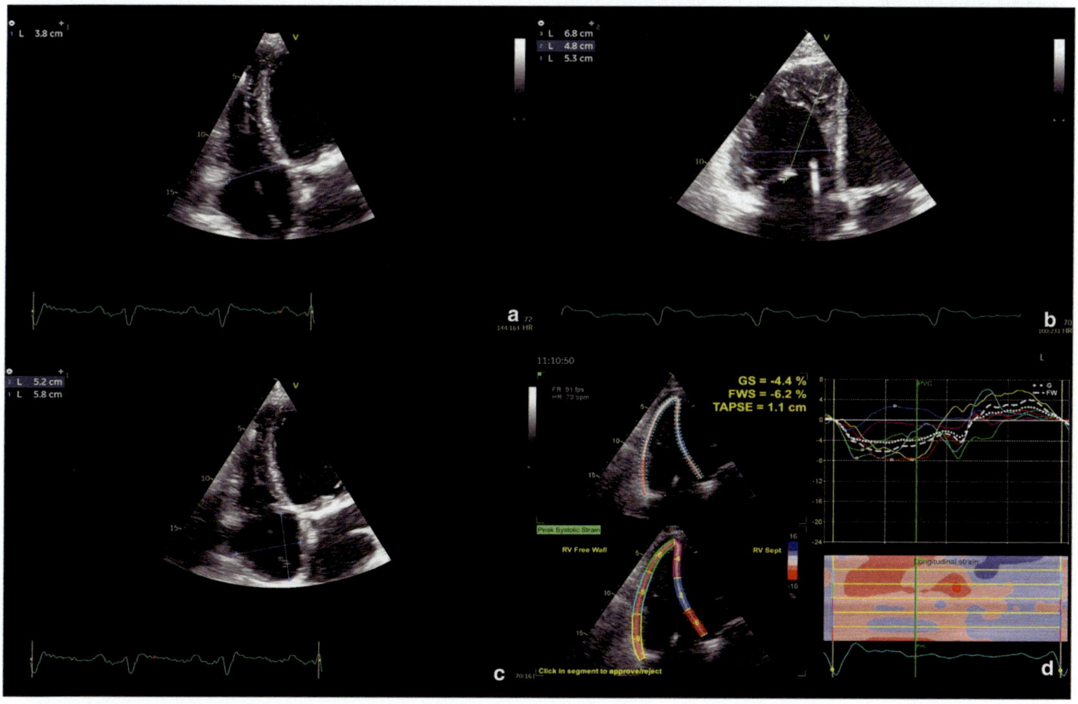

Fig. 7.10 Right chamber dimension measurement: **a** tricuspid annulus; **b** right ventricle; **c** right atrium; **d** right ventricle global strain measurement by speckle tracking echocardiography

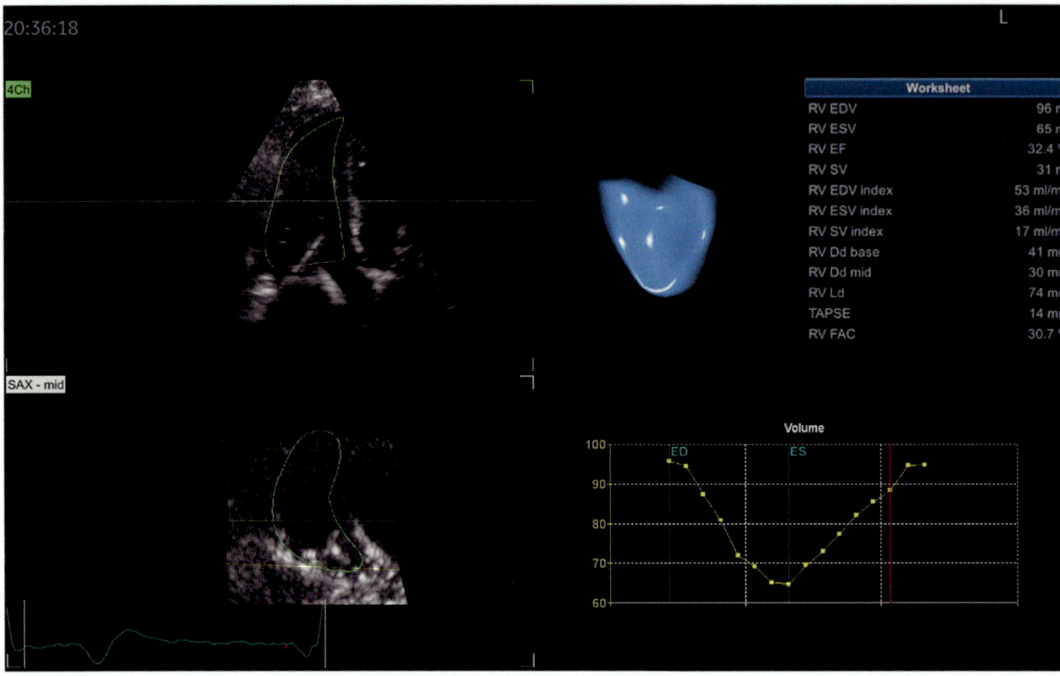

Fig. 7.11 Three-dimensional echocardiographic measurements of RV volumes and EF measurement

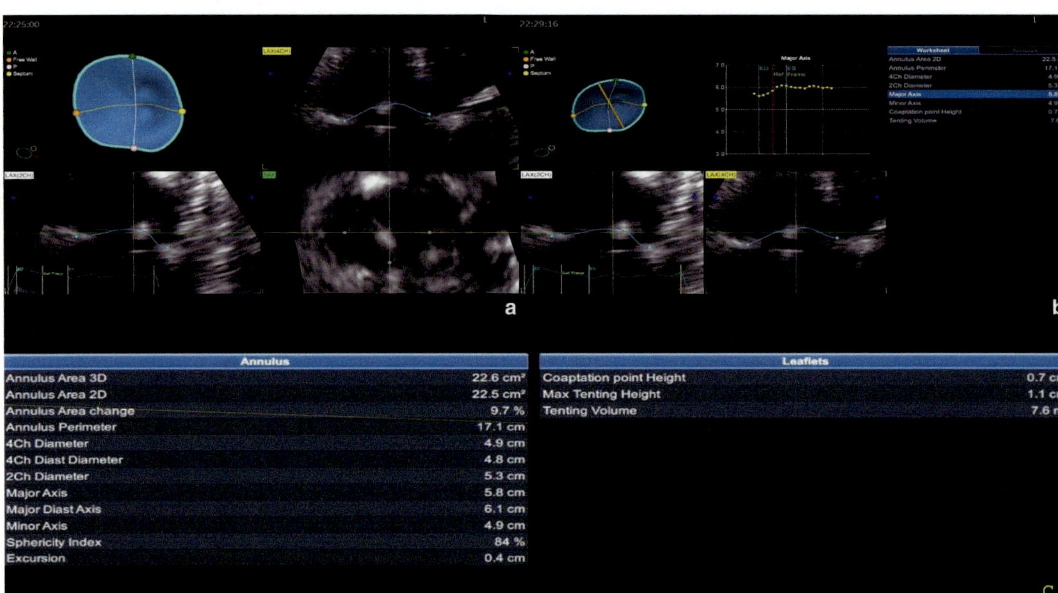

Fig. 7.12 Tricuspid complex parameters evaluation by three-dimensional echocardiographic—(tricuspid valve quantification)

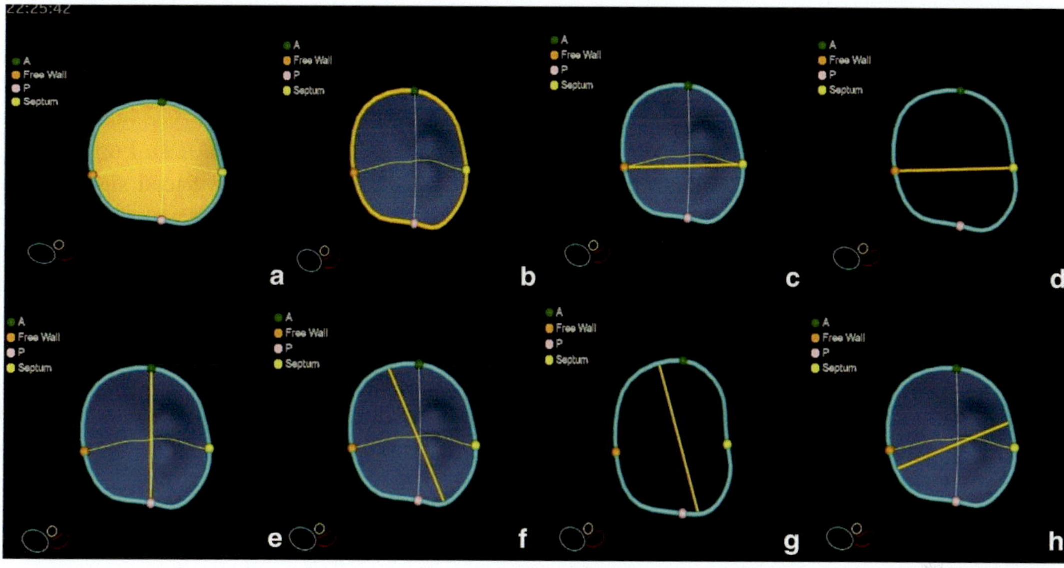

Fig. 7.13 Tricuspid annulus parameters evaluation by TV: **a** annulus area 3D; **b** annulus perimeter; **c** 4Ch diameter; **d** 4Ch diastolic diameter, **e** 2Ch diameter, **f** major axis, **g** major diastolic axis, **h** minor axis

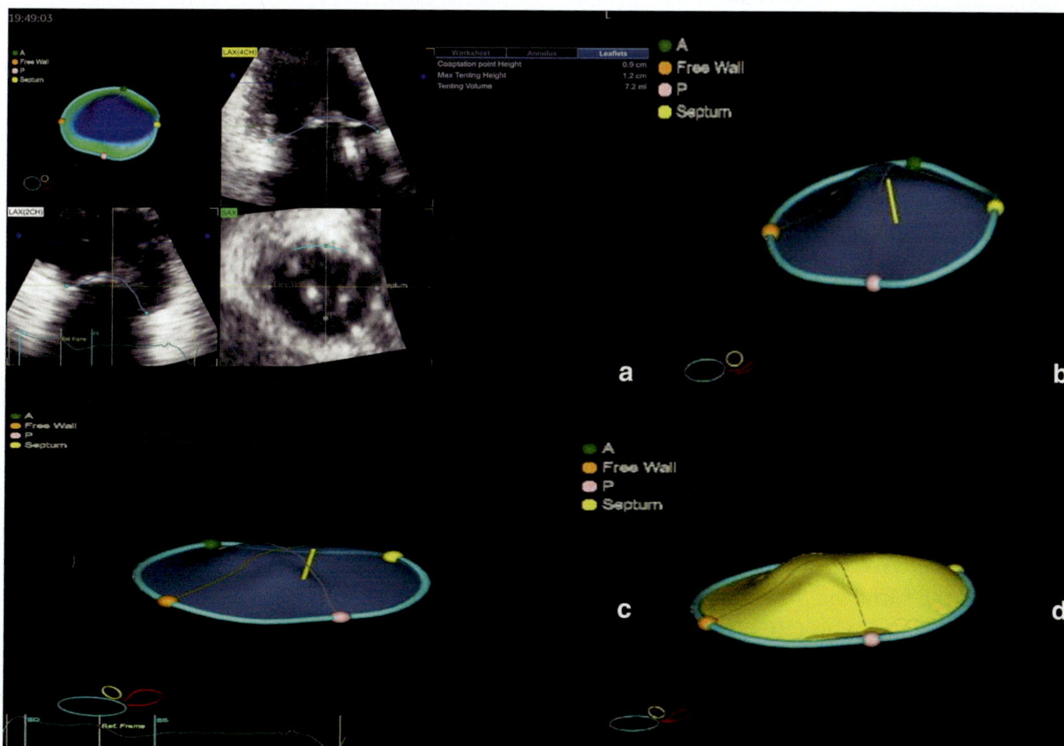

Fig. 7.14 Tricuspid valve leaflets parameters (A) measured by TVQ: **a** measurement; **b** coaptation point height; **c** maxim tenting height, **d** tenting volume

Outcomes of CIED-induced tricuspid regurgitation

CIED-induced TR is associated with a poorer prognosis (Hoke et al. 2014; Najib et al. 2013; Seo et al. 2020; Al-Bawardy et al. 2013). It is widely acknowledged that significant TR is linked to heightened morbidity and mortality as more than moderate TR is correlated with a decrease in one-year survival rates, ranging from 65 to 80%. (Hoke et al. 2014; Al-Bawardy et al. 2013; Delling et al. 2016; Nath et al. 2004) TR related to CIEDs has been demonstrated to induce remodeling of the right heart, leading to enlargement of right atrial and ventricular volumes and deterioration in RV function (Arabi et al. 2015; Hoke et al. 2014). In severe cases, TR due to leads may clinically manifest as symptoms of right heart failure, such as hepatomegaly and ascites. Notably, approximately half of patients necessitating tricuspid valve surgery due to severe lead-related TR primarily present with severe symptoms of right heart failure. Additionally, severe lead-related TR has been associated with a higher incidence of heart failure-related events, including hospitalizations, tricuspid valve surgeries, or upgrades to CRT, along with a decline in long-term survival rates (Hoke et al. 2014).

The prevalence of significant TR in over six years in patients with implanted devices carries a heightened risk of mortality, even after adjusting for factors like left ventricular dysfunction and pulmonary hypertension (Addetia et al. 2014). Initial studies on implantable cardioverter-defibrillators (ICDs) revealed a reduction in sudden death among recipients, yet a rise in heart failure-related hospitalizations and deaths was observed (Arabi et al. 2015; Seo et al. 2020). Several variables were identified as significantly correlated with CIED-related TR upon multivariate analysis. These included advancing age, lower body mass index, elevated heart rate, a history of mitral valve repair or replacement, significant mitral regurgitation, increased pulmonary pressure (pulmonary artery systolic pressure > 37 mm Hg), and dilation of the RV (Al-Bawardy et al. 2013). Quantitative methods like TR VC demonstrated that placing a device lead in a patient already experiencing TR raises the chances of developing moderate or severe TR by 54% and 43% for every 2 mm increase in VC width (Muraru et al. 2019). Furthermore, the presence of an obstructive lead significantly amplifies the probability of developing significant TR by a factor of 10. When using the VC and PISA evaluation, TR is worsened by 1 grade in 70.8% of the patients and 2 grades in 17.1% of the patients in the follow-up period, with an increase in PISA and VC values progressively and significantly in the follow-up period, as well as RA volumes and RV diameters and a decrease of the RV ejection fraction (Arabi et al. 2015).

Treatment of tricuspid valve damage or dysfunction associated with CIED leads

The management of CIED-related severe TR hinges on several factors (Sugeng et al. 2010; Addetia et al. 2019; Chang et al. 2017), including the presence of symptoms related to right-sided heart failure, the severity of TR, the extent of damage to the tricuspid valve due to leads, the degree of RV dysfunction, and dilation of the tricuspid annulus. Additionally, distinguishing between lead-related primary and secondary functional TR is crucial yet often challenging, understanding that these two conditions are frequently intertwined. Moreover, if left untreated, severe primary TR induced by leads can lead to the development of a superimposed secondary TR, which often persists even after lead removal and restoration of leaflet function. Management approaches may involve medical therapy, considering transvenous lead extraction and potential tricuspid valve repair or replacement (Chang et al. 2017).

Medical therapy. Loop diuretics are frequently prescribed (Nishimura et al. 2014), while aldosterone antagonists are considered beneficial additional agents, especially in instances involving hepatic congestion and secondary aldosterone elevation.

Transvenous lead extraction (TLE). The primary reasons for considering TLE are device-related infections, accounting for about two-thirds of cases, and lead dysfunction, which constitutes about one-third of cases (Park et al. 2018; Seo et al. 2020). However, there is not a formal guideline indication for TLE precisely due to lead-related TR.

The term "lead extraction" refers to a procedure aimed at removing a lead implanted for over a year, requiring specialized techniques and technology. Generally, lead extraction is considered a relatively safe procedure, with perioperative mortality rates between 0.4% and 0.8% (Hoke et al. 2014; Addetia et al. 2014; Yu et al. 2020; Monaco et al. 2014). However, inherent risks are involved regardless of the technique employed for lead removal. These risks include bleeding, laceration, or perforation of major venous and cardiac structures, hemopericardium, infection, injury to the tricuspid valve, pulmonary embolism, and potentially fatal arrhythmias. Intraoperative monitoring with TEE holds particular significance, as it allows the operator to monitor for injuries to the tricuspid valve, papillary muscles, and tendinous cords, where partial muscle rupture could progress to complete rupture. Furthermore, when lead extraction becomes necessary, it is vital to reassess the clinical indication for pacing or stimulation and explore alternative approaches for CIEDs. These alternatives may include epicardial stimulation, His-bundle pacing, leadless pacemakers, subcutaneous ICDs, or positioning leads in the coronary sinus (Beurskens et al. 2019).

Surgical treatment. Failure to promptly detect and address TR induced by CIEDs poses an increased risk for progressive dilation of the tricuspid annulus, enlargement or dysfunction of the RV, and eventual RV heart failure. Additionally, there is a high likelihood of severe and irreversible damage to the TV leaflets. Surgical intervention for valve repair or replacement may be necessary in such cases. Whether to repair or replace the valve depends on carefully considering the risk of recurrent TR following TV annuloplasty and the associated surgical risks. The reported 30-day mortality rate following surgical TV repair is approximately 6%. (Nishimura et al. 2014; Taramasso et al. 2019). During surgical TV replacement, which becomes necessary due to extensive valve damage or significant remodeling or dysfunction of the RV, securing the cardiac implantable CIED lead becomes imperative. Typically, the lead is fastened in the commissure between two leaflets, often the posterior and septal leaflets, using suture approximation (Raman et al. 2016).

Percutaneous treatment. Other options may be explored when medical treatment proves ineffective, and the patient is not eligible for surgery. Currently, only one notable study is available that investigates transcatheter tricuspid valve intervention (TTVI) in patients with CIEDs. The studies, including patients with severe TR, with and without CIEDs undergoing TTVI, revealed similar outcomes in both groups, including procedural success rates, residual TR, symptomatic improvement, and survival (Taramasso et al. 2019).

7.1 Conclusion

Lead-related TR is a common condition requiring meticulous echocardiographic evaluation using various imaging modalities to determine the mechanism underlying tricuspid valve dysfunction precisely. When severe regurgitation is diagnosed too late after the tricuspid annulus has expanded, irreversible changes may occur, and merely extracting the lead may not resolve the issue. Early diagnosis and treatment of TR enable timely intervention, helping to circumvent cardiac surgery and potential complications, including heart failure.

These findings underscore the importance of adopting a preventive approach and conducting echocardiographic monitoring to anticipate the onset or exacerbation of tricuspid regurgitation following cardiac implantable electronic device implantation. This proactive strategy aims to reduce hospital admissions and mortality rates.

Three-dimensional echocardiography provides the severity assessment of new or worsening TR at various time points post-implantation or determining the need for lead extraction or valve repair but also evaluates the likelihood of minimizing lead-induced tricuspid valve damage and dysfunction.

References

Addetia K, Maffessanti F, Mediratta A, et al. Impact of implantable transvenous device lead location on severity of tricuspid regurgitation. J Am Soc Echocardiogr. 2014;27(11):1164–75.

Addetia K, Harb SC, Hahn et al. Cardiac implantable electronic device lead-induced tricuspid regurgitation. *JACC Cardiovasc Imaging* 2019;12:622–636.

Addetia K, Harb SC, Hahn RT et al. Cardiac Implantable Electronic Device Lead-Induced Tricuspid Regurgitation. JACC Cardiovasc Imaging. 2019 Apr;12(4): 622-636.

Al-Bawardy R, Krishnaswamy A, Bhargava M, et al. Tricuspid regurgitation in patients with pacemakers and implantable cardiac defibrillators: a comprehensive review. Clin Cardiol. 2013;36(5):249–54.

Anvardeen K, Rao R, Hazra S, Hay K, Dai H, Stoyanov N, Birnie D, Dwivedi G, Chan KL. Prevalence and significance of tricuspid regurgitation post-endocardial lead placement. JACC Cardiovasc Imaging. 2019;12:562–4.

Arabi P, Özer N, Ateş AH, et al. Effects of pacemaker and implantable cardioverter defibrillator electrodes on tricuspid regurgitation and right sided heart functions. Cardiol J. 2015;22(6):637–44.

Benfari G, Antoine C, Miller WL, et al. Excess mortality associated with functional tricuspid regurgitation complicating heart failure with reduced ejection fraction. Circulation. 2019;140:196–206.

Beurskens NEG, Tjong FVY, De Bruin-Bon RHA, Dasselaar KJ, Kuijt WJ, Wilde AAM, et al. Impact of leadless pacemaker therapy on cardiac and atrioventricular valve function through 12 months of follow-up. Circ Arrhythm Electrophysiol. 2019;12: e007124.

Chang JD, Manning WJ, Ebrille E et al. Tricuspid Valve Dysfunction Following Pacemaker or Cardioverter-Defibrillator Implantation. *J Am Coll Cardiol.* 2017;9;69(18):2331–2341.

Delling FN, Hassan ZK, Piatkowski G, et al. Tricuspid regurgitation and mortality in patients with transvenous permanent pacemaker leads. Am J Cardiol. 2016;117:988–92.

Di Monaco A, Pelargonio G, Narducci ML, et al. Safety of transvenous lead extraction according to centre volume: a systematic review and meta-analysis. Europace. 2014;16:1496–507.

Dietz MF, Prihadi EA, van der Bijl P, et al. Prognostic implications of right ventricular remodeling and function in patients with significant secondary tricuspid regurgitation. Circulation. 2019;140:836–45.

Faletra FF, Leo LA, Paiocchi VL, et al. Imaging-based tricuspid valve anatomy by computed tomography, magnetic resonance imaging, two and three-dimensional echocardiography: correlation with anatomic specimen. Eur Heart J - Cardiovasc Imaging. 2019;20:1–13.

Fukuda S, Saracino G, Matsumura Y, et al. Three-dimensional geometry of the tricuspid annulus in healthy subjects and in patients with functional tricuspid regurgitation: a real-time, 3-dimensional echocardiographic study. Circulation. 2006;114:I492-498.

Gelves-Meza J, Lang RM, Valderrama-Achury MD, et al. Tricuspid Regurgitation Related to Cardiac Implantable Electronic Devices: An Integrative Review. J Am Soc Echocardiogr. 2022;35(11):1107–22.

Gmeiner J, Sadoni S, Orban M, et al. Prevention of pacemaker lead-induced tricuspid regurgitation by transesophageal echocardiography guided implantation. JACC Cardiovasc Interv. 2021;14:2636–8.

Hahn RT, Zamorano JL. The need for a new tricuspid regurgitation grading scheme. Eur Heart J Cardiovasc Imaging. 2017;18(12):1342–3.

Hahn RT, Weckbach LT, Noack T, et al. Proposal for a Standard Echocardiographic Tricuspid Valve Nomenclature. JACC Cardiovasc Imaging. 2021;14(7): 1299–305.

Hahn RT, Meduri CU, Davidson CJ and al. Early feasibility study of a transcatheter tricuspid valve annuloplasty: SCOUT trial 30- day results. *J Am Coll Cardiol 2017;*69:1795–806.

Hoke U, Auger D, Thijssen J, et al. Significant lead-induced tricuspid regurgitation is associated with poor prognosis at long-term follow-up. Heart. 2014;100:960–8.

Hoke U, Auger D, Thijssen et al. Significant lead-induced tricuspid regurgitation is associated with poor prognosis at long-term follow-up. *Heart* 2014;100:960–968.

Mateusz K. Hołda, Jorge D. Zhingre Sanchez et al. Right Atrioventricular Valve Leaflet Morphology Redefined: Implications for Transcatheter Repair Procedures, *JACC: Cardiovascular Interventions,* 2019;12(2):169–178.

Hua L, Handscumacher MD, Chandrasekaran K, et al. Guidelines for the echocardiographic assessment of the right heart in adults: a report from the American society of echocardiography endorsed by the European association of echocardiography, a registered branch of the European society of cardiology, and the Canadian society of echocardiography. J Am Soc Echocardiogr. 2010;23:685–713.

Hua L, Handscumacher MD, Chandrasekaran K, et al. Guidelines for the echocardiographic assessment of the right heart in adults: a report from the American society of echocardiography endorsed by the European association of echocardiography, a registered branch of the European society of cardiology, and the Canadian society of echocardiography. J Am Soc Echocardiogr. 2010;23:685–713.

Kim JB, Spevack DM, Tunick PA, et al. The effect of transvenous pacemaker and implantable cardioverter defibrillator lead placement on tricuspid valve function: an observational study. J Am Soc Echocardiogr. 2008;21:284–7.

Lang RM, Badano LP, Mor-Avi V, et al. Recommendations for cardiac chamber quantification by echocardiography in adults: an update from the American Society of Echocardiography and the European Association of Cardiovascular Imaging. Eur Heart J Cardiovasc Imaging. 2015;16:233–70.

Lin G, Nishimura RA, Connolly HM, et al. Severe symptomatic tricuspid valve regurgitation due to permanent pacemaker or implantable cardioverter-defibrillator leads. J Am Coll Cardiol. 2005;45:1672–5.

Mediratta A, Addetia K, Yamat M et al. 3D echocardiographic location of implantable device leads and mechanism of associated tricuspid regurgitation. JACC Cardiovasc Imaging. 2014 Apr;7(4):337-347.

Muraru D, Hahn RT, Soliman OI, et al. 3-Dimensional Echocardiography in Imaging the Tricuspid Valve. JACC Cardiovasc Imaging. 2019;12(3):500–15.

Muraru D, Maisano F, Zamorano JL, et al. Tricuspid regurgitation: recent advances in understanding pathophysiology, severity grading and outcome. Eur Heart J Cardiovasc Imaging. 2022;23:913–29.

Najib MQ, Vittala SS, Challa S, et al. Predictors of severe tricuspid regurgitation in patients with permanent pacemaker or automatic implantable cardioverter-defibrillator leads. Tex Heart Inst J. 2013;40(5):529–33.

Nath J, Foster E, Heidenreich PA. Impact of tricuspid regurgitation on long-term survival. J Am Coll Cardiol. 2004;43:405–9.

Nishimura RA, Otto CM, Bonow RO, et al. 2014 AHA/ACC guideline for the management of patients with valvular heart disease: a report of the American College of Cardiology/American Heart Association Task Force on Practice Guidelines. J Am Coll Cardiol. 2014;63:e57-185.

Park JB, Lee SP, Lee JH, et al. Quantification of right ventricular volume and function using single-beat three-dimensional echocardiography: a validation study with cardiac magnetic resonance. J Am Soc Echocardiogr. 2016;29:392–401.

Park SJ, Gentry JL 3rd, Varma N, et al. Transvenous Extraction of Pacemaker and Defibrillator Leads and the Risk of Tricuspid Valve Regurgitation. JACC Clin Electrophysiol. 2018;4(11):1421–8.

Patel B, Daraghmeh A, Machado C. Severe Tricuspid Valve Regurgitation Requiring Surgical Intervention as a Result of Pacemaker Lead Extraction: A Case Series. The Journal of Innovations in Cardiac Rhythm Management. 2014;5:1525–9.

Prihadi EA, van der Bijl P, Dietz M, et al. Prognostic implications of right ventricular free wall longitudinal strain in patients with significant functional tricuspid (Muraru D, Badano LP, Nagata Y, et al. Development and prognostic validation of partition values to grade right ventricular dysfunction severity using 3D echocardiography. Eur Heart J Cardiovasc Imaging. 2020;21:10–21regurgitation. *Circ Cardiovasc Imaging*. 2019;12: e008666

Raman J, Sugeng L, Lai DT, Jeevanandam V. Complex tricuspid valve repair in patients with pacer defibrillator-related tricuspid regurgitation. Ann Thorac Surg. 2016;101:1599–601.

Riesenhuber M, Spannbauer A, Gwechenberger M, et al. Pacemaker lead-associated tricuspid regurgitation in patients with or without pre-existing right ventricular dilatation. Clin Res Cardiol. 2021;110(6):884–94.

Seo Y, Ishizu T, Nakajima H, et al. Clinical utility of 3-dimensional echocardiography in the evaluation of tricuspid regurgitation caused by pacemaker leads. Circ J. 2008;72(9):1465–70.

Seo J, Kim DY, Cho I et al. Prevalence, predictors, and prognosis of tricuspid regurgitation following permanent pacemaker implantation. *PLoS One*. 2020;26;15(6):e0235230.

Shimada YJ, Shiota M, Siegel RJ, et al. Accuracy of right ventricular volumes and function determined by three-dimensional echocardiography in comparison with magnetic resonance imaging: a meta-analysis study. J Am Soc Echocardiogr. 2010;23(9):943–53.

Smolarek D, Gruchala, et al. Echocardiographic evaluation of right ventricular systolic function: The traditional and innovative approach. Cardiol J. 2013;2013:24. https://doi.org/10.5603/CJ.a2017.0051.

Spinner EM, Shannon P, Buice D, et al. In vitro characterization of the mechanisms responsible for functional tricuspid regurgitation. Circulation. 2011;124:920–9.

Sugeng L, Mor-Avi V, Weinert L, et al. Multimodality comparison of quantitative volumetric analysis of the right ventricle. JACC Cardiovasc Imaging. 2010;3(1):10–8.

Taramasso M, Gavazzoni M, Pozzoli A, et al. Tricuspid regurgitation: predicting the need for intervention, procedural success, and recurrence of disease. JACC Cardiovasc Imaging. 2019;12:605–21.

Vahanian A, Beyersdorf F, Praz F, et al, 2021 ESC/EACTS Guidelines for the management of valvular heart disease: Developed by the Task Force for the management of valvular heart disease of the European Society of Cardiology (ESC) and the European Association for Cardio-Thoracic Surgery (EACTS), *Eur Heart J*, 2021

Volpato V, Badano LP, Figliozzi S, et al. Multimodality cardiac imaging and new display options to broaden our understanding of the tricuspid valve. Curr Opin Cardiol. 2021;36(5):513–24.

Yu YJ, Chen Y, Lau CP, et al. Nonapical Right Ventricular Pacing Is Associated with Less Tricuspid Valve Interference and Long-Term Progress of Tricuspid Regurgitation. J Am Soc Echocardiogr. 2020;33(11):1375–83.

Zoghbi WA, Adams D, Bonow RO, et al. Recommendations for noninvasive evaluation of native valvular regurgitation: a report from the American Society of Echocardiography developed in collaboration with the Society for Cardiovascular Magnetic Resonance. J Am Soc Echocardiogr. 2017;30:303–71.

Echocardiographic Follow-Up the Patients with Implanted Devices

8

Abstract

Besides classical systolic function parameters and valvular pathology, patients with implanted devices need a particular evaluation. *Patients with pacemaker/ implanted cardioverter (ICD) +/− PM.* (1) Mechanical dyssynchrony induced by the high burden of right ventricle apical (RVA) pacing, influencing the long-term evolution. (2) Subclinical left ventricle (LV) systolic dysfunction identification using advanced echocardiographic techniques. (3) Pacemaker-induced cardiomyopathy (PIMC) criteria identification and the timing of up Grade at cardiac resynchronization therapy (CRT). *Patients with CRT*: Revers remodeling identification.

8.1 Patients with Pacemakers Evaluation After the Implant

1. *Mechanical dyssynchrony induced by RV apical pacing*

The prevalence of intra-ventricular dyssynchrony in patients with RVA pacing is up to 45–50% of cases with normal left ventricle ejection fraction (LVEF) and increases parallel with a decrease of LV function (Pastore et al. 2008; Fang et al. 2010).

Pacing the RV apex (Fig. 8.1a) can cause abnormal electrical activation of the ventricles, manifested on an electrocardiogram as a widening of the QRS with a pattern of left ventricle branch block (LBBB) and mechanical dyssynchrony (Sarvari et al. 2017). This electrical abnormality may deleterious affect LV function (Manolis 2006; Sweeney and Prinzen 2006). RVA pacing produces an electrical wavefront propagated directly from the myocardium, not the His–Purkinje conduction system. Early activation of the interventricular septum and late activation of the LV lateral wall follow the abnormal sequence activation (Prinzen et al. 1999). As a consequence, septal flush (SF) is usually present in most patients with conventional RV pacing, and its magnitude was inversely related to LV function and directly related to end-systolic volume (Sarvari et al. 2017) (Fig. 8.1b) (Supplementary material 1).

RVA pacing can induce interventricular dyssynchrony (between the RV and the LV), and intraventricular dyssynchrony (within the LV) (Tops et al. 2006). RV apical pacing produces a mechanical delay between the septum and the posterior wall (Lupi et al. 2006; Liu et al. 2008; Albertsen et al. 2008; Ypenburg et al. 2009). Echocardiographic techniques available for dyssynchrony assessment includes Doppler

Supplementary Information The online version contains supplementary material available at https://doi.org/10.1007/978-3-031-64079-7_8.

D.-M. Toader, *Echocardiographic Evaluation of Patients with Implanted Devices*, https://doi.org/10.1007/978-3-031-64079-7_8

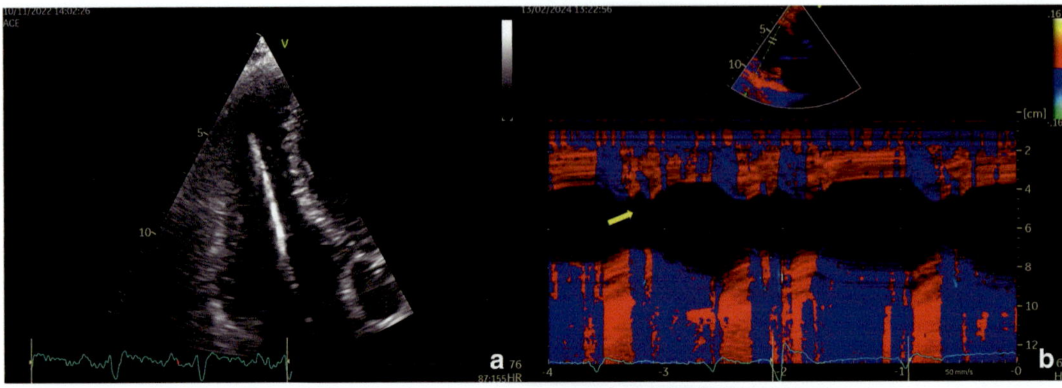

Fig. 8.1 **a** RV apical pacing viewed from apical four-chamber view right ventricle focused; **b** Septal flush viewed from Mode echocardiography

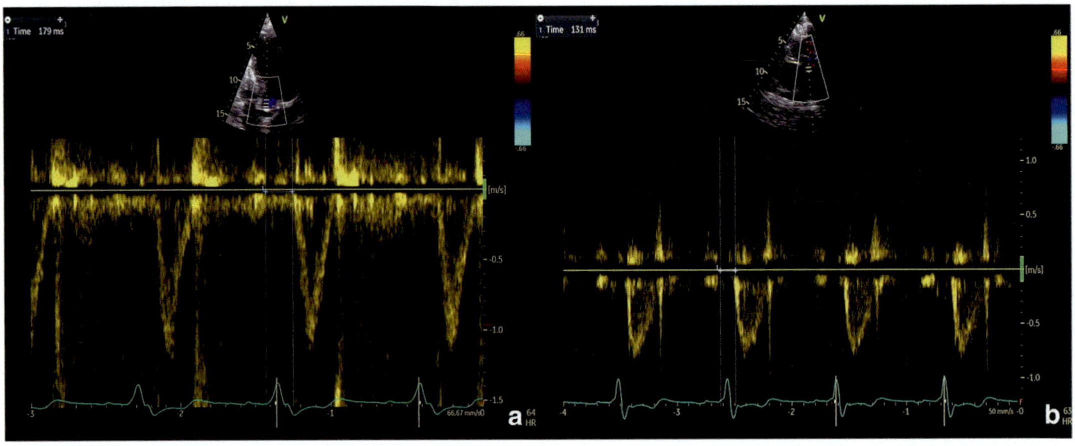

Fig. 8.2 Interventricular mechanical delay calculation: **a** left ventricle pre-ejection period obtained from apical 5-chamber view: **b** right ventricle pre-ejection period obtained from parasternal short-axis view of the great vessels

techniques, tissue Doppler imaging, speckle tracking echocardiography (STE) and three-dimensional echocardiography (3DE).

The electromechanical delay or interventricular dyssynchrony is calculated as the difference between the time from the onset of the QRS complex to the onset of pulmonary systolic flow (RV electromechanical delay) or aortic systolic flow (LV electromechanical delay) (Tops et al. 2006; Schmidt et al. 2007). Interventricular dyssynchrony is measured by interventricular mechanical delay (IVMD) (Fig. 8.2), representing the difference between the times of right ventricular (RV) and LV contraction. Pulsed wave (PW) Doppler images of aortic and pulmonary flow velocities recording of LV outflow tract (apical 5-chamber view) and RV outflow tract (parasternal short-axis view of the great vessels) allow the calculation of the difference in time between the LV pre-ejection period (LVEP) (Fig. 8.2A) (ECG-derived Q wave onset and the onset of LV outflow) and RV pre-ejection period (PEP) (Fig. 8.2b). Pathological values and indicators of interventricular dyssynchrony are IVMD values of>40 ms and LVPEP of>140 ms (Waggoner et al. 2007; Agler et al. 2007).

LV dyssynchrony represents the delay in mechanical activation between the interventricular septum and the posterior or lateral wall (Tops et al. 2009).

Intraventricular dyssynchrony can be evaluated by M-mode-derived septal-to-posterior wall motion delay (SPWMD) (Fig. 8.3a) or by systolic time interval measurement by Tissue Velocity Imaging (TVI) technique (Fig. 8.3b). SPWMD represents the difference between the time from the onset of ECG-derived Q wave to the initial peak posterior displacement of the septum and the time from the onset of QRS to the peak systolic displacement of the posterior wall. Pathological SPWMD value is > 130 ms (Agler et al. 2007). Other imaging techniques for intraventricular dyssynchrony evaluation are strain analysis and real-time 3-dimensional echocardiography (Fig. 8.3 C) (Marsan et al. 2008). Systolic dyssynchrony index (SDI) is calculated by STE or Real-Time Three-Dimensional Echocardiography (RT3DE). SDI is quantified by calculating the standard deviation of time to peak systolic strain (TP-SD) of six segments A-3ch, A4ch, and A-2ch view. Pathological value is > 60 ms (Mele et al. 2006; Teima et al. 2019; Cho et al. 2005; Tops et al. 2007; Dai et al. 2013; Kapetanakis et al. 2005). Sustained RVA pacing may have a deleterious effect on left ventricular (LV) systolic function in some patients (Tops et al. 2009; Tantengco et al. 2001; Zhang et al. 2008), resulting in LV remodelling, with the decrease of EF, and an increase of end-systolic volumes (Sarvari et al. 2017; Curtis et al. 2013; Wilkoff 2003).

The patients with RV apical pacing need careful follow-up with ventricular dyssynchrony assessment (Tops et al. 2009). One-year follow-up non-RVA pacing was not inferior to RVA pacing. However, the variables, such as the paced period longer than one year, the lead position, percentage of pacing, and baseline LV function, favor non-RVA pacing (Shimony et al. 2012). The changes in LV function might occur within one year of RV apical pacing (Hillock and Mond 2012; Molina et al. 2013). Long-term consequence of RVA, most frequent after four years of follow-up is the LVEF reduction by 5–15% in patients with normal baseline LV function (Tops et al. 2006). The lead on the anterior RV wall, away from the septum, may produce similar effects to RVA pacing (Lieberman et al. 2004).

EF and GLS decrease with permanent RV pacing in patients with normal LV function at implantation (Saito et al. 2015; Yu et al. 2009).

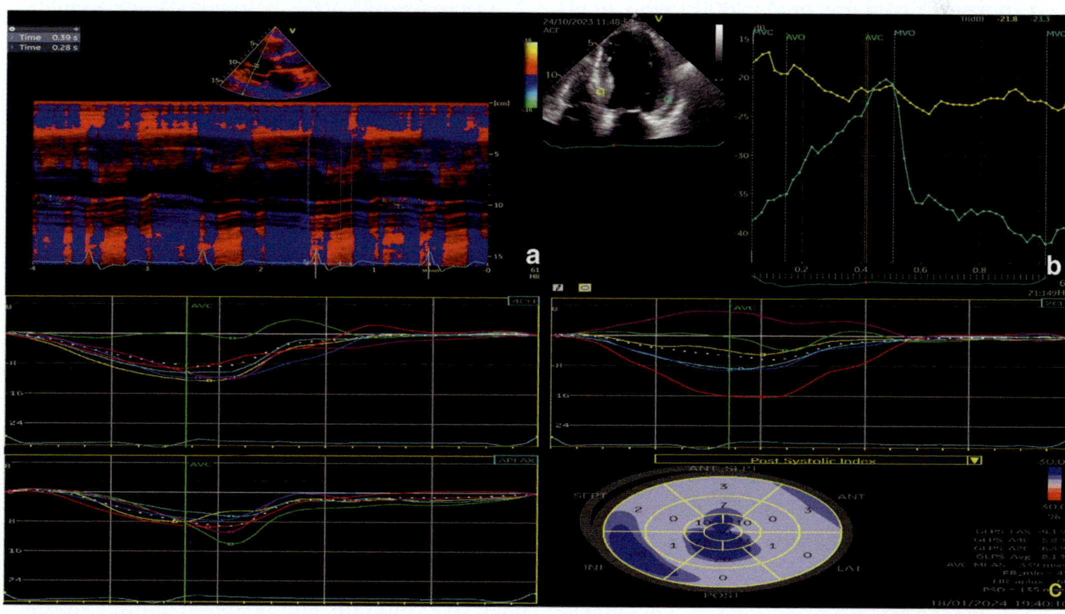

Fig. 8.3 Intraventricular dyssynchrony calculation: **a** M-mode-derived septal-to-posterior wall motion delay; **b** systolic time interval evaluated by tissue velocity imaging technique

Biventricular pacing can prevent these adverse effects (Yu et al. 2009).

In long-term RVA pacing, the patient might present myocardial perfusion defects, identified even in the absence of coronary disease, in up to 65% of the patients, usually near the pacing site (Tse et al. 2002; Skalidis et al. 2001) changes in LV wall thickness (Oosterhout et al. 1998) and LV remodelling (Vernooy et al. 2006) functional mitral regurgitation (Barold and Ovsyshcher 2005), and left atrial remodeling (Maurer et al. 1984), diastolic dysfunction, and hemodynamic changes (Lieberman et al. 2006).

Nonischemic patients with RV apical pacing are more likely to improve clinically and functionally after CRT upgrading (Bommel et al. 2009; Sutton et al. 2006).

Hiper responders, the patients who show complete functional recovery up to normalization of LV function after CRT, are almost exclusively seen in nonischemic cardiomyopathy (Ypenburg et al. 2009; Castellant et al. 2008). The LV activation pattern induced by extended areas of myocardial scar in ischemic cardiomyopathy is not correctable by the CRT (Sweeney and Prinzen 2008). Prognosis after CRT depends on the LV reverse remodeling rather than clinical response (Ypenburg et al. 2009; Woo et al. 2005).

Long-term follow-up of patients with RVA must identify the viability/contractility and adequately select those patients who may benefit from upgrading to CRT (Ciampi et al. 2010; Moonen et al. 2008).

Subclinical LV dysfunction in RVA-paced patients

2D STE can help detect subclinical left ventricular dysfunction in patients with RVA pacing (Teima et al. 2019). The speckle tracking radial strain cut-off for dyssynchrony is the time difference in peak anteroseptal to posterior wall strain more than or equal to 130 ms (Suffoletto et al. 2006) (Fig. 8.4).

GLS decreases after permanent pacemaker 1 and 3 months after implantation (Teima et al. 2019). GLS predicts subclinical LV dysfunction and outcome (Nahum et al. 2010). LV GLS measured by STE is significantly preserved in RVS compared to RVA, underlying the advantage of RVS (Fig. 8.5a) over RVA pacing (Inoue et al. 2011) (Fig. 8.5b). Compared with RVS, the RVA also has an unfavorable effect on LV untwisting (Inoue et al. 2010).

PIMC criteria identification and timing of CRT upgrading

Patients with a high burden of RVA pacing (> 90%) for sick sinus node dysfunction or atrioventricular (AV) block may present a long-term risk of cardiac morbidity and mortality due to LV dyssynchrony (Baronaitė-Dūdonienė et al. 2014). Most of the patients with RVA pacing present SF, with LV dysfunction and adverse remodeling (Sarvari et al. 2017; Delgado et al. 2009).

There is not a standardized definition of PICM. The most often used diagnostic criteria for PICM are:

1. Decrease of LVEF below 50%, regardless of patients' symptoms, or a reduction of LVEF by>/10%
2. Decrease of LVEF below 45%, or reduction of LVEF by>/10% or more after pacemaker implantation.
3. A decrease of LVEF below 40% indicates upgrading to CRT.
4. Reduction of LVEF by>/5% or more, with signs and symptoms of heart failure, without other etiology of heart failure (Mizner et al. 2022; Kim et al. 2018).

A group of patients with RV pacing may present symptoms of HF with LVEF-preserved EF, raising the problem of PIMC using LVEF as the sole parameter for disease definition (Yu et al. 2014). Some studies have also included a reduction of 15% in global GLS from baseline as criteria of PIMC (Babu et al. 2018). Another requirement for diagnosis is the presence of symptoms and hospitalization (Sweeney et al. 2003). The development of atrial fibrillation (AF) might be a potential manifestation

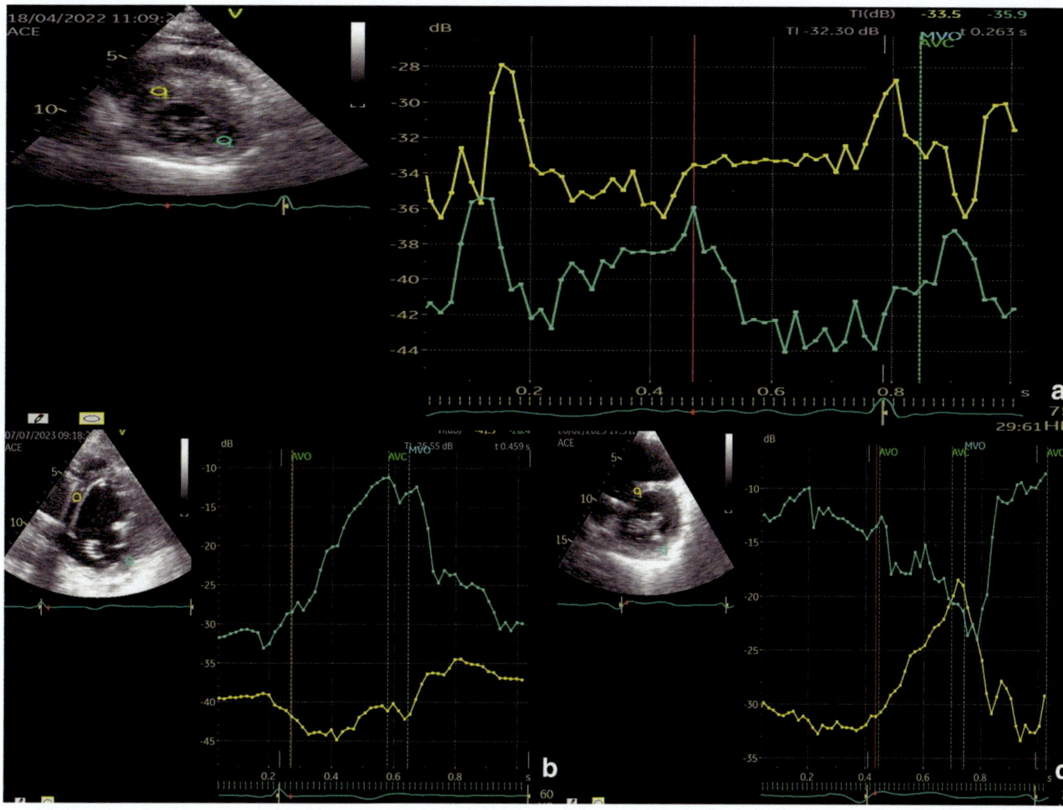

Fig. 8.4 Radial strain in patients with right ventricular pacing: **a** Healthy volunteer; **b** septal right ventricle lead position, **c** apical right ventricular lead position

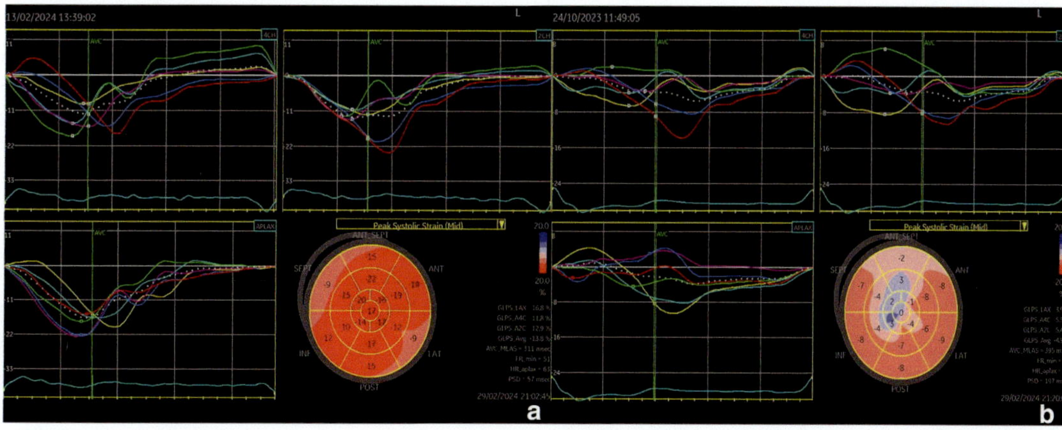

Fig. 8.5 GLS in patients with pacemaker: **a** a patient with a VVI pacemaker and septal (Hiss bundle) lead position; **b** a patient with a double chamber pacemaker and right ventricular apical lead position, before upgrading to CRT

of PICM (Fleischmann et al. 2006). When compared to atrial vs. dual chamber pacing for sinus node dysfunction, the patients with a high pacing burden were at a significantly increased risk of developing AF at 2.9 years follow-up. A high percent of pacing correlated with increased left atrial and ventricular volumes, explaining the link to the development of AF in these patients (Nielsen et al. 2003). PIMC is a consequence of pacing burden > 20% (Khurshid et al. 2014). The variables associated with an increased risk of PICM are older age, wider QRS pre-implantation on ECG, wider paced QRS on ECG, male gender, history of myocardial infarction, atrioventricular block, AF, and decreased LVEF before implantation (Kiehl et al. 2016; Lee et al. 2016; Khurshid et al. 2014; Merchant et al. 2017; Cho et al. 2019; Abdin et al. 2019; Safak et al. 2019; Naqvi and Chao 2023). The patients with baseline LVEF < 55% before pacing, paced QRS duration > 160 ms, and pacing burden more than 33% have a higher risk of developing PICM (Laksono et al. 2023).

Management for patients with PICM

The percentage of ventricular pacing should be kept to a minimum to avoid the detrimental effects of RVA pacing (Sweeney and Prinzen 2006), or an alternative strategy such as upgrading RV pacing to CRT, "de novo" CRT, or an alternative pacing site (Tops et al. 2009). Patients with depressed LVEF before implantation, patients with complete AV block or congenital AV block and need for an extended period of pacing necessitate alternatives for RVA pacing (Tops et al. 2009).

CRT ESC guidelines recommend upgrading to CRTs in patients with conventional pacemakers or an ICD who develop refractory heart failure and LVEF ≤ 35% and for those with significant RV pacing burden (Class IIa level B) (Glikson et al. 2021).

CRT can prevent PICM and is superior to RV pacing in relieving symptoms. Biventricular pacing is effective and safe in patients with LBBB and remains first-line therapy (Glikson et al. 2021).

HBP can be superior to BVP because it activates the ventricle via the native conduction system, avoiding PIMC (Archontakis et al. 2022; Gardas et al. 2022). HBP presents some disadvantages, such as technical difficulties, reduced R wave amplitudes, and high and unstable thresholds (Archontakis et al. 2022; Yuan et al. 2022)

Left Bundle Branch Pacing (LBBP) This technique might be an option for patients with signs of PICM after a long time of use of RV pacing (Ye et al. 2021; Wang et al. 2022; Hua et al. 2022).

72.2–84% of patients with severe PICM (LVEF < 35%) who were upgraded to CRT improved LVEF to > 35% over a median of 7 months, with the most critical improvement after the first three months post-device upgrade (Kiehl et al. 2016; Khurshid et al. 2014; Lu et al. 2022; Gwag et al. 2017; Schwerg et al. 2015). The researchers suggest a window of opportunity for the upgrading of patients with PICM, indicating the best time from diagnosis to upgrade of up to 144 months (Kerley et al. 2023). Effects expected after upgrading are reverse remodeling of the LV (defined as a reduction in LV end-diastolic or end-systolic volume) (Tops et al. 2007; Vatankulu et al. 2009; Witte et al. 2006), the mitral regurgitation severity improvement (Leclercq et al. 2007), and LVEF improvement (Valls-Bertault et al. 2004).

The effect of CRT on ventricular dyssynchrony is: acute reduction in the LV pre-ejection interval after onset of CRT (Witte et al. 2006; Horwich et al. 2004; Eldadah et al. 2006) decreasing in time-to-peak strain difference of various LV segments (Tops et al. 2009). Patients with moderate to severe LV dysfunction and a standard pacemaker indication will receive CRT instead of RV apical pacing alone.

Factors influencing response to CRT up-grading

A typical LBBB strain pattern is characterized by an early shortening of the septal wall before the opening of the aortic valve, with a concomitant stretch in the lateral wall. Immediate lengthening (rebound stretch) follows early septal activation, causing a delayed lateral wall peak contraction (Galli et al. 2023) (Fig. 8.6). This activation pattern is a predictor of LV reverse remodelling and prognosis after CRT (Risum et al. 2015).

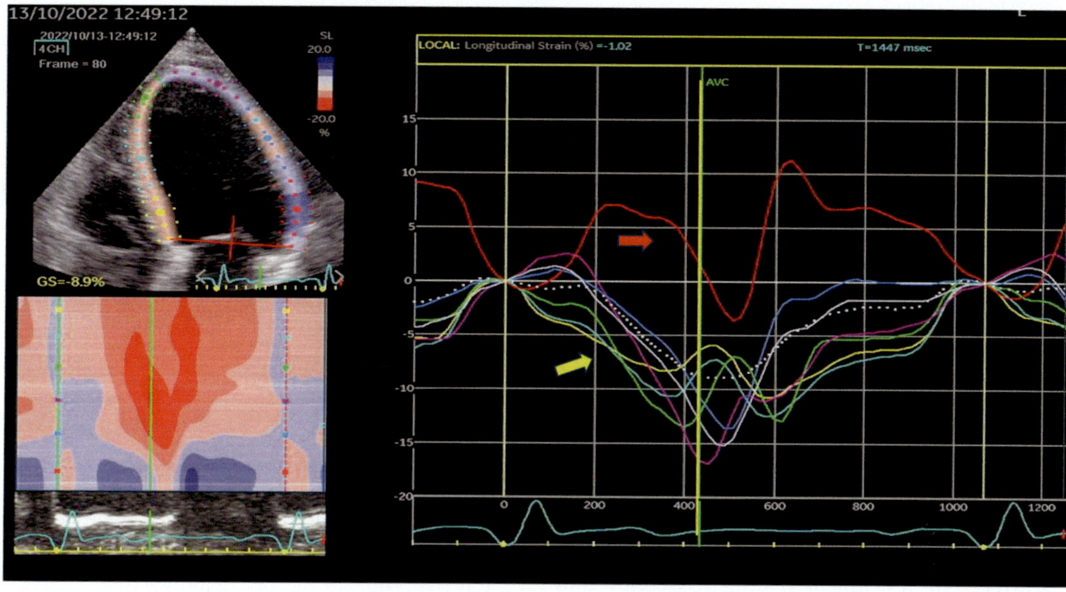

Fig. 8.6 Strain traces from the septum and lateral wall in a patient with left bundle branch block before CRT; yellow arrow: septal curve, red arrow: lateral wall curve

The localization of myocardial scar can impact septal motion in LBBB patients and should be considered in LV dyssynchrony evaluation. The presence of lateral wall scar leads to the loss of septal rebound stretch, *whereas extensive* anterior ischemia increases rebound stretch (Aalen et al. 2019). The septal flash and/or apical rocking have also proven to predict CRT response in patients with right ventricular pacing needing an upgrade to CRT (Stankovic et al. 2017).

Other pacing strategies and alternative pacing sites

Minimal ventricular pacing algorithms promote normal AV conduction, maintaining intrinsic ventricular conduction (Olshansky et al. 2007; Sweeney et al. 2007).

Atrial-based pacing maintains normal ventricular electrical activation and prevents cardiac desynchronization. This pacing modality is recommended in patients with sinus node disease without AV conduction abnormalities (Epstein et al. 2008). AV sequential pacing is superior to single-ventricular pacing (Ventricle pacing and sensing -VVI, or Ventricle pacing and sensing with rate response enabled—VVIR), producing a 10% to 53% improvement in cardiac output, Compared with VVI pacing (Sweeney and Prinzen 2006), dual-pacing dual-sensing dual-response rate-adaptive pacemaker (DDDR) is the most physiological pacing mode. Studies revealed that LA and LV diameters were increasing, and LV fractional shortening decreased in the DDDR groups, and no changes in the atrial-pacing atrial-sensing inhibited-response rate-adaptive pacemaker (AAIR) groups. In long-term follow-up (2,9 $\pm$ 1.1 years), AF was less common in the AAIR group than in the DDDR group (Nielson et al. 2003).

Alternative RV pacing sites, the RV outflow tract, septal pacing, and direct His bundle (HB) pacing result in less electrical activation delay (a shorter QRS duration) and less mechanical dyssynchrony (Tops et al. 2009). In the short term, RV outflow tract pacing favors hemodynamics and LV dyssynchrony (Cock et al. 2003). Right ventricle septal (RVS) pacing is a better alternative than RV apical pacing in short-term follow-up (Victor et al. 2006; Kypta et al. 2008). In patients with permanent atrial fibrillation and AV node ablation, presenting a narrow QRS before implantation, RVS pacing is a better strategy compared with RVA pacing (Takemoto et al. 2009). RVS pacing guided by the paced QRS morphology preserves long-term LV function via minimizing LV dyssynchrony and preserves LV function in long-term follow-up (Takemoto et al. 2009).

RV non-apical pacing is associated with a higher LVEF at follow-up (Wezong, et al. 2013). In patients with impaired LV function, patients with ongoing pathology such as ischemia, poorly controlled systemic hypertension, or diabetes, pacing outside the RVA may be desirable (Curtis et al. 2013). Patients with depressed LV function at baseline who require permanent pacemaker are more susceptible to the deleterious effects of RV apical pacing (Sweeney and Prinzen 2006).

RVS pacing in most patients is effective and well tolerated, suggesting that the exact place of the lead in the septal wall would be of great importance in LV deterioration (Sarvari et al. 2017). Pacing from the right ventricle (RV) septum provides more physiological LV activation because of its closer location to the specialized conduction system (Molina et al. 2013; Saito et al. 2015; Zhang et al. 2012). RVS or HB pacing induce more synchronous LV contraction than RVA pacing, resulting in better electromechanical synchrony than RVA pacing (Kronborg et al. 2014; Zhuang et al. 2018).

Patients with RVA pacing have a lower LVEF at mid- and long-term follow-up, with a decrease as the follow-up period increases compared with the patients with RVS pacing (Zhuang et al. 2018). HB pacing is considered more physiological than RVA pacing (Weizong et al. 2013). In HB or para-Hisian pacing, after 23.4 ± 8.3 months, patients presented a decrease in LV end-diastolic diameter and an increase in LVEF (Deshmukh et al. 2000). Intraventricular (Zanon et al. 2008; Occhetta et al. 2006) and interventricular dyssynchrony (Occhetta et al. 2006) during para-Hisian pacing.

8.2 CRT Patients Evaluation After Implant

Qualitative parameters of CRT response are:

- The disappearance of septal flush and apical rocking
- MR improvement.

Quantitative parameters of CRT response are:

- Decrease in LVSV/LVDV
- Improvement in LVEF, 2D, and 3D strain parameters.

A substantial number of patients have a poor response to CRT (Daubert et al. 2012).

CRT predicting factors response are:

- Baseline mechanical dyssynchrony
- The presence of a scar
- Position of the LV lead (Delgado et al. 2011).

The follow-up of patients treated with CRT is generally performed using echocardiography (Mele et al. 2017). Different imaging techniques are not interchangeable in assessing LV dimensions and function in patients with CRT (Greupner et al. 2012; Wood et al. 2014).

Evaluation of CRT response

As a general rule, if echocardiography is used before CRT implantation, it should be used also during patient follow-up (Verhaert et al. 2010). The definition of reverse remodeling after CRT implantation is different. The echocardiography has an essential role in assessing myocardial performance after CRT (Galli et al. 2017).

Response to CRT depends on electrical conduction delay and myocardial viability (Aalen et al. 2019; Gorcsan and Lumens 2019). Parameters used to assess the response to CRT are LV-EF, end-systolic volume (ESV), and dyssynchrony.

1. Ejection fraction: In most studies, LVEF following CRT improvement is 4–5%. The non-deterioration of the EF can be considered a favorable effect of CRT, given the progressive nature of LV remodelling in heart failure (HF) (Liuba et al. 2014; Friedman et al. 2014).
2. End-systolic volume: Most studies used a decrease in LVESV>/15% at the end of the follow-up period of 6 months as a CRT response (Chung et al. 2008). The reduction in ≥ 15% LVESV is an independent predictor of all-cause mortality in heart failure patients treated with CRT (Bertini et al. 2013). LVESV can be best measured using 3D echocardiography (Lang et al. 2012). The reduction in LV ESV of about 10% 3–6 months after CRT predicts survival after one year; Significant mitral regurgitation six months after CRT associates an adverse clinical outcome at four years (Onishi et al. 2013).
3. Mechanical dyssynchrony: Changes in dyssynchrony are essential for the response to CRT (Bleeker and Mollema 2007; Gorcsan and Yu 2012). Some authors consider the reduction of LV mechanical dyssynchrony to be directly linked to pacing rather than a marker of the biological response triggered by the CRT (Greupner et al. 2012).

Dyssynchrony after CRT and risk for ventricular arrhythmias

Dyssynchrony at baseline before CRT is generally a marker for a good prognosis, but dyssynchrony on follow-up echocardiography after CRT is associated with an increased risk for ventricular arrhythmias (Gorcsan and Yu 2012). In patients with mild HF and persistent dyssynchrony after CRT, SD of time-to-peak transverse strain in 12 LV myocardial segments can be used to predict the risk of arrhythmias (Kutyifa et al. 2013). Dyssynchrony by speckle tracking radial strain at the level of anteroseptal to posterior wall delay ≥ 130 ms after CRT associates appropriate anti-tachycardia pacing or shock after CRT (Haugaa et al. 2014) (Fig. 8.4c).

It is not easy to find a single dyssynchrony parameter. Currently, the LVEF and ESV measurements represent the best approach (Greupner et al. 2012).

The reverse LV remodelling after CRT is more significant in patients with non-ischemic HF etiology and greater mechanical dyssynchrony prior to implantation (Bommel et al. 2009).

CRT produces a 15% decrease in end-systolic volume in 54% of patients in short and mid-term follow-up (3–6 months) (Stellbrink et al. 2001; Bleeker and Box 2006).

Six month of follow-up is the best moment to evaluate the effect of CRT on LV remodeling. The maximum reduction of LVESV in patients considered responders is in the first six months (Galli et al. 2017).

In CRT responders, who also showed clinical response, LVEFs increased to>35% from baseline at *one-year follow-up,* and LV volumes decreased by 10–16% from baseline. Values of LV diameters and volumes were lower, and LVEF was higher compared with non-responders (Vidal et al. 2006).

The beneficial effect of CRT on LV remodeling seems to be maximal in the first 3–9 months of treatment (Ghio et al. 2009b). The echocardiographic evaluation of CRT patients at 9– 12 months provides also significant prognostic information. The patients with LVEF normalization at 12 months (> 50%) have a low risk of ventricular tachyarrhythmias and a favorable clinical course at 2.2 years (Ruwald et al. 2014). Patients with an EF>35% at one year from the implant have a better outcome in the long term (Frigerio et al. 2014).

LV reverse remodeling assessed by ΔLV-ESV is a strong predictor of outcome following CRT during a median follow-up of 32 months and is better than ΔLV-EF and ΔGLS (Menet and Guyomar 2016). The predictors of clinical prognosis and CRT response in HF patients are LVESV reduction ≥ 15% and/or absolute value of LVEF increase ≥ 5% at 6–12 months follow-up (Stellbrink et al. 2001; St John Sutton et al. 2003; Abraham et al. 2004). Clinical trials have demonstrated these benefits in the first year after

CRT implantation (Bristow et al. 2004; Cleland et al. 2005; Moss et al. 2009; Linde et al. 2008; Ponikowski et al. 2016).

Super responders represent the patients with > 30% reduction in end-systolic volume at six months follow-up. These patients showed a more considerable end-systolic volume before CRT (Ypenburg et al. 2009; António et al. 2009). The patients with improvement of EF > 50% are "super responders" and have a favorable outcome (Manne et al. 2013). Some researchers can also consider non-deterioration of the EF to be a favorable effect of CRT (Liuba et al. 2014).

The definition of no responders has been proposed to be the lack of clinical response or the absence of LV reverse remodeling at six months follow-up (Stellbrink et al. 2001; Abraham et al. 2002).

60–70% of patients with HF receiving CRT demonstrate a favorable response on echocardiogram and favorable outcomes (Ypenburg et al. 2009).

Patients with non-ischemic cardiomyopathy, longer HF duration, and a lower increased LVEF at initial CRT response should be carefully monitored because they may present a re-worsening of LVEF. This phenomenon is described in one-third of CRT responders (Oki et al. 2022). A shorter HF duration is associated with a favorable CRT echocardiographic response (Wang et al. 2018; Greene et al. 2017; Loyaga-Rendon et al. 2015). The presence of arrhythmia and low biventricular pacing also associates with an absence of response to CRT (Mullens et al. 2009).

The prognosis of patients with re-worsening LVEF after CRT response might have a wrong course (Oka et al. 2017). The trajectory of LVEF in HF is related to prognosis (Lupón et al. 2018). A slow increase in LVEF at initial recovery was related to subsequent LVEF re-worsening in patients with dilated cardiomyopathy (Nabeta et al. 2021).

Follow-up echocardiography has to be performed at fixed intervals (Sarvari et al. 2017; Prinzen et al. 1999; Ypenburg et al. 2009; Oka et al. 2017; Ichibori et al. 2017): one year and two years (Oki et al. 2022). The sixth month of follow-up is the best moment to evaluate the effect of CRT on LV remodeling (Galli et al. 2017). CARE-HF study sub-analysis showed the most beneficial effect of CRT on LV remodeling in the first 3–9 months of treatment (Ghio et al. 2009b). Some studies showed that assessments made after 3–6 months of CRT have prognostic significance (Yu et al. 2015). The REVERSE study showed that reducing LVESV after six months of CRT is an independent predictor of long-term survival (Gold et al. 2015). The persistence of a mitral regurgitation more significant than mild after six months of CRT is associated with an adverse clinical outcome at four years of follow-up (Onishi et al. 2013). In the MADIT-CRT trial, patients with normalization of LVEF at 12 months (> 50%) have a very low risk of ventricular tachyarrhythmias and a favorable clinical course at 2.2 years (Ruwald et al. 2014). An EF > 35% at one year from the implant has a better outcome in the long term (Frigerio et al. 2014). Regular follow-up echocardiography must be performed in patients with an initial CRT response despite initial improvements in LVEF. Therefore, appropriately evaluating the timing of CRT implantation is essential to avoid LVEF re-worsening after CRT (Oki et al. 2022).

A decrease of ESV of 10–15% with 2DE and 5–10% with 3DE is a positive biological effect of CRT. A reduction by ≥ 9.5% of LVESV has a sensitivity and specificity of 70% in predicting all-cause mortality (Foley et al. 2009). LV reverse remodeling after six months of CRT is a better predictor of long-term survival than the clinical response (Bertini et al. 2013). There is not always a concordance between clinical and echocardiographic CRT response. Some patients with an improvement in clinical endpoints did not show any improvement in echocardiographic parameters (Chung et al. 2008; Auger et al. 2010). Following CRT implant, synchrony is restored (with the disappearance of SF), and the septal wall thickness and contractility are markedly improved (Sze and Daubert 2018). This achievement might be explained by the electrical activation of the septum, irrespective of the modality of ventricle pacing biventricular or LV pacing only (Sharma et al. 2018).

LV pacing can only restore SF-dyssynchrony because it prevents the leftward motion of the septum in contrast to RV pacing. There is no absolute requirement for biventricular pacing to restore SF-dyssynchrony and septal function. HB pacing may become the alternative for an LV lead in the future (Sharma et al. 2018). Pacing could also be deleterious in right-to-left septal activation, producing SF and septal hypercontractility (Sarvari et al. 2017). A deep septal RV lead or His-bundle pacing will produce a normal left-to-right septal activation, SF, and septal hypofunction prevention (Mafi-Red et al. 2016). From these points of view, RV pacing is not per se deleterious, as long as the LV conduction system is quickly activated after the electrical impulse of the RV lead (Calle et al. 2020). The HPCSP is a simple procedure that avoids coronary sinus catheterization difficulties for LV electrodes (Pujol-López et al. 2022).

8.3 Conclusions

Patients with implanted devices need a special echocardiographic follow-up.

In pacemaker patients with RVA lead, echocardiography provides essential data regarding PIMC criteria identification and the moment of CRT–upgrade. Echocardiographic techniques available for dyssynchrony assessment include Doppler techniques, tissue Doppler imaging, strain analysis, and three-dimensional echocardiography.

Echocardiography is an important imaging tool to measure patients' short-time and long-time response to CRT and optimize the device in non-responders. Speckle tracking echocardiography and three-dimensional echocardiography provide novel parameters that could measure dyssynchrony persistence in this group of patients.

References

Aalen JM, Remme EW, Larsen CK, et al. Mechanism of abnormal septal motion in left bundle branch block: role of left ventricular wall interactions and myocardial scar. JACC Cardiovasc Imaging. 2019;12(12):2402–13.

Abdin A, Yalin K, Zink MD, et al. Incidence and predictors of pacemaker induced cardiomyopathy: a single-center experience. J Electrocardiol. 2019;57:31–4.

Abraham WT, Fisher WG, Smith AL, et al. Cardiac resynchronization in chronic heart failure. N Engl J Med. 2002;346:1845–53.

Abraham WT, Young JB, Leon AR, et al. On behalf of the Multicenter InSync ICD II Study Group. Effects of cardiac resynchronization on disease progression in patients with left ventricular systolic dysfunction, an indication for an implantable cardioverter-defibrillator, and middly symptomatic chronic heart failure. Circulation. 2004;110:2864–68.

Agler DA, Adams DB, Waggoner AD. Cardiac resynchronization therapy and the emerging role of echocardiography (Part 2); the comprehensive examination. J Am Soc Echocardiogr. 2007;20:76–90.

Albertsen AE, Nielsen JC, Poulsen SH, et al. DDD(R)-pacing, but not AAI(R)-pacing induces left ventricular desynchronization in patients with sick sinus syndrome: tissue-Doppler and 3D echocardiographic evaluation in a randomized controlled comparison. Europace. 2008;10:127–33.

António N, Teixeira R, Coelho L, et al. Identification of "super-responders" to cardiac resynchronization therapy: the importance of symptom duration and left ventricular geometry. Europace. 2009;11:343–9.

Archontakis S, Sideris K, Laina A, et al. His bundle pacing: a promising alternative strategy for anti-bradycardic pacing—report of a single center experience. Hellenic J Cardiol. 2022;64:77–86.

Auger D, van Bommel RJ, Bertini M, et al. Prevalence and characteristics of patients with clinical improvement but not significant left ventricular reverse remodeling after cardiac resynchronization therapy. Am Heart J. 2010;160:737–43.

Babu NMS, Srinath SC, Lahiri A, et al. Three-dimensional echocardiography with left ventricular strain analyses helps earlier prediction of right ventricular pacing-induced cardiomyopathy. J Saudi Heart Assoc. 2018;30(2):102–7.

Barold SS, Ovsyshcher IE. Pacemaker-induced mitral regurgitation. Pacing Clin Electrophysiol. 2005;28:357–60.

Baronaitė-Dūdonienė K, Vaškelytė J, Puodžiukynas A, et al. Evaluation of left ventricular longitudinal function and synchrony after dual chamber pacemaker implantation. Medicina. 2014;50:330–44.

Bertini M, Hoke U, van Bommel RJ, et al. Impact of clinical and echocardiographic response to cardiac resynchronization therapy on long-term survival. Cardiovasc. Imaging. 2013;14:774–81.
Birnie DH, Tang ASL. The problem of non-response to cardiac resynchronization therapy. Curr Opin Cardiol. 2006;21(1):20–6.
Bleeker GB, Bax JJ, Fung JW-H, et al. Clinical versus echocardiographic parameters to assess response to cardiac resynchronization therapy. Am J Cardiol. 2006;97:260–63.
Bleeker GB, Mollema SA. Holman ER et al Left ventricular resynchronization is mandatory for response to cardiac resynchronization therapy: analysis in patients with echocardiographic evidence of left ventricular dyssynchrony at baseline. Circulation. 2007;116:1440–8.
Bristow MR, Saxon LA, Boehmer J, et al. For the Comparison of Medical Therapy, Pacing and Defibrillation in Heart Failure (COMPANION) investigators. Cardiac resynchronization therapy with or without an implantable defibrillator in advanced heart failure. N Engl J Med. 2004;350:2140–50.
Calle S, Delens C, Kamoen V, De Pooter J, Timmermans F. Septal flash: at the heart of cardiac dyssynchrony. Trends Cardiovasc Med. 2020;30:115–22.
Castellant P, Fatemi M, Bertault-Valls V, Etienne Y, Blanc JJ. Cardiac resynchronization therapy: "nonresponders" and "hyperresponders." Heart Rhythm. 2008;5:193–7.
Cho GY, Song JK, Park WJ. Mechanical dyssynchrony assessed by tissue Doppler imaging is a powerful predictor of mortality in congestive heart failure with normal QRS duration. J Am Coll Cardiol. 2005;46:2237–43.
Cho SW, Gwag HB, Hwang JK, et al. Clinical features, predictors, and long-term prognosis of pacing-induced cardiomyopathy. Eur J Heart Fail. 2019;21(5):643–51.
Chung ES, Leon AR, Tavazzi L, et al. Results of the predictors of response to CRT (PROSPECT) trial. Circulation. 2008;117:2608–16.
Ciampi Q, Pratali L, Citro R, et al. Clinical and prognostic role of pressure-volume relationship in the identification of responders to cardiac resynchronization therapy. Am Heart J. 2010;160(5):906–914.
Cleland J, Daubert J, Eerdmann E, et al. The effect of cardiac resynchronization therapy on morbidity and mortality in heart failure. N Engl J Med. 2005;352:1539–49.
Curtis AB, Worley SJ, Adamson PB, et al. Biventricular pacing for atrioventricular block and systolic dysfunction. N Engl J Med. 2013;368:1585–93.
Dai M, Lu J, Qian D. Assessment of left ventricular dyssynchrony and cardiac function in patients with different pacing modes using real-time three-dimensional echocardiography: Comparison with tissue Doppler imaging. Exp Ther Med. 2013;6:1213–9.
Daubert JC, Saxon L, Adamson PB, et al. 2012 EHRA/HRS expert consensus statement on cardiac resynchronization therapy in heart failure: implant and follow-up recommendations and management. Heart Rhythm. 2012;9:1524–76.
de Cock CC, Giudici MC, Twisk JW. Comparison of the haemodynamic effects of right ventricular outflow-tract pacing with right ventricular apex pacing: a quantitative review. Europace. 2003;5:275–8.
Delgado V, Tops LF, Trines SA, et al. Acute effects of right ventricular apical pacing on left ventricular synchrony and mechanics. Circ Arrhythm Electrophysiol. 2009;2:135–45.
Delgado V, van Bommel RJ, Bertini M, et al. Relative merits of left ventricular dyssynchrony, left ventricular lead position, and myocardial scar to predict long-term survival of ischemic heart failure patients undergoing cardiac resynchronization therapy. Circulation. 2011;123(1):70–8.
Deshmukh P, Casavant DA, Romanyshyn M, Anderson K. Permanent, direct His-bundle pacing: a novel approach to cardiac pacing in patients with normal His-Purkinje activation. Circulation. 2000;101:869–77.
Eldadah ZA, Rosen B, Hay I, et al. The benefit of upgrading chronically right ventricle-paced heart failure patients to resynchronization therapy demonstrated by strain rate imaging. Heart Rhythm. 2006;3:435–42.
Epstein AE, DiMarco JP, Ellenbogen KA, et al. ACC/AHA/HRS 2008 guidelines for device-based therapy of cardiac rhythm abnormalities: a report of the American College of Cardiology/American Heart Association Task Force on Practice Guidelines (Writing Committee to Revise the ACC/AHA/NASPE 2002 Guideline Update for Implantation of Cardiac Pacemakers and Antiarrhythmia Devices). J Am Coll Cardiol. 2008;51:e1-62.
Fang F, Chan JY, Yip GW, et al. Prevalence and determinants of left ventricular systolic dyssynchrony in patients with normal ejection fraction received right ventricular apical pacing: a real-time three-dimensional echocardiographic study. Eur J Echocardiogr. 2010;11:109–18.
Fleischmann KE, Orav EJ, Lamas GA, et al. Pacemaker implantation and quality of life in the Mode Selection Trial (MOST). Heart Rhythm. 2006;3(6):653–9.
Foley PW, Leyva F, Frenneaux MP. What is treatment success in cardiac resynchronization therapy? Europace. 2009;11:v58–65.
Freudenberger RS, Wilson AC, Lawrence-Nelson J, Hare JM, Kostis JB. Myocardial infarction Data Acquisition Study Group (MIDAS 9). Permanent pacing is a risk factor for the development of heart failure. Am J Cardiol. 2005;95:671–4.
Friedman DJ, Upadhyay GA, Rajabali A, et al. Progressive ventricular dysfunction among nonresponders to cardiac resynchronization therapy: baseline predictors and associated clinical outcomes. Heart Rhythm. 2014;11:1991–8.
Frigerio M, Lunati M, Pasqualucci D, et al. Left ventricular ejection fraction overcrossing 35% after one year of cardiac resynchronization therapy predicts long-term survival and freedom from sudden cardiac

death: single center observational experience. Int J Cardiol. 2014;172:64–71.

Galli E, Leclercq C, Donal E. Mechanical dyssynchrony in heart failure: still a valid concept for optimizing treatment? Arch Cardiovasc Dis. 2017;110(1):60–8.

Galli E, Galand V, Le Rolle V, et al. The saga of dyssynchrony imaging: are we getting to the point. Front Cardiovasc Med. 2023.

Gardas R, Golba KS, Soral T, et al. The effects of his bundle pacing compared to classic resynchronization therapy in patients with pacing-induced cardiomyopathy. J Clin Med. 2022;11(19):5723.

Ghio S, Freemantle N, Scelsi L, et al. Long-term ventricular reverse remodelling with cardiac resynchronization therapy: results from the CARE-HF trial. Eur J Heart Fail. 2009a;1:480–8.

Ghio S, Freemantle N, Scelsi L, et al. Long-term left ventricular reverse remodelling with cardiac resynchronization therapy: results from the CARE-HF trial. Eur J Heart Fail. 2009b;11(5):480–8.

Glikson M, Nielsen JC, Kronborg MB, et al. 2021 ESC Guidelines on cardiac pacing and cardiac resynchronization therapy. Eur Heart J. 2021;42(35):3427–520.

Gold MR, Daubert C, Abraham WT, et al. The impact of reverse remodeling on long-term survival in mildly symptomatic heart failure patients receiving cardiac resynchronization therapy: results of the REVERSE study. Heart Rhythm. 2015;12:524–30.

Gorcsan J III, Lumens J, Opposing wall pushing and stretching response to cardiac resynchronization therapy requires electrical delay and viability, JACC: Cardiovasc Imaging. 2019;1212:2414–16.

Gorcsan J 3rd, Yu CM. Sanderson JE (2012) Ventricular resynchronization is the principle mechanism of benefit with cardiac resynchronization therapy. Heart Fail Rev. 2012;17:737–46.

Greene SJ, Hernandez AF, Dunning A, Ambrosy AP, Armstrong PW, Butler J, et al. Hospitalization for recently diagnosed versus worsening chronic heart failure: from the ASCEND-HF Trial. J Am Coll Cardiol. 2017;69:3029–39.

Greupner J, Zimmermann E, Grohmann A, et al. Headtohead comparison of left ventricular function assessment with 64- row computed tomography, biplane left cineventriculography, and both 2- and 3-dimensional transthoracic echocardiography: comparison with magnetic resonance imaging as the reference standard. J Am Coll Cardiol. 2012;59:1897–907.

Gwag HB, Chun KJ, Hwang JK, et al. Comparison of de novo versus upgrade cardiac resynchronization therapy; focused on the upgrade for pacing-induced cardiomyopathy. Yonsei Med J. 2017;58:703–9.

Haugaa KH, Marek JJ, Ahmed M, Ryo K, Adelstein EC, Schwartzman D, et al. Mechanical dyssynchrony after cardiac resynchronization therapy for severely symptomatic heart failure is associated with risk for ventricular arrhythmias. J Am Soc Echocardiogr. 2014;27:872–9.

Hillock RJ, Mond HG. Pacing the right ventricular outflow tract septum: time to embrace the future. Europace. 2012;14:28–35.

Horwich T, Foster E, De Marco T, Tseng Z, Saxon L. Effects of resynchronization therapy on cardiac function in pacemaker patients "upgraded" to biventricular devices. J Cardiovasc Electrophysiol. 2004;15:1284–9.

Hua J, Wang C, Kong Q, et al. Comparative effects of left bundle branch area pacing, His bundle pacing, biventricular pacing in patients requiring cardiac resynchronization therapy: A network meta-analysis. Clin Cardiol. 2022;45(2):214–23.

Ichibori H, Fukuzawa K, Kiuchi FHRS. Predictors and clinical outcomes of transient responders to cardiac resynchronization therapy, paced and clinical electrophysiology. 2017;40(3):301–9.

Inoue K, Okayama H, Nishimura K, et al. Right ventricular pacing from the septum avoids the acute exacerbation in left ventricular dyssynchrony and torsional behavior seen with pacing from the apex. J Am Soc Echocardiogr. 2010;23:195–2000.

Inoue K, Okayama H, Nishimura K, et al. Right ventricular septal pacing preserves global left ventricular longitudinal function in comparison with apical pacing—analysis of speckle tracking. Circ J. 2011;75:1609–15.

Kapetanakis S, Kearney MT, Siva A, et al. Real-time three-dimensional echocardiography: a novel technique to quantify global left ventricular mechanical dyssynchrony. Circulation. 2005;112:992–1000.

Kaye G, Ng JY, Ahmed S, et al. The prevalence of pacing-induced cardiomyopathy (PICM) in patients with long-term right ventricular pacing—is it a matter of definition? Heart Lung Circ. 2019;28.

Kerley RN, O'Dowling C, Campos F, et al. The therapeutic benefit of upgrade to cardiac resynchronization therapy in patients with pacing-induced cardiomyopathy, Heart Rhythm O_2. 2023;4(4):225–31.

Khurshid S, Epstein AE, Verdino RJ, et al. Incidence and predictors of right ventricular pacing-induced cardiomyopathy. Heart Rhythm. 2014;11(9):1619–25.

Khurshid S, Obeng-Gyimah E, Supple GE, et al. Reversal of pacing-induced cardiomyopathy following cardiac resynchronization therapy. JACC Clin Electrophysiol. 2018;4(2):168–77.

Khurshid S, Epstein AE, Verdino RJ, et al. Incidence and predictors of right ventricular pacing-induced cardiomyopathy. Heart Rhythm. 2014; 11(9):1619–25.

Kiehl EL, Makki T, Kumar R, et al. Incidence and predictors of right ventricular pacing-induced cardiomyopathy in patients with complete atrioventricular block and preserved left ventricular systolic function. Heart Rhythm. 2016;13(12):2272–8.

Kim JH, Kang K-W, Chin JY, et al. Major determinant of the occurrence of pacing-induced cardiomyopathy in complete atrioventricular block: a multicenter, retrospective analysis over a 15-year period in South Korea. BMJ Open. 2018;8:e019048.

Kronborg MB, Mortensen PT, Poulsen SH, et al. His or para-His pacing preserves left ventricular function in atrioventricular block: a double-blind, randomized, crossover study. Europace. 2014;16:1189–96.

Kutyifa V, Pouleur AC, Knappe D, Al-Ahmad A, Gibinski M, Wang PJ, et al. Dyssynchrony and the risk of ventricular arrhythmias. JACC Cardiovasc Imaging. 2013;6:432–44.

Kypta A, Steinwender C, Kammler J, Leisch F, Hofmann R. Long-term outcomes in patients with atrioventricular block septal ventricular lead implantation compared with standard apical pacing. Europace. 2008;10:574–9.

Laksono S, Angkasa IS, Hosanna C. Pacing induced cardiomyopathy: diagnosis and management. AHJ. 2023;32(3):4–8.

Lang RM, Badano LP, Tsang W, et al. EAE/ASE recommendations for image acquisition and display using three-dimensional echocardiography. J Am Soc Echocardiogr. 2012;25:3–46.

Leclercq C, Cazeau S, Lellouche D, et al. Upgrading from single chamber right ventricular to biventricular pacing in permanently paced patients with worsening heart failure: the RD-CHF study. Pacing Clin Electrophysiol. 2007;30(Suppl 1):S23-30.

Lee SA, Cha MJ, Cho Y, et al. Paced QRS duration and myocardial scar amount: predictors of long-term outcome of right ventricular apical pacing. Heart Vessels. 2016;31(7):1131–9.

Lieberman R, Grenz D, Mond HG, Gammage M. Selective site pacing: defining and reaching the selected site. Pacing Clin Electrophysiol. 2004;27:883–6.

Lieberman R, Padeletti L, Schreuder J, et al. Ventricular pacing lead location alters systemic hemodynamics and left ventricular function in patients with and without reduced ejection fraction. J Am Coll Cardiol. 2006;48:1634–41.

Linde C, Abraham WT, Gold MR, et al. For the REVERSE (REsynchronization reVErses Remodeling in Systolic left vEntricular dysfunction) Study Group. Randomized trial of cardiac resynchronization in mildly symptomatic heart failure patients and in a asymptomatic patients with left ventricular dysfunction and previous heart failure symptoms. J Am Coll Cardiol. 2008;52:1834–43.

Liu WH, Chen MC, Chen YL, et al. Right ventricular apical pacing acutely impairs left ventricular function and induces mechanical dyssynchrony in patients with sick sinus syndrome: a real-time three-dimensional echocardiographic study. J Am Soc Echocardiogr. 2008;21:224–9.

Liuba I, Frankel DS, Riley MP, et al. Scar progression in patients with nonischemic cardiomyopathy and ventricular arrhythmias. Heart Rhythm. 2014;11:755–62.

Loyaga-Rendon RY, Acharya D, Pamboukian SV, Tallaj JA, Cantor R, Starling RC, et al. Duration of heart failure is an important predictor of outcomes after mechanical circulatory support. Circ Heart Fail. 2015;8:953–9.

Lu W, Lin J, Dai Y, Chen K, Zhang S. The therapeutic effects of upgrade to cardiac resynchronization therapy in pacing-induced cardiomyopathy or chronic right ventricular pacing patients: a meta-analysis. Heart Fail Rev. 2022;27:507–16.

Lupi G, Sassone B, Badano L, et al. Effects of right ventricular pacing on intra-left ventricular electromechanical activation in patients with native narrow QRS. Am J Cardiol. 2006;98:219–22.

Lupón J, Gavidia-Bovadilla G, Ferrer E, De Antonio M, Perera-Lluna A, López-Ayerbe J, et al. Dynamic trajectories of left ventricular ejection fraction in heart failure. J Am Coll Cardiol. 2018;72:591–601.

Mafi-Rad M, Luermans JGLM, Blaauw Y. Feasibility and acute hemodynamic effect of left ventricular septal pacing by transvenous approach through the interventricular septum. Circ Arrhythm Electrophysiol. 2016;9(3):e003344.

Manne M, Rickard J, Varma N, et al. Normalization of left ventricular ejection fraction after cardiac resynchronization therapy also normalizes survival. Pacing Clin Electrophysiol. 2013;36:970–7.

Manolis AS. The deleterious consequences of right ventricular apical pacing: time to seek alternate site pacing. Pacing Clin Electrophysiol. 2006;29:298–315.

Marsan NA, Breithardt OA, Delgado V, Bertini M, Tops LF. Predicting response to CRT. The value of two- and three-dimensional echocardiography. Europace. 2008;10 Suppl 3:iii73–79.

Maurer G, Torres MA, Corday E, Haendchen RV, Meerbaum S. Two-dimensional echocardiographic contrast assessment of pacing-induced mitral regurgitation: relation to altered regional left ventricular function. J Am Coll Cardiol. 1984;3:986–91.

Mele D, Pasanisi G, Capasso F, et al. Left ventricular myocardial deformation dyssynchrony identifies responders to cardiac resynchronization therapy in patients with heart failure. Eur Heart J. 2006;27:1070–8.

Mele D, Bertini M, Malagù M. Current role of echocardiography in cardiac resynchronization therapy. Heart Fail Rev. 2017;22:699–722.

Menet A, Guyomar Y. Ennezat PV al, Prognostic value of left ventricular reverse remodeling and performance improvement after cardiac resynchronization therapy: a prospective study. Int J Cardiol. 2016;204:6–11.

Merchant FM, Hoskins MH, Musat DL, et al. Incidence and time course for developing heart failure with high-burden right ventricular pacing. Circ Cardiovasc Qual Outcomes. 2017;10(6):e003564.

Mizner J, Jurak P, Linkova H, Smisek R, Curila K. Ventricular dyssynchrony and pacing-induced cardiomyopathy in patients with pacemakers, the utility of ultra-high-frequency ECG and other dyssynchrony assessment tools. Arrhythmia and Electrophysiology Review. Radcliffe Medical Media; 2022, vol. 11.

Molina L, Sutton R, Gandoy W, et al. Medium-Term effects of septal and apical pacing in pacemaker dependent patients: a double-blind prospective randomized study. Pacing Clin Electrophysiol. 2013;00:1–8.

Moonen M, Senechal M, Cosyns B, et al. Impact of contractile reserve on acute response to cardiac resynchronization therapy. Cardiovasc Ultrasound. 2008;6:65

Moss AJ, Hall WJ, Cannom DS, Klein H, Brown MW, Daubert JP, et al. For the MADIT-CRT Trial Investigators. Cardiac Resynchronization therapy for the prevention of heart failure events. N Engl J Med. 2009;361:1329–38.

Mullens W, Grimm RA, Verga T, Dresing T, Starling RC, Wilkoff BL, et al. Insights from a cardiac resynchronization optimization clinic as part of a heart failure disease management program. J Am Coll Cardiol. 2009;53:765–73.

Nabeta T, Ishii S, Ikeda Y, et al. Late gadolinium enhancement for re-worsening left ventricular ejection fraction in patients with dilated cardiomyopathy. ESC Heart Fail. 2021;8:615–24.

Nahum J, Bensaid A, Dussault C, et al. Impact of longitudinal myocardial deformation on the prognosis of chronic heart failure patients. Circ Cardiovasc Imaging. 2010;3:249–56.

Naqvi TZ, Chao CJ. Adverse effects of right ventricular pacing on cardiac function: prevalence, prevention and treatment with physiologic pacing. Trends Cardiovasc Med. 2023;33(2):109–22.

Nielsen JC, Kristensen L, Andersen HR, et al. A randomized comparison of atrial and dual-chamber pacing in 177 consecutive patients with sick sinus syndrome: echocardiographic and clinical outcome. J Am Coll Cardiol. 2003;42(4):614–23.

Occhetta E, Bortnik M, Magnani A, et al. Prevention of ventricular desynchronization by permanent para-Hisian pacing after atrioventricular node ablation in chronic atrial fibrillation: a crossover, blinded, randomized study versus apical right ventricular pacing. J Am Coll Cardiol. 2006;47:1938–45.

Oka T, Inoue K, Toyoshima Y, et al. Duration of reverse remodeling response to cardiac resynchronization therapy: Rates, predictors, and clinical outcomes. Int j Cardiol. 2017;243(15):340–6.

Oki T, Ishii S, Takigami Y, Eda Y, Maemura K. Re-worsening left ventricular ejection fraction after response to cardiac resynchronization therapy. J Cardiol. 2022;79:358–64.

Oki T, Ishii S, Takigami Y, Eda Y, Maemura K, Re-worsening left ventricular ejection fraction after response to cardiac resynchronization therapy. J Cardiol. 2022;79:358–64.

Olshansky B, Day JD, Moore S, et al. Is dual-chamber programming inferior to single-chamber programming in an implantable cardioverterdefibrillator? Results of the INTRINSIC RV (Inhibition of Unnecessary RV Pacing With AVSH in ICDs) study. Circulation. 2007;115:9–16.

Onishi T, Onishi Y, Marek JJ, et al. Mechanistic features associated with improvement in mitral regurgitation after cardiac resynchronization therapy and their relation to long-term patient outcome. Circ Heart Fail. 2013;6:685–93.

Pastore G, Noventa F, Piovesana P, et al. Left ventricular dyssynchrony resulting from right ventricular apical pacing: relevance of baseline assessment. Pacing Clin Electrophysiol. 2008;31:1456–62.

Ponikowski P, Voors A, Anker S. On behalf of authors/task force members. 2016 ESC guidelines for the diagnosis and treatment of acute and chronic heart failure. Eur Heart J. 2016;37(27):2129–200.

Prinzen FW, Hunter WC, Wyman BT, McVeigh ER. Mapping of regional myocardial strain and work during ventricular pacing: experimental study using magnetic resonance imaging tagging. J Am Coll Cardiol. 1999;33:1735–42.

Pujol-López M, Arjona RJ, Guasch E. Septal flash correction with His-Purkinje pacing predicts echocardiographic response in resynchronization therapy. Pacing Clin Electrophysiol. 2022;45:374–83.

Risum N, Tayal B, Hansen TF, et al. Identification of typical left bundle branch block contraction by strain echocardiography is additive to electrocardiography in the prediction of long-term outcome after cardiac resynchronization therapy. J Am Coll Cardiol. 2015;66(6):631–41.

Ruwald MH, Solomon SD, Foster E, et al. Left ventricular ejection fraction normalization in cardiac resynchronization therapy and risk of ventricular arrhythmias and clinical outcomes: results from the multicenter automatic defibrillator implantation trial with cardiac resynchronization therapy (MADIT-CRT) trial. Circulation. 2014;130:2278–86.

Safak E, Ince H, Gkouvatsou L, et al. Pacing-induced cardiomyopathy in chronic right ventricular apical pacing: a midterm follow-up study. Eur J Med Res. 2019;24(1):23.

Saito M, Kaye G, Negishi K, et al. Dyssynchrony, contraction efficiency and regional function with apical and non-apical RV pacing. Heart. 2015;101:600–8.

Sarvari SI, Sitges M, Sanz M, et al. Left ventricular dysfunction is related to the presence and extent of a septal flash in patients with right ventricular pacing. Europace. 2017;19:289–96.

Schmidt M, Bromsen J, Herholz C, et al. Evidence of left ventricular dyssynchrony resulting from right ventricular pacing in patients with severely depressed left ventricular ejection fraction. Europace. 2007;9:34–40.

Schwerg M, Dreger H, Poller WC, Dust B, Melzer C. Efficacy of optimal medical therapy and cardiac resynchronization therapy upgrade in patients with pacemaker-induced cardiomyopathy. J Interv Card Electrophysiol. 2015;44:289–96.

Sharma PS, Dandamudi G, Herweg B, et al. Permanent His-bundle pacing as an alternative to biventricular pacing for cardiac resynchronization therapy: a multicenter experience. Heart Rhythm. 2018;15(3):413–20.

Shimony A, Eisenberg MJ, Filion KB, Amit G. Beneficial effects of right ventricular non-apical vs. apical pacing: a systematic review and meta-analysis of randomized controlled trials. Europace 2012;14:81–91.

Skalidis EI, Kochiadakis GE, Koukouraki SI, et al. Myocardial perfusion in patients with permanent ventricular pacing and normal coronary arteries. J Am Coll Cardiol. 2001;37:124–9.

St John Sutton MG, Plappert T, Abraham WT, Smith AL, DeLurgio DB, Leon AR, et al. For the multicenter InSync Randomized Clinical Evaluation (MIRACLE) study group. Effect of cardiac resynchronization therapy on left ventricular size and function in chronic heart failure. Circulation. 2003;107:1985–90.

Stankovic I, Prinz C, Ciarka A, et al. Long-term outcome after CRT in the presence of mechanical dyssynchrony seen with chronic RV pacing or intrinsic LBBB. JACC Cardiovasc Imaging. 2017;10(10 Pt A):1091–99.

Stellbrink C, Breithardt OA, Franke A, et al. Impact of cardiac resynchronization therapy using hemodynamically optimized pacing on left ventricular remodeling in patients with congestive heart failure and ventricular conduction disturbances. J Am Coll Cardiol. 2001;38:1957–65.

Suffoletto MS, Dohi K, Cannesson M, Saba S, Gorcsan J. 3 rd: Novel speckle-tracking radial strain from routine black-and-white echocardiographic images to quantify dyssynchrony and predict response to cardiac resynchronization therapy. Circulation. 2006;113:960–8.

Sutton MG, Plappert T, Hilpisch KE, et al. Sustained reverse left ventricular structural remodeling with cardiac resynchronization at one year is a function of etiology: quantitative Doppler echocardiographic evidence from the Multicenter InSync Randomized Clinical Evaluation (MIRACLE). Circulation. 2006;113:266–72.

Sweeney MO, Prinzen FW. A new paradigm for physiologic ventricular pacing. J Am Coll Cardiol. 2006;47:282–8.

Sweeney MO, Prinzen FW. Ventricular pump function and pacing: physiological and clinical integration. Circ Arrhythm Electrophysiol. 2008;1:127–39.

Sweeney MO, Hellkamp AS, Ellenbogen KA, et al. Adverse effect of ventricular pacing on heart failure and atrial fibrillation among patients with normal baseline QRS duration in a clinical trial of pacemaker therapy for sinus node dysfunction. Circulation. 2003;107(23):2932–7.

Sweeney MO, Bank AJ, Nsah E, et al. Minimizing ventricular pacing to reduce atrial fibrillation in sinus-node disease. N Engl J Med. 2007;357:1000–8.

Sze E, Daubert EJ. Left bundle branch block-induced left ventricular remodeling and its potential for reverse remodeling. J Interv Card Electrophysiol. 2018;52:343–52.

Takemoto Y, Hasebe H, Osaka T, et al. Right ventricular septal pacing preserves long-term left ventricular function via minimizing pacing-induced left ventricular dyssynchrony in patients with normal baseline QRS duration. Circ J. 2009;73:1829–35.

Tantengco MV, Thomas RL, Karpawich PP. Left ventricular dysfunction after long term right ventricular apical pacing in the young. J Am Coll Cardiol. 2001;37:2093–2100.

Teima SM, Mahfouz EME, Maaty ARA, Eladawy AH. Assessment of left ventricular asynchrony after permanent cardiac pacing by using speckle tracking echocardiography. Med J Cairo Univ. 2019;7(87):4579–86.

Teima SM, Mahfouz EME, Maaty ARA, Eladawy AH. Assessment of left ventricular asynchrony after permanent cardiac pacing by using speckle tracking echocardiography. Med J Cairo Univ. 2019;7(87):4579–4586.

Tops LF, Schalij MJ, Holman ER, et al. Right ventricular pacing can induce ventricular dyssynchrony in patients with atrial fibrillation after atrioventricular node ablation. J Am Coll Cardiol. 2006;48:1642–8.

Tops LF, Suffoletto MS, Bleeker GB. Speckle-tracking radial strain reveals left ventricular dyssynchrony in patients with permanent right ventricular pacing. J Am Coll Cardiol. 2007;50(12):1180–8.

Tops LF, Schalij MJ, Bax JJ, et al. The effects of right ventricular apical pacing on ventricular function and dyssynchrony implications for therapy. J Am Coll Cardiol. 2009;54:764–6.

Tse HF, Yu C, Wong KK, Tsang V, Leung YL, Ho WY, Lau CP: functional abnormalities in patients with permanent right ventricular pacing. The effect of sites of electrical stimulation. J Am Coll Cardiol. 2002;40:1451–1458.

Valls-Bertault V, Fatemi M, Gilard M, et al. Assessment of upgrading to biventricular pacing in patients with right ventricular pacing and congestive heart failure after atrioventricular junctional ablation for chronic atrial fibrillation. Europace. 2004;6:438–43.

van Bommel RJ, Bax JJ, Abraham WT, et al. Characteristic of heart failure patients associated with good and poor response to CRT: a PROSPECT sub-analysis. Eur Heart J. 2009;30:2470–7.

van Oosterhout MF, Prinzen FW, Arts T, et al. Asynchronous electrical activation induces asymmetrical hypertrophy of the left ventricular wall. Circulation. 1998;98:588–95.

Vatankulu MA, Goktekin O, Gurkan KM, et al. Effect of long-term resynchronization therapy on left ventricular remodeling in pacemaker patients upgraded to biventricular devices. Am J Cardiol. 2009;103:1280–4.

Verhaert D, Grimm RA, Puntawangkoon C, et al. Long-term reverse remodeling with cardiac resynchronization therapy: results of extended echocardiographic follow-up. J Am Coll Cardio. 2010;55(10):1788–95.

Vernooy K, Dijkman B, Cheriex EC, Prinzen FW, Crijns HJ. Ventricular remodeling during long-term right ventricular pacing following His bundle ablation. Am J Cardiol. 2006;97:1223–7.

Victor F, Mabo P, Mansour H, et al. A randomized comparison of permanent septal versus apical right ventricular pacing: short-term results. J Cardiovasc Electrophysiol. 2006;17:238–42.

Vidal B, Sitges M, Marigliano A, et al. Relation of response to cardiac resynchronization therapy to left ventricular reverse remodeling. Am J Cardiol. 2006;97:876–81.

Waggoner AD, Agler DA, Adamds DB. Cardiac resynchronization therapy and the emerging role of echocardiography (Part 1): indications and results from current studies. J Am Soc Echocardiogr. 2007;20:70–5.

Wang NC, Li JZ, Adelstein EC, Althouse AD, Sharbaugh MS, Jain SK, et al. New-onset left bundle branch block-associated idiopathic nonischemic cardiomyopathy and time from diagnosis to cardiac resynchronization therapy: the NEOLITH II study. Pacing Clin Electrophysiol. 2018;41:143–54.

Wang Y, Zhu H, Hou X, et al. Randomized Trial of Left Bundle Branch Vs Biventricular Pacing for Cardiac Resynchronization Therapy. J Am Coll Cardiol. 2022;80(13):1205–16.

Weizong W, Zhongsu W, Yujiao Z, et al. Effects of right ventricular nonapical pacing on cardiac function: a meta-analysis of randomized controlled trials. Pacing Clin Electrophysiol. 2013;36:1032–51.

Wilkoff BL. The dual chamber and VVI implantable defibrillator (DAVID) trial: rationale, design, results, clinical implications and lessons for future trials. Card Electrophysiol Rev. 2003;7:468–72.

Witte KK, Pipes RR, Nanthakumar K, Parker JD. Biventricular pacemaker upgrade in previously paced heart failure patients—improvements in ventricular dyssynchrony. J Card Fail. 2006;12:199–204.

Woo GW, Petersen-Stejskal S, Johnson JW, et al. Ventricular reverse remodeling and 6-month outcomes in patients receiving cardiac resynchronization therapy: analysis of the MIRACLE study. J Interv Card Electrophysiol. 2005;12:107–13.

Wood PW, Choy JB, Nanda NC, et al. Left ventricular ejection fraction and volumes: it depends on the imaging method. Echocardiography. 2014;31:87–100.

Ye Y, Wu S, Su L, et al. Feasibility and outcomes of upgrading to left bundle branch pacing in patients with pacing-induced cardiomyopathy and infranodal atrioventricular block. Front Cardiovasc Med. 2021;14(8):674452.

Ypenburg C, van Bommel RJ, Borleffs CJ, et al. Long-term prognosis after cardiac resynchronization therapy is related to the extent of left ventricular reverse remodeling at midterm follow-up. J Am Coll Cardiol. 2009;53:483–90.

Yu CM, Chan JY, Zhang Q, et al. Biventricular pacing in patients with bradycardia and normal ejection fraction. N Engl J Med. 2009;361:2123–34.

Yu CM, Fang F, Luo XX, et al. Long-term follow-up results of the pacing to avoid cardiac enlargement (PACE) trial. Eur J Heart Fail. 2014;16(9):1016–25.

Yu CM, Bleeker GB, Fung JW, et al. Left ventricular reverse remodeling but not clinical improvement predicts long-term survival after cardiac resynchronization therapy. Circulation. 2015;112:1580–6.

Yuan Z, Cheng L, Wu Y. Meta-analysis comparing safety and efficacy of left bundle branch area pacing versus his bundle pacing. Am J Cardiol. 2022;164:64–72.

Zanon F, Bacchiega E, Rampin L, et al. Direct His bundle pacing preserves coronary perfusion compared with right ventricular apical pacing: a prospective, cross-over mid-term study. Europace. 2008;10:580–7.

Zhang XH, Chen H, Siu CW, et al. New onset heart failure after permanent right ventricular pacing in patients with acquired high grade atrioventricular block and normal left ventricular function. J Cardiovasc Electrophysiol. 2008;19:136–41.

Zhang HX, Qian J, Hou FQ, et al. Comparison of right ventricular apex and right ventricular outflow tract septum pacing in the elderly with normal left ventricular ejection fraction: long-term followup. Kardiol Pol. 2012;70:1130–9.

Zhuang L, Mao Y, Wu L, Niu W, Chen K. Effects of right ventricular septum or His-bundle pacing versus right ventricular apical pacing on cardiac function: a systematic review and meta-analysis of randomized controlled trials. Int J Med Res. 2018;46(9):3848–60.

9 Echocardiography-Guided Optimization of Atrioventricular and Interventricular Delay in Patients with Implanted Devices

Abstract

Echocardiography is the primary imaging technique performed for optimal settings using many parameters. Following cardiac resynchronization therapy, optimization of the atrioventricular and intraventricular intervals provides additional benefits, improving mechanical dyssynchrony and left ventricular performance. The optimization of pacing parameters refers to the atrioventricular interval and the interventricular interval. Atrioventricular optimization is usually necessary in cardiac resynchronization therapy patients with stage two (pseudonormal) or stage three (restrictive) diastolic dysfunction. In patients with atrioventricular block, the adequate setting of the atrioventricular interval will maintain the contractile ventricular function and long-term prognosis. The interventricular optimization is less often necessary than the atrioventricular interval optimization.

The optimization of pacing parameters refers to the atrioventricular (AV) interval (atrioventricular activation delay) and the intraventricular (VV) interval (interventricular activation delay) (Cobb and Gold 2017; Mele et al. 2017).

Following cardiac resynchronization therapy (CRT), optimization of the AV and VV intervals provides additional benefits, improving mechanical dyssynchrony and left ventricular (LV) performance (Bertini et al. 2010) 30–40% of patients do not respond to CRT (AAbraham et al. 2002). Echocardiographic pacemaker optimization in resting conditions includes:

1. The baseline echocardiogram
2. Atrioventricular delay (AVD) optimization
3. Interventricular delay (VVD) optimization
4. Determination of rate-adaptive AVD
5. Determination of appropriate sensitivity for rate response (Naqvi 2010).

1. *Baseline Echocardiogram*

An echocardiogram should be performed at the baseline pacemaker settings (Sern et al. 2008; Ronaszeki et al. 2007). Doppler filter, gain, scale, and sweep speed settings are essential for adequate measurement and best temporal and spatial resolution (Lang et al. 2015).

2. *AV Delay optimization*

The AVD represents the time from the beginning of paced or sensed atrial activity to the impulse of ventricle stimulation or sensed ventricular activity (Aboulenein et al. 2016). From a hemodynamic point of view, the optimal programmed AVD depends on the interval between LA and LV contraction, which in turn depends on the interatrial conduction delay (Wish et al. 1987).

D.-M. Toader, *Echocardiographic Evaluation of Patients with Implanted Devices*,
https://doi.org/10.1007/978-3-031-64079-7_9

The AV interval optimization has two purposes:

1. to ensure the best filling, the optimal atrial contribution to the diastolic filling will produce an adequate ventricular preload and, consequently, greater stroke volume.
2. to allow the LV to be captured by the artificial stimulus and, consequently, an effective ventricular resynchronization (Ronaszeki 1989).

An optimal AVD must also reduce the presystolic mitral regurgitation. Because of this appropriate setting, the patients will present LV reverse remodeling in long-term follow-up (Aboulenein et al. 2016; Bleeker et al. 2007). In patients with atrioventricular block, the adequate setting of AVD will benefit the contractile ventricular function and long-term prognosis (Morales et al. 2006).

AVD optimization uses LV diastolic filling time intervals, indices of LV systolic function, or both (Bleeker et al. 2007; Gorcsan et al. 2008). The majority of methods used to optimize the AV interval utilize the Doppler techniques (Cobb and Gold 2017).

The parameters measured by echocardiography for AVD optimization in different studies were:

- *aortic velocity-time integral (VTI)* (Kerlan et al. 2006; Thomas et al. 2009; Jansen et al. 2006). This parameter represents the distance that blood travels in one heartbeat. For VTI measurement, the pulse wave (PW) Doppler gate will be positioned at the left ventricular outflow tract (LVOT) in the apical 5-chamber (A5ch)view, and then the systolic waveform will be outlined 8 (Fig. 9.1a).
- *diastolic mitral flow pattern* (Ritter et al. 1999; Lane 2004) evaluated by PW Doppler from apical four- chamber (A4ch) view, with the sample volume placed at the tips of the mitral valve leaflets during diastole. Measured are acquired at a sweep speed of 100 mm/s averaging three values (Lang et al. 2015).

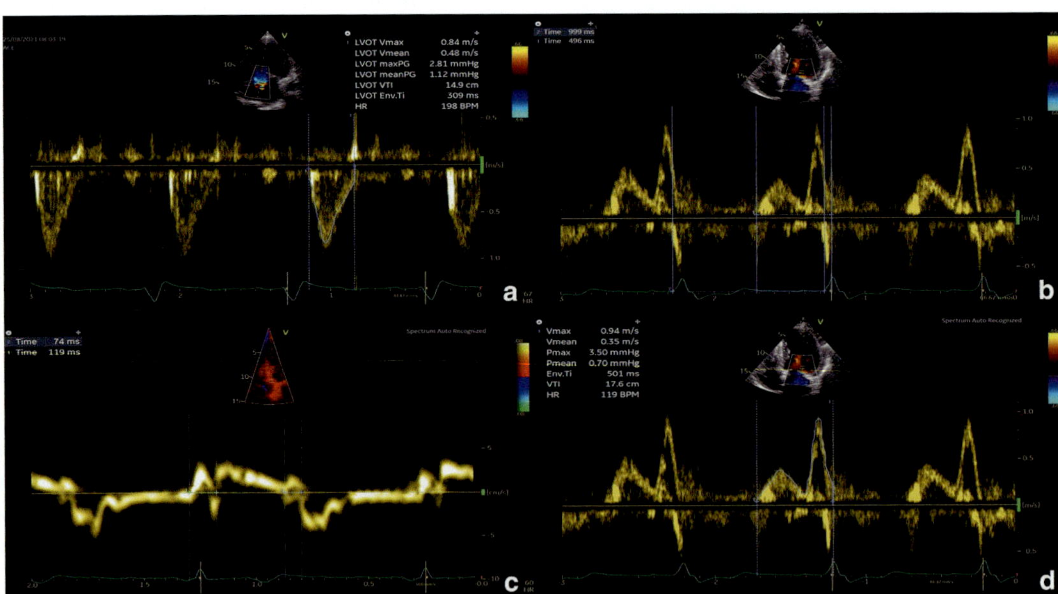

Fig. 9.1 **a** Left ventricle velocity time integral measurement by pulsed Doppler echocardiography from apical five-chamber view; **b** Diastolic filing time measurement from apical four-chamber view; **c** Myocardial performance index measurement by tissue Doppler echocardiography; **d** Mitral inflow velocity time integral measurement by pulsed Doppler echocardiography from apical four-chamber view

- *diastolic filling time* represents the difference between the cycle length and the interval between an A wave and the subsequent E wave. This parameter is obtained from the PW Doppler diastolic mitral inflow signal in the A4ch view (Thomas et al. 2009; Stockburger et al. 2006) (Fig. 9.1b).
- *myocardial performance index* (Stockburger et al. 2006) (Fig. 9.1c)
- *VTI of mitral inflow* (Jansen et al. 2006) (Fig. 9.1d)
- *dP/dt* measured from CW Doppler mitral regurgitant envelope (Morales et al. 2006)
- *tissue Doppler imaging*: index of LV dyssynchrony (Thomas et al. 2009; Bordachar et al. 2004) (Fig. 9.2a–c).
- *Left ventricular global longitudinal peak systolic strain (LVGLS)* assessed from the A4ch-, 2ch-, and 3 ch- view by speckle tracking echocardiography (STE) (Bordachar et al. 2004; Mortensen et al. 2004) (Fig. 9.2d) *Peak systolic left atrial strain* calculated from the A4ch view: the global left atrial strain (LA GLPSS), the reservoir phase (LASr), the conduit phase (LAScd), and the contraction phase (LASct) of the left atrium using dedicated speckle tracking software (Blessberger 2023) (Fig. 9.3).
- *LV and right ventricular (RV) pre-ejection delays, interventricular mechanical delay (IVD),* The pulsed wave Doppler spectral from aortic and pulmonary valves are analyzed at a sweep speed of 100 mm/s, averaging three values. The left ventricular pre-ejection time (LVET) (Fig. 9.4a) represents the QRS onset and the beginning of the transaortic ejection signal. The right ventricular pre-ejection interval (RVPEI) represents the time from the QRS onset to the beginning of the transpulmonary ejection signal. The difference between LVPEI and RVPEI is referred to as IVD (Stockburger et al. 2006) (Fig. 9.4b).
- *LVEF measured by biplane Simpson method* (Statescu et al. 2011) (Fig. 9.5) *and stroke volume* the left ventricular outflow tract (LVOT) diameter, is measured by 2D TTE in the parasternal long axis during mid-systole. This value will be multiplied by the LVOT volume time integral (VTI), measured on PW-Doppler traced during systole, from the A5c view (Mortensen et al. 2004; Blessberger 2023).

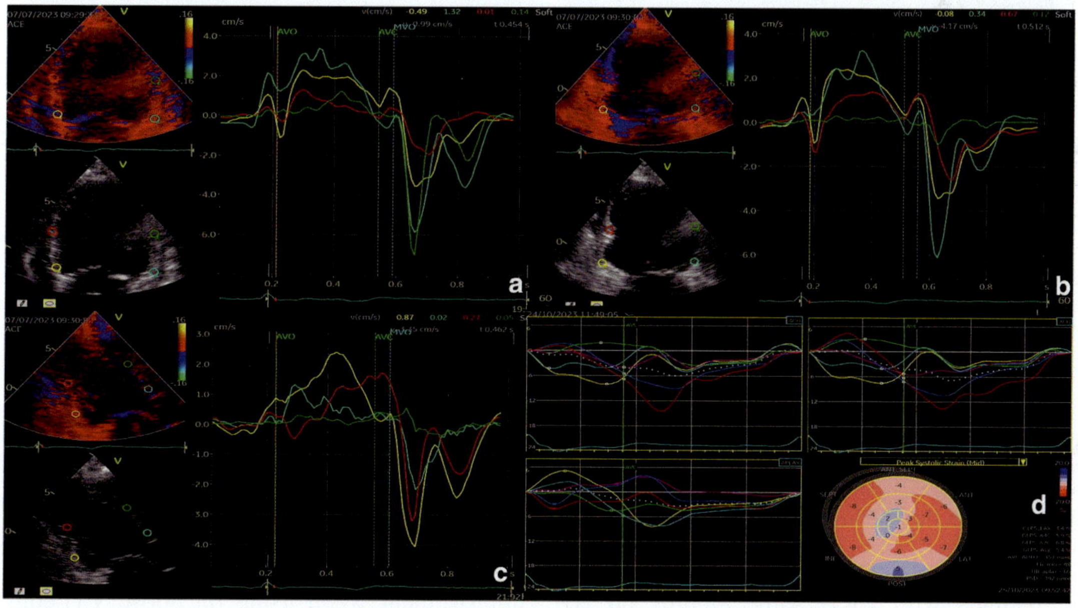

Fig. 9.2 Index of left ventricle dyssynchrony measured by tissue Doppler imaging from **a** apical for-chamber view, **b** two-chamber view, **c** three-chamber view; **d** Left ventricle global longitudinal strain measurement

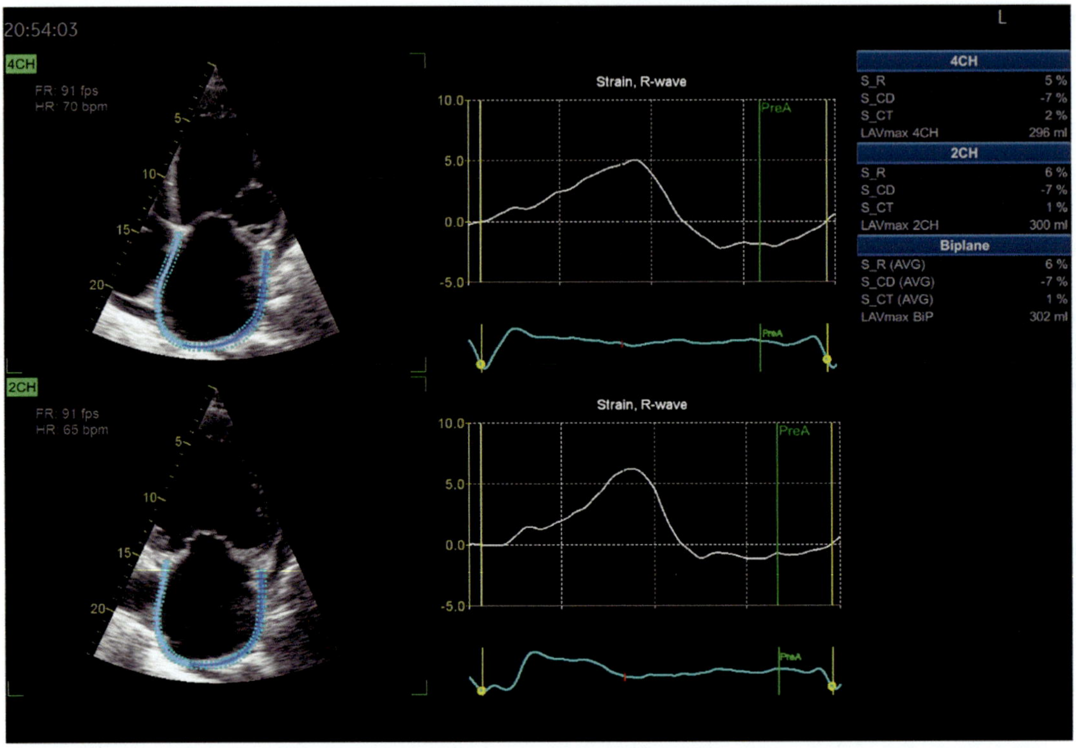

Fig. 9.3 Left atrial strain calculation using dedicated speckle tracking software

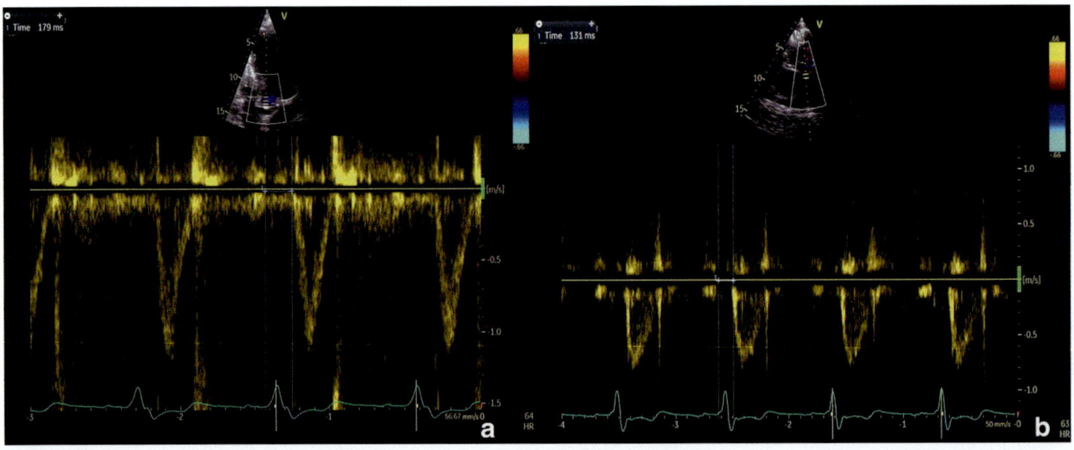

Fig. 9.4 Interventricular mechanical delay measurement: **a** Left ventricular pre-ejection time measurement by pulsed Doppler echocardiography from apical five-chamber view; **b** The right ventricular pre-ejection interval measurement by pulsed Doppler echocardiography from parasternal short-chamber view at the level of great arteries

In patients with CRT, some studies on AV delay optimization by Doppler echocardiography found a more remarkable systolic improvement when using the aortic VTI compared with the mitral diastolic inflow (Kerlan et al. 2006).

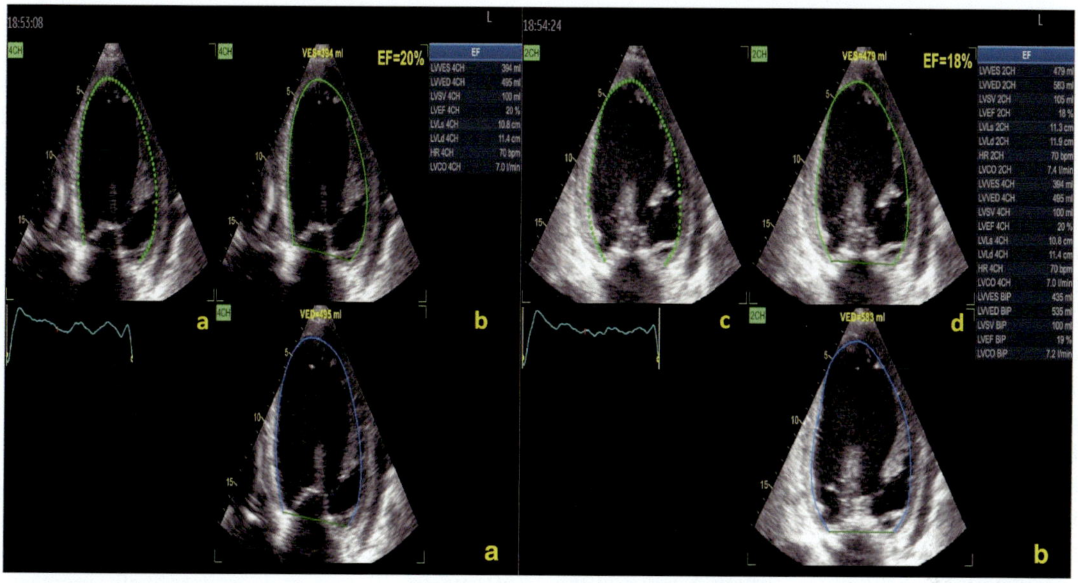

Fig. 9.5 Left ventricle ejection fraction measured by biplane Simpson method from apical four-chamber and apical two-chamber view

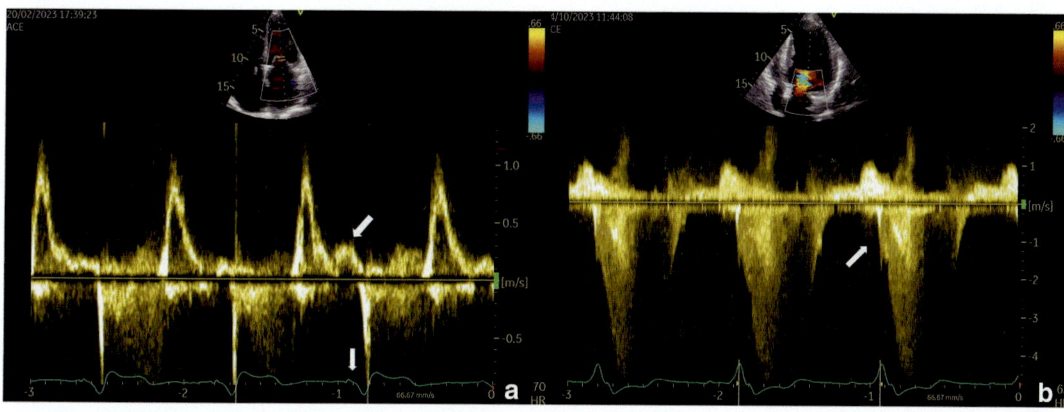

Fig. 9.6 **a** The beginning of ventricular contraction before the ending of atrial systole in a patient with too-short AVD (arrows); **b** diastolic mitral regurgitation in a patient with a too-long AVD (arrow)

The optimal AV interval must promote ventricular pacing without (1) truncation of the A-wave or (2) E- and A-wave fusion on PW Doppler diastolic mitral inflow tracing at the baseline sinus rate. (Blessberger 2023)

A too-short AVD will produce the beginning of ventricular contraction before the ending of atrial systole, resulting in underfilling of the ventricle (Fig. 9.6a), while a too-long AVD will produce diastolic mitral regurgitation (Fig. 9.6b). The main consequence will be a decrease in cardiac output (CO). A long AV delay may also allow native LV conduction, with deleterious effects in CRT patients (Janosik et al. 1989; Pearson et al. 1988).

AV synchrony is essential for hemodynamics, but there has yet to be a consensus regarding how the echocardiographic Doppler AV timing optimization would match the electrophysiology (Auricchio et al. 1999). Many centers currently use an empiric AV delay set at approximately 100 to 130milliseconds; other centers use the AV delay optimization algorithms based on ECG data: AV delay optimal as [PR(ms)X 0.50], if QRS is>150ms or [PR(ms)X 0.70] if QRS is < 150 ms (Stelbrink et al. 2001).

Acute improvements during AV optimization are demonstrated by LV dP/dt increasing by 13%–34% (Auricchio et al. 1999; Kass et al. 1999; Perego et al. 2003; Gelder et al. 2004) and stroke volume (Porciani et al. 2005).

Not all patients show hemodynamic benefit after optimization (Sawhney et al. 2004). Patients with intra-atrial conduction delay at baseline benefit most from the AV delay optimization. These patients belong to an empiric set with too short an A-V delay and present a complete loss of the mitral inflow A wave at the echocardiographic examination (Kedia et al. 2006).

Echocardiography methods for optimization of atrioventricular delay (AVD) used in clinical trials are:

1. Ritter's method in MIRACLE (Multicenter InSync Randomized Clinical Evaluation) Study (Abraham et al. 2002)
2. iterative method in CARE-HF (Cardiac Resynchronization-Heart Failure) study (Cleland 2005)
3. device-based algorithm in COMPANION (Comparison of Medical Therapy, Pacing and Defibrillation in Chronic Heart Failure) study (Bristow et al. 2004).

The Ritter and iterative AVD optimization protocols use PW Doppler interrogation of mitral inflow to assess LV filling and PW Doppler of the LV outflow tract to assess LV ejection (Ritter et al. 1999; Waggoner et al. 2005).

The Ritter method—was proposed for patients with complete heart block treated with dual-chamber pacing and used the mitral inflow technique (Ritter et al. 1999). It consists of synchronizing atrial contraction termination with the onset of ventricular systole. This method uses *the* interval from the pacing spike to the end of the A wave on mitral inflow at short and long AV delays.

Long AV delay is measured when there is a partial fusion of E and A waves on mitral Doppler inflow. Short AV delay is measured when ventricular contraction before completion of A wave produces a truncated A wave on mitral Doppler inflow. The time difference between the QRS onset on ECG and the completion of the A wave on Dopler mitral inflow is measured at each AV interval. According to the formula, the optimal AV delay is the time-shifted from short and long

Optimal AV interval= Avshort +[(AVlong+QAlong)-(AVshort+QAshort)] (Naqvi 2010; Ritter et al. 1999).

Ritter's method starts with a short AVD (50 ms to 70 ms) and progressively increases in 10-20 ms increments (Fig. 9.7). The shortest AVD is the interval at which mitral inflow A-wave can be well identified. The next step is a long AVD setting, usually 250 ms (Fig. 9.8). If the patient presents a native AV conduction at this value, AVD is decreased in 20-ms decrements until the fusion pattern on mitral inflow. The mitral inflow will be measured by Doppler echocardiography at this AVD. AVD higher than 250 ms needs to be tested. QRS morphology at the shortest AVD, identical to QRS morphology at the highest AVD, confirms biventricular pacing. It is also essential to identify the transition in QRS morphology (Naqvi 2010) (Fig. 9.9).

AVD above and below Ritter's optimal AVD will be tested until the best echo-Doppler parameters are achieved. Optimal mitral inflow associates an LV VTI and ejection duration improvement, a minimum isovolumic contraction time, MR, and pulmonary artery pressure. Pulmonary vein flow allows indirect assessment of left atrial pressure (Naqvi 2010).

This method must be used cautiously in CRT patients because the loading conditions may significantly alter LV filling pressures. Also, the mitral A wave may be severely attenuated or abbreviated, limiting the mitral A wave truncation identification (Bleeker et al. 2007).

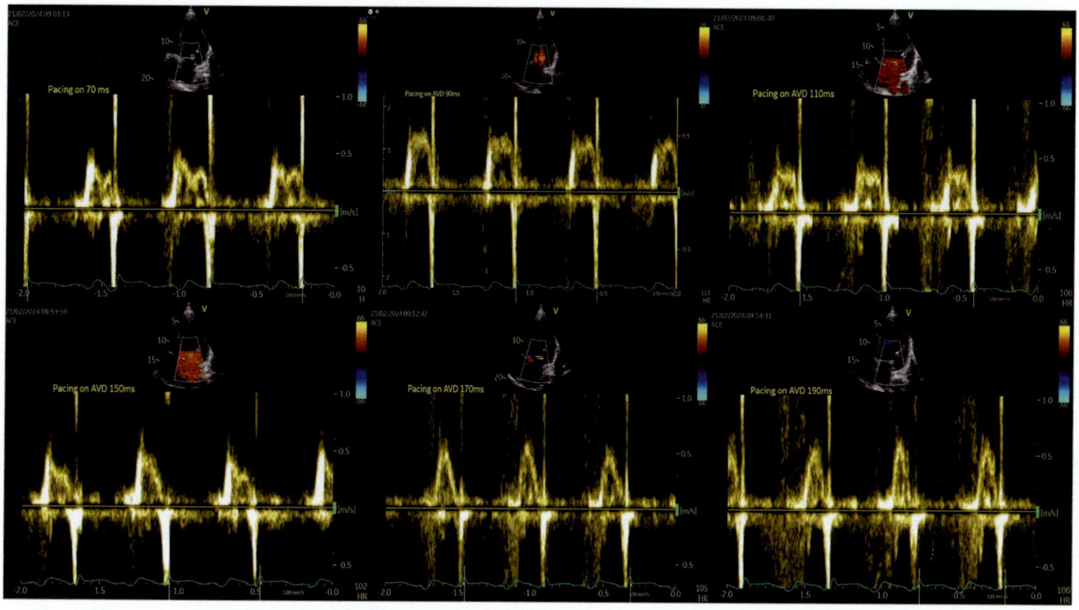

Fig. 9.7 Ritter method principle: a short AVD (70 ms) progressively increasing in 20 ms increments and diastolic mitral inflow evaluation by pulsed Doppler echocardiography

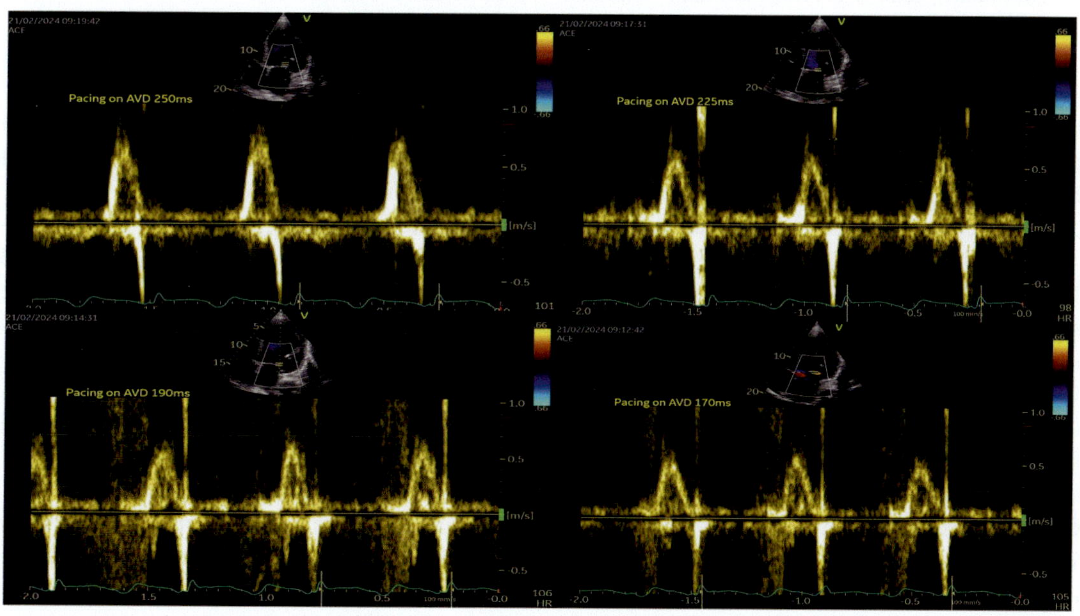

Fig. 9.8 Ritter method principle: a long AVD (250 ms) progressively decreases in 20 ms increments and diastolic mitral inflow evaluation by pulsed Doppler echocardiography

The most used approach is the "iterative" method, which consists of repetition of the measurement of the ventricular filling time (or VTI) on the Doppler trace at the AV interval and then progressively decreasing at 20 ms (Mele et al. 2017). But not all authors agree on the trans mitral Doppler method for the AV interval optimization (Valeur et al. 2010).

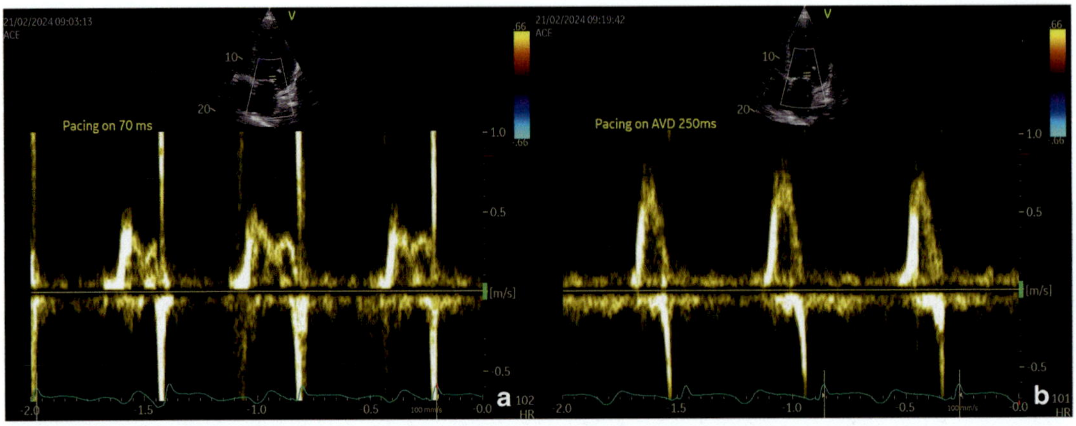

Fig. 9.9 Ritter method principle: A QRS morphology at the shortest AVD (70 ms) is identical to B QRS morphology at the highest AVD (250 ms), confirming biventricular pacing and diastolic mitral inflow evaluation by pulsed Doppler echocardiography

The iterative method uses pulsed-wave Doppler trans mitral inflow (for A wave truncation identification and the diastolic filling time measurement) and VTI measurement (Bleeker et al. 2007). It consists of programming the CRT device in atrial synchronous V pacing mode testing a series of AV intervals sequentially. With high sweep speeds, low filters, and adequate ECG monitoring, the pulsed wave sample volume will be placed deep into the left atrium for mitral valve closure click detection (Oh et al. 2006).

The AVD will be initially set at between 160 and 200 milliseconds. This value must be shorter than the intrinsic PR for capture ensuring (Bleeker et al. 2007; Oh et al. 2006). ADV will be *p*rogressively reduced in 10- to 25-ms decrements from the longest AVD that provides biventricular capture without fusion until the optimal mitral inflow pattern is obtained, without atrial truncation or E and A fusion (Fig. 9.10) (Naqvi 2010). The minimal AVD that allows for adequate E and A wave separation and termination of the A wave at approximately 40 to 60 milliseconds before the onset of the QRS represents an optimal AV delay usually corresponds with a stage I diastolic filling pattern (Oh et al. 2006). The optimal AVD corresponds to the longest diastolic filling time or the highest aortic VTI. An optimal aortic VTI evaluation will use a fast sweep speed, a large velocity scale, and a low filter. At least ten beats have to be followed before recording the aortic VTI (Bleeker et al. 2007).

A variation on the iterative method for AV optimization uses transaortic Doppler velocities as a surrogate for stroke volume. The optimal sensed and paced AV delay depends on the maximum aortic time-velocity integral value measured during six paced and sensed AV delays. The protocol includes Ao VTI measurements at AV delays of 60, 80, 100, 120, 140, and 160 ms. Each paced and sensed AV delay setting will be separated by a rest period of at least 10 to 15 beats.

Simplified Doppler method for AV optimization is a step-by-step approach and uses pulsed Doppler mitral inflow (Kedia et al. 2006):

Step 1: Optimize the ECG signal.

Step 2: Optimize pulsed Doppler mitral inflow velocities: high sweep speeds, low filters, and the sample volume set at a mitral annular level for closure clicks identification.

Step 3: Examine the mitral inflow pattern.

No AV optimization protocol is required if:

a. E and A waves are separated and identified on the Doppler envelope.
b. Termination of the A wave occurs at least 40 milliseconds before QRS onset or mitral

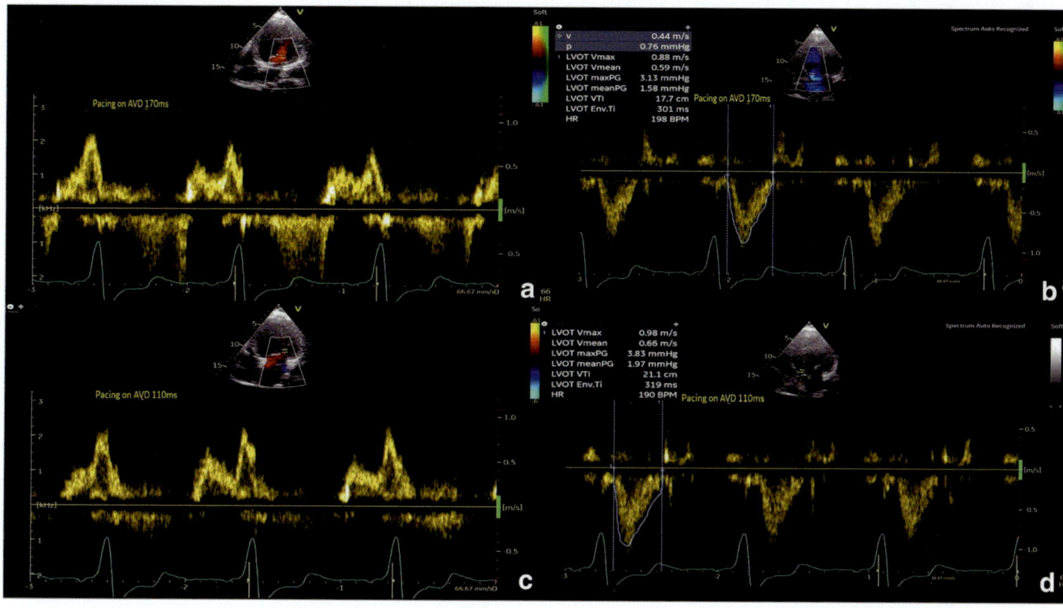

Fig. 9.10 Iterative method principle: Diastolic mitral inflow (**a**) and LV VTI (**b**) measurement by pulsed Doppler echocardiography at 170ms; Optimal Diastolic mitral inflow without atrial truncation or E and A fusion (**c**) and optimal LV VTI (**d**) measurement by pulsed Doppler echocardiography at 110 ms

valve closure click. The mitral valve closure click alignment with the QRS complex is a surrogate for the beginning of LV systole. The stage I diastolic of filling pattern (E wave lower than A wave) does not require optimization (Kedia et al. 2006).

AV optimization is recommended if:

A wave is missing, orE and A waves are merged, or A wave is truncated by mitral valve closure.

AV optimization is necessary in patients with stage II (pseudonormal) or stage III (restrictive) diastolic dysfunction (Kedia et al. 2006; Oh et al. 2006).

A wave may be missing in patients with intra-atrial conduction delay and usually requires a longer AV pacing delay, but if the AV pacing delay is set too long, E and A waves might merge. A truncated A wave by mitral valve closure requires lengthening of the AV delay. These situations need iterative or Ritter methods (2008). Patients with AF, frequent ventricular ectopy, tachycardia, or mitral prosthetic valves may be problematic (2008).

An *optimized diastolic filling* allows E and A separation, and the end of mitral inflow A-wave coincides with the R-wave of the electrocardiogram without A wave truncation (Fig. 9.1) or diastolic MR. Abnormal relaxation mitral inflow pattern is usually an indicator of adequate AVD programming (Naqvi 2010, 2008). Pseudonormal or restrictive mitral inflow pattern, truncation, or absence of A-wave in sinus rhythm patients, E, and A fusion suggest an inappropriate AVD (2008). Prominent atrial reversal during pulmonary venous flow interrogation suggests a too-short AVD (Ronaszeki 1989). Diastolic MR and E and A fusion on mitral inflow indicates an AVD that is too long (Fig. 9.5). Patients with advanced LV dysfunction present nonspecific markers of increased LV end-diastolic and left atrial pressure: decreased dP/dt, increased aortic pre-ejection time, restrictive mitral pattern of mitral inflow and pulmonary venous flow, MR, and increased pulmonary artery systolic pressure. These parameters are helpful to guide during pacemaker optimization (Naqvi 2010; Taha et al. 2010).

Biventricular (VV) optimization

The VV optimization consists of an "optimal" interventricular (VV) interval selection that further improves inter- and intraventricular dyssynchrony and, thus, mechanical efficiency or stroke volume (Bleeker et al. 2007).

The VV interval selection represents the sequence identification and the contraction delay between the LV and RV. The VV optimization is performed less often than the AV interval optimization. The methods proposed are based mainly on conventional Doppler, tissue Doppler, and dyssynchrony indices (Cobb and Gold 2017; Bordachar et al. 2003, 2000).

V-V optimization consists of changing the V-V sequence, starting with the LV activation before the RV, and then stepwise lengthening or shortening the V-V interval with 20 milliseconds and measuring the highest aortic time-velocity integral (Thomas et al. 2009; Stockburger et al. 2006, 2008; Leon et al. 2005).

VV optimization also prolongs LV filling time and reduces inter- and intra-LV dyssynchrony, with an increase in stroke volume (Vanderheyden et al. 2005).

VVD-only optimization, such as atrial fibrillation, is used when AVD cannot be optimized. VVD optimization after AVD optimization has incremental benefits (Mortensen et al. 2004; Porciani et al. 2005; Bordachar et al. 2000; Sogaard et al. 2002).

Mitral inflow needs re-evaluation after optimal VV programming and AVD modification if required (Naqvi 2010). V-V optimization usually results in a significant reduction in MR (Bordachar et al. 2000).

Acute VV optimization results in the dP/dt improvement (Perego et al. 2003; Gelder et al. 2004).

Reduced longitudinal contraction with a further increase in diastolic filling time results in sequential VV activation, compared with simultaneous biventricular activation (Sogaard et al. 2002). The highest aortic VTI is obtained when the left ventricle is paced before the right ventricle (Parreira et al. 2005).

Inter- and intra-LV dyssynchrony by pulsed-wave TDI and stroke volume by aortic VTI are the most appropriate echocardiographic parameters measured during VV optimization (Vanderheyden et al. 2005).

Exercise and pacemaker optimization

Patients with dilated cardiomyopathy have a long LV systole and short LV diastole at rest, with increased left atrial pressures accentuated during exercise (Plehn et al. 2007, 2008; Sheppard et al. 1993). Modern pacemaker devices allow rate-response and rate-adaptive AVD shortening during exercise. It is unclear whether AVD should be adapted to heart rate in patients with heart failure (Valzania et al. 2008; Melzer et al. 2008; Scharf et al. 2005).

The issues about pacing optimization are:

1. Optimized AV and VV delays vary over time. The AV delay tends to increase and the VV to reduce, making their re-evaluation necessary (O'Donnell et al. 2005).
2. Optimization by echocardiography is typically performed at rest and may be different in the exercise condition. Programming a fixed, optimized AV and VV interval at the time of implantation might not be physiologic (Shanmugam et al. 2012; Schueler et al. 2012).
3. The sequence of AV and VV optimization remains an unsolved issue (Zuber et al. 2008).
4. The optimization of the AV and VV intervals will not fully compensate for a suboptimal position of the LV lead (Khan and Virdee 2011).
5. In patients with ischemia or scars, optimizing the VV interval can compensate for the negative effects of lead position in a scar area (Jansen et al. 2006; Marsan and Bleeker 2009).
6. The effect of supine body position versus sitting on the optimal AV delay is unknown.
7. Optimized intervals resulted in acute improvements in LV diastolic and systolic function but without improvements in clinical

outcomes or response rates to CRT (Cobb and Gold 2017) sustaining the recommendation of AV and VV intervals optimization routinely in specific subgroups:

- patients who do not respond to CRT
- those with ischemic etiology of the HF, and
- those who need atrial pacing.

Patients without response to CRT might have additional clinical benefits from the optimization of the VV interval over the only AV interval optimization (Weiss and Malik 2010). All the other patients will have a fixed AV delay is empirically set at 100–120 ms with a simultaneous VV interval (Ponikowski and Voors 2016). The AV and VV interval optimization will use the transaortic and transmitral Doppler techniques (Mele et al. 2017).

Sequential pacing is better than simultaneous pacing, having additional clinical benefit over the only AV interval optimization (Cobb and Gold 2017). The AV versus VV optimization sequence must be clarified, but better results are obtained when AVD is optimized first. This technique allows mitral valve closure immediately after completion of atrial contraction and, in consequence, permits an improved LV filling and cardiac output (Naqvi 2010; Zuber et al. 2008).

A suboptimal optimization of the intervals is a predictor of poor CRT response (Chandraprakasam and Mentzer 2015; Gold et al. 2013; Gold 2013).

CRT optimization increases cardiac output in patients with a scar-adjacent LV lead position. The optimization is not necessary in the concordant or remote LV lead position. This approach sustains the importance of an optimally positioned achievement of the LV pacing lead. If this is not possible by the transvenous approach, an alternative technique will be used. Lead repositioning should be considered in patients with suboptimal lead positions and without LV remodeling response after CRT (Khan and Virdee 2011).

9.1 Conclusion

AV and VV interval optimization is routinely necessary in CRT non-responders, patients with ischemic etiology of the HF, and patients who need atrial pacing. Patients without response to CRT might have additional clinical benefits from the optimization of the VV interval over the only AV interval optimization. The AV and VV interval optimization will usually use the transaortic and transmitral Doppler techniques. Ritter's method, iterative method, and device-based algorithm have been used in clinical trials for CRT device optimization. At the moment there is no consensus regarding the best approach to interval optimizations in CRT patients.

In patients with double chamber pacemakers, the adequate setting of atrioventricular interval will maintain the contractile ventricular function and long-term prognosis.

References

Aboulenein J, Tawfik M, Maaty A, Wali H, Refaei W, et al. Optimizing the atrioventricular delay in dual chamber pacemakers; is it worth? J Cardiol Curr Res. 2016;5(3):14–12.

Abraham WT, Fisher WG, Smith AL, et al. Cardiac resynchronization in chronic heart failure. N Engl J Med. 2002;346:1845–53.

Auricchio A, Stellbrink C, Block M, et al. Effect of pacing chamber and atrio-ventricular delay on acute systolic function of paced patients with congestive heart failure: the Pacing Therapies for Congestive Heart Failure Study Group: the Guidant Congestive Heart Failure Research Group. Circulation Circulation. 1999;99:2993–3001.

Bertini M, Valzania C, Biffi M, et al. Interventricular delay optimization: a comparisonamong three different echocardiographic methods. Echocardiography. 2010;27(1):38–43.

Bleeker GB, Yu C-M, Nihoyannopoulos P, de Sutter J, de Veire NV. Optimal use of echocardiography in cardiac resynchronization therapy. Heart. 2007;93:1339–50.

Bordachar P, Garrigue S, Reuter S, et al. Hemodynamic assessment of right, left, and biventricular pacing by peak endocardial acceleration and echocardiography in patients with end-stage heart failure. Pacing Clin Electrophysiol. 2000;23:1726–30.

Bordachar P, Garrigue S, Lafitte S, et al. Interventricular and intra-left ventricular electromechanical delays in right ventricular paced patients with heart failure: implications for upgrading to biventricular stimulation. Heart. 2003;89:1401–5.

Bordachar P, Stephane L, Sylvain R, et al. Biventricular pacing and left ventricular pacing in heart failure. J Cardiovasc Electrophysiol. 2004;15(12):1342–7.

Bristow MR, Saxon LA, Boehmer J, et al. Cardiac resynchronization therapy with or without an implantable defibrillator in advanced chronic heart failure. N Engl J Med. 2004;350:2140–50.

Blessberger H, Kammler J, Kellermair J, Kiblboeck D, Nahler A et al. Impact of pacing mode and different echocardiographic parameters on cardiac output (PADIAC) Front. Cardiovasc. Med. 2023;10:1185518.

Cleland JGF, Daubert J-C, Erdmann E, et al. for the Cardiac resynchronization-heart failure (CARE-HF) study investigators. The effect of cardiac resynchronization on morbidity andmortality in heart failure. N Engl J Med 2005; 352:1539–1549.

Chandraprakasam S, Mentzer GG. Recent advances in the optimization of cardiac resynchronization therapy. Curr Heart Fail Rep. 2015;12:48–60.

Donazzan L, Rigolli M, De Simone V, et al. Cardiac resynchronization therapy: Twelve-month effects of echocardiographic atrioventricular and inter-ventricular delay optimization. Rationale and design of the CARTEDO trial. Int J Cardiol. 2016;202:185–187.

Cobb DB, Gold MR. The role of atrioventricular and interventricular optimization forcardiac resynchronization therapy. Heart Failure Clin. 2017;13:209–23.

Gold MR, Yu Y, Singh JP, et al. The effect of left ventricular electrical delay on AV optimization for cardiac resynchronization therapy. Heart Rhythm. 2013;10:988–93.

Gorcsan III J, Abraham T, Agler DA, Echocardiography for cardiac resynchronization therapy: recommendations for performance and reporting–a report from the american society of echocardiography Dyssynchrony Writing Group Endorsed by the Heart Rhythm Soc J Am Soc Echocardiography, 2008,21(3):192–213.

Gorcsan J, Abraham T, Agler DA, et al. Echocardiography for cardiac resynchronization therapy: recommendations for performance and reporting-a report from the American society of echocardiography dyssynchrony writing group endorsed by the heart rhythm society. J Am Soc Echocardiogr. 2008;21(3):191–213.

Janosik DL, Pearson AC, Buckingham TA, et al. The hemodynamic benefit of differential atrioventricular delay intervals for sensed and paced atrial events during physiologic pacing. J Am Coll Cardiol. 1989;14(2):499–507.

Jansen AH, Bracke FA, van Dantzig JM, et al. Correlation of echo-Doppler optimization of atrioventricular delay in cardiac resynchronization therapy with invasive hemodynamics in patients with heart failure secondary to ischemic or idiopathic dilated cardiomyopathy. Am J Cardiol. 2006;97(4):552–7.

Kass DA, Chen CH, Curry C, et al. Improved left ventricular mechanics from acute VDD pacing in patients with dilated cardiomyopathy and ventricular conduction delay. Circulation. 1999;99:1567–73.

Kedia N, Ng K, Apperson-Hansen C, et al. Usefulness of atrioventricular delay optimization using Doppler assessment of mitral inflow in patients undergoing cardiac resynchronizationtherapy. Am J Cardiol. 2006;98:780–5.

Kerlan JE, Sawhney NS, Waggoner AD, et al. Prospective comparison of echocardiographic atrioventricular delay optimization methods for cardiac resynchronization therapy. Heart Rhythm. 2006;3(2):148–54.

Khan FZ, Virdee MS. Read PA et al Impact of VV optimization in relation to left ventricular lead position: an acute haemodynamic study. Europace. 2011;13:845–52.

Lang RM, Badano LP, Mor-Avi V. Recommendations for cardiac chamber quantification by echocardiography in adults: an update from the American society of echocardiography and the European association of cardiovascular imaging. J Am SocEchocardiogr. 2015;28:1–39.

Lane R, Chow AW, Chin D, et al. Selection and optimisation of biventricular pacing: the role of echocardiography. Heart. 2004;90(suppl 6):vi10–vi16.

Leon AR, Abraham WT, Brozena S, et al. Cardiac resynchronization with sequential biventricular pacing for the treatment of moderate to severe heart failure. J Am Coll Cardiol. 2005;46:2298–304.

Marsan NA, Bleeker GB. Van Bommel RJ et al Cardiac resynchronization therapy in patients with ischemic versus nonischemic heart failure: differential effect of optimizing interventricularpacing interval. Am Heart J. 2009;158:769–76.

Mele D, Bertini M, Malagù M. Current role of echocardiography in cardiac resynchronization therapy. Heart Fail Rev. 2017;22:699–722.

Melzer C, Bondke H, Thomas K, Nienaber CA, Baumann G, Ismer B. Should we use the rate-adaptive AV delay in cardiac resynchronization therapy-pacing? Europace. 2008;10:53–8.

Morales MA, Startari U, Panchetti L, et al. Atrioventricular delay optimization by doppler-derived left ventricular dP/dt improves 6-month outcome of resynchronized patients. Pacing and Clin Electrophysiol. 2006;29(6):564–8.

Mortensen PT, Peter S, Hassan M, et al. Sequential biventricular pacing. Pacing Clin Electrophysiol. 2004;27(3):339–45.

Naqvi TZ. Echocardiography-guided biventricular pacemaker optimization. J Am Coll Cardiol Img. 2010;3:1168–80.

O'Donnell D, Nadurata V, Hamer A, et al. Long-term variations in optimal programming of cardiac

resynchronization therapy devices. Pacing Clin Electrophysiol. 2005;28:S24–6.
Oh JK, Hatle L, Tajik AJ, Little WC. Diastolic heart failure can be diagnosed by comprehensive two-dimensional and Doppler echocardi ography. J Am Coll Cardiol. 2006;47:500–6.
Parreira L, Santos JF, Madeira J, et al. Cardiac resynchronization therapy with sequential biventricular pacing: impact of echocardiography guided VV delay optimization on acute results. Rev Port Cardiol. 2005;24:1355–65.
Pearson AC, Janosik DL, Redd RR, et al. Doppler echocardiographic assessment of the effect of varying atrioventricular delay and pacemaker mode on left ventricular filling. Am Heart J. 1988;115(3):611–21.
Perego GB, Chianca R, Facchini M, et al. Simultaneous versus sequential biventricular pacing in dilated cardiomyopathy: an acute hemodynamic study. Eur J Heart Fail. 2003;5:305–13.
Plehn G, Vormbrock J, Zühlke C, et al. Disproportionate shortening of left ventricular diastolic duration in patients with dilated cardiomyopathy. Med Klin (Munich). 2007;102:707–13.
Plehn G, Vormbrock J, Perings C, et al. Loss of diastolic time as a mechanism of exercise-induced diastolic dysfunction in dilated cardiomyopathy. Am Heart J. 2008;155:1013–9.
Ponikowski P, Voors AA. Anker SD et al ESC guidelines for the diagnosis and treatment of acute and chronic heart failure: the task force for the diagnosis and treatment of acute and chronic heart failure of the European society of cardiology. Eur J Heart Fail. 2016;18:891–975.
Porciani MC, Dondina C, Macioce R, et al. Echocardiographic examinination of atrioventricular and interventricular delay optimization in cardiac resynchronization therapy. Am J Cardiol. 2005;95:1108–10.
Ritter P, Padeletti L, Gillio-Meina L, et al. Determination of the optimal atrioventricular delay in DDD pacing. Europace. 1999;1(2):126–30.
Ronaszeki A, Ector H, Denef B, Aubert AE, De Werf V, De Geest H. Effect of short AV delay on cardiac output. Pacing Clin Electrophysiol. 2007;13:1728–31.
Ronaszeki A. Hemodynamic consequences of the timing of atrial contraction during complete AV block. Acta Biomedica Lovaniensia 1989;15.
Sawhney NS, Waggoner AD, Garhwal S, et al. Randomized prospective trial of atrioventricular delay programming for cardiac resynchronization therapy. Heart Rhythm. 2004;1(5):562–7.
Scharf C, Li P, Muntwyler JR, et al. Rate-dependent AV delay optimization in cardiac resynchronization therapy. Pacing Clin Electrophysiol. 2005;28:279–84.
Schueler M, Voss F, Bauer A, et al. Atrioventricular delay programming in cardiac resynchronization therapy devices: fixed or adaptive? A randomized monocenter trial. J Electrocardiol. 2012;45:783–6.
Sern H, Lim SH, Lip GYH, Sanderson JE. Ventricular optimization of biventricular pacing: a systematic review. Europace. 2008;10:901–6.
Shanmugam N, Prada-Delgado O, Campos AG, et al. Rate adaptive AV delay and exercise performance following cardiac resynchronization therapy. Heart Rhythm. 2012;9:1815–21.
Sheppard R, Ren JF, Ross J, McAllister M, Chandrasekaran K, Kutalek SP. Doppler echocardiographic assessment of the hemodynamic benefits of rate adaptive AV delay during exercise in paced patients with complete heart block. Pacing Clin Electrophysiol. 1993;16:2157–60.
Sogaard P, Egeblad H, Pedersen AK, et al. Sequential versus simultaneous biventricular resynchronization for severe heart failure evaluation by tissue doppler imaging. Circulation. 2002;106:2078–84.
Statescu C, Sascau RA, Maciuc V, et al. Programming an optimal atrioventricular interval in a dual chamber pacemaker regional population. Maedica. 2011;6(4):272–6.
Stelbrink C, Breithardt OA, Franke A. Impact of cardiac resychronization therapy using hemodynamically optimized pacing on left ventricular remodeling in patients with congestive heart failure and ventricular conduction disturbances. J Am Coll Cardiol. 2001;38:1957–60.
Stockburger M, Fateh-Moghadam S, Nitardy A, et al. Optimization of cardiac resynchronization guided by Doppler echocardiography: haemodynamic improvement and intraindividual variability with different pacing configurations and atrioventricular delays. Europace. 2006;8(10):881–6.
Taha N, Zhang J, Ranjan R, et al. Biventricular pacemaker optimization guided by comprehensive echocardiography—preliminary observations regarding the effects on systolic and diastolic ventricular function and third heart sound. J Am Soc Echocardiogr. 2010;23:857–66.
Thomas DE, Yousef ZR, Fraser AG. A critical comparison of echocardiographic measurements used for optimizing cardiac resynchronization therapy: stroke distance is best. Eur J Heart Fail. 2009;11(8):779–88.
Valeur N, Fritz-Hansen T, Risum N, et al. Echocardiographic effects of changing atrioventricular delay in cardiac resynchronization therapy based on displacement. J Am Soc Echocardiogr. 2010;23:621–7.
Valzania C, Eriksson MJ, Boriani G, Gadler F. Cardiac resynchronization therapy during rest and exercise: comparison of two optimization methods. Europace. 2008;10:1161–9.
van Gelder BM, Bracke FA, Meijer A, et al. Effect of optimizing the VV interval on left ventricular contractility in cardiac resynchronization therapy. Am J Cardiol. 2004;93:1500–3.
Vanderheyden M, De Backer T, Rivero-Ayzera M, et al. Tailored echocardiographic interventricular delay programming further optimizes left ventricular performance after cardiacresynchronization therapy. Heart Rhythm. 2005;2:1066–72.
Waggoner A, Faddis M, Osborn J, et al. AV delay programming and cardiac resynchronization

therapy: left ventricular diastolic filling indices and relation to stroke volume. J Am Coll Cardiol. 2005;45(3A):99A.

Weiss R, Malik R. Wish M et al V-Voptimization in car diac resynchronization therapy non-responders: RESPONSE-HF trial results. Heart Rhythm. 2010;7(Suppl):S26.

Wish M, Fletcher RD, Gottdiener JS, et al. Importance of left atrial timing in the programming of dual-chamber pacemakers. Am J Cardiol. 1987;60(7):566–71.

Zuber M, Toggweiler S, Roos M, et al. Comparison of different approaches for optimization of atrioventricular and interventricular delay in biventricular pacing. Europace. 2008;10:367–73.

Echocardiographic Evaluation of Complications After Intracardiac Devices Implantation

10

Abstract

Complications after device implantation are more frequent during the first month and more rare in long-term follow-up. Many factors are involved in the appearance of complications in patients with implanted devices. In short-term follow-up, the most frequent are pericardial effusions and infection. In long-term follow-up, the complications are linked to the lead's presence: pacemaker-induced cardiomyopathy in patients with right ventricle apical lead and tricuspid regurgitation in patients with implanted cardioverter because of a high dimension of the lead. It is essential to diagnose and adequately treat this pathology because of the negative prognosis. Transthoracic and transesophageal echocardiography are the main imaging techniques used in this approach. 1–2% of patients present complications in the first 30 days after pacemaker insertion and progressively decrease during long-term follow-up. Complication risks generally increase with the complexity of the device and comorbidities, are more common in device upgrading or lead revisions, and are lower in patients with de novo implantation. The decision to upgrade to more complex systems or prophylactic replacement of CIED generators and leads must be carefully weighted. Complication rates are related to individual and center implantation volumes.

Supplementary Information The online version contains supplementary material available at https://doi.org/10.1007/978-3-031-64079-7_10.

10.1 Myocardial Perforation

15% of patients with cardiac pacemakers or ICDs may develop lead perforation (Knopp et al. 2022). The incidence of lead perforation ranges from 0.09 to 1.5% (Kirkfeldt et al. 2011; Udo et al. 2012; Cano et al. 2017; Hsu et al. 2013; Gadler et al. 2015; Migliore et al. 2014; Ohlow et al. 2013; Mahapatra et al. 2005; Sterlinski et al. 2008; Lin et al. 2014). The incidence of myocardial perforation (MP) after a pacemaker implant ranges from 0.1 to 1% and from 0.6 to 5.2% with implantable cardiac defibrillators (ICD) (Welch et al. 2011). The prevalence is 15% in ventricles, 6% in the atria, 14% in patients with ICD devices, and 3% in those with pacemakers (Hirschl et al. 2007).

Cardiac consequences of myocardial perforation from pacemaker leads may be pericarditis, a pericardial effusion, or cardiac tamponade (Kirkfeldt et al. 2011; Cano et al. 2017; Hsu et al. 2013; Gadler et al. 2015; Migliore et al. 2014; Ohlow et al. 2013; Shingaki et al. 2015; Allouche et al. 2021; Chlabicz et al. 2021; Agarwal et al. 2017). Acute (< 24 h) myocardial perforation after pacemaker implantation occurs in 1–7% of patients (Haq et al. 2008; Sanoussi

D.-M. Toader, *Echocardiographic Evaluation of Patients with Implanted Devices*, https://doi.org/10.1007/978-3-031-64079-7_10

et al. 2005; Madershahian et al. 2010; Issa and Issa 2021). In the subacute phase (1–30 days), MP occurs in 0.03–0.4% of treated patients/ year (Cano et al. 2017; Sterlinski et al. 2008). Delayed cardiac perforation due to cardiac devices ranges between 0.1 and 0.8% for pacemaker leads and from 0.6 to 5.2% for implantable cardiac defibrillators (Issa and Issa 2021; Shariff et al. 2021). Most reported cases present weeks to months after the device implant (Rajkumar et al. 2017; Xiong et al. 2018).

MP may be acute within the first 24 h, subacute between 1 and 30 days, and chronic > 30 days after implantation (Allouche et al. 2021; Haq et al. 2008; Sadamatsu et al. 2009; Liang et al. 2013; Laborderi et al. 2008). Pericardial effusion, consequently of the lead migration, usually occurs within 5–21 days after the implantation and is generally self-limited (Chlabicz et al. 2021), and few patients may present delayed progression to cardiac tamponade (Shingaki et al. 2015b; Buszkiewicz et al. 2021). The magnitude of the trauma is the main cause of the syndrome (Imazio and Hoit 2013).

The predictors for the development of MP are old age (> 80 years), female sex, steroid use, and active fixation (Cano et al. 2017; Sterlinski et al. 2008; Laborderi et al. 2008; Stefanidis et al. 2009; Lopez et al. 2007; Tziakas et al. 2009). The incidence of perforation is also higher when the lead is placed on the right ventricular free wall or the apex where the myocardium is thinner and is lower when the lead is placed on the septal wall or in the right ventricular outflow tract where the ventricular wall is thicker (Laborderi et al. 2008; Boriani et al. 2008; Khan et al. 2005; Haghjoo et al. 2010; Singhal et al. 2007).

Transthoracic echocardiography (TTE) is the first-line imaging test in patients with suspected myocardial perforation and reveals the presence, size, and hemodynamic importance of the pericardial effusion (Adler et al. 2015). Two-dimensional echocardiography with Doppler detects pericardial effusion and hemodynamic impact (Imazio and Hoit 2013; Klein et al. 2013; Cosyns et al. 2014). The standard echocardiographic windows for pericardial effusion diagnosis are parasternal long (ps lax) (Fig. 10.1a) (Supplementary material 1), parasternal short (ps sax) (Fig. 10.1b) (Supplementary material 2), apical four-chamber (A4ch) (Fig. 10.1c) (Supplementary material 3), and the subxiphoid view (Fig. 10.1d) (Supplementary material 4) (Kumar et al. 2022). A pericardial effusion feature is an anechoic zone surrounding the heart, usually circumferential (unless loculated) in large pericardial effusions (Goodman et al. 2012). The subxiphoid view is the most reliable incidence of pericardial effusion. Echocardiographic diagnosis of cardiac tamponade includes right atrial collapse in systole (the earliest sign) (Fig. 10.2a) (Supplementary material 5), the right ventricular collapse in diastole (Fig. 10.2b, c) (Supplementary material 6, 7), and the presence of a plethoric inferior vena cava with minimal respiratory variation (Hanson and Chan 2021) (Fig. 10.2d).

Echocardiography performed in the first 24 h after implantation may identify mild (</10 mm in diastole) (Fig. 10.3a), moderate (11–20 mm) (Fig. 10.3b), or large pericardial effusion (> 20 mm) (Imazio and Hoit 2013; Ohlow et al. 2013) (Fig. 10.3c). The images must be digitally stored for follow-up studies.

Echocardiography accuracy has only 41.2% sensitivity and 84.2% specificity in myocardial perforation detection, revealing the presence of the RV lead in the pericardial space with or without pericardial effusion (Rajkumar et al. 2017).

The effusion size will be detailed and described in the echocardiographic report, including the extent and the location of each measurement. The hemodynamic significance parameter is the rapidity of the effusion accumulation (Imazio and Hoit 2013; Shabetai 2004). Loculated pericardial effusions or pericardial effusions that contain clots, which a transthoracic approach cannot diagnose, require transoesophageal echocardiography (TEE) (Imazio and Hoit 2013; Cosyns et al. 2014).

Mild or moderate effusions should be echocardiographic monitored. In patients with hemodynamic compromise or large effusions, pericardiocentesis should be performed (Ohlow et al. 2013) (Supplementary Material 8).

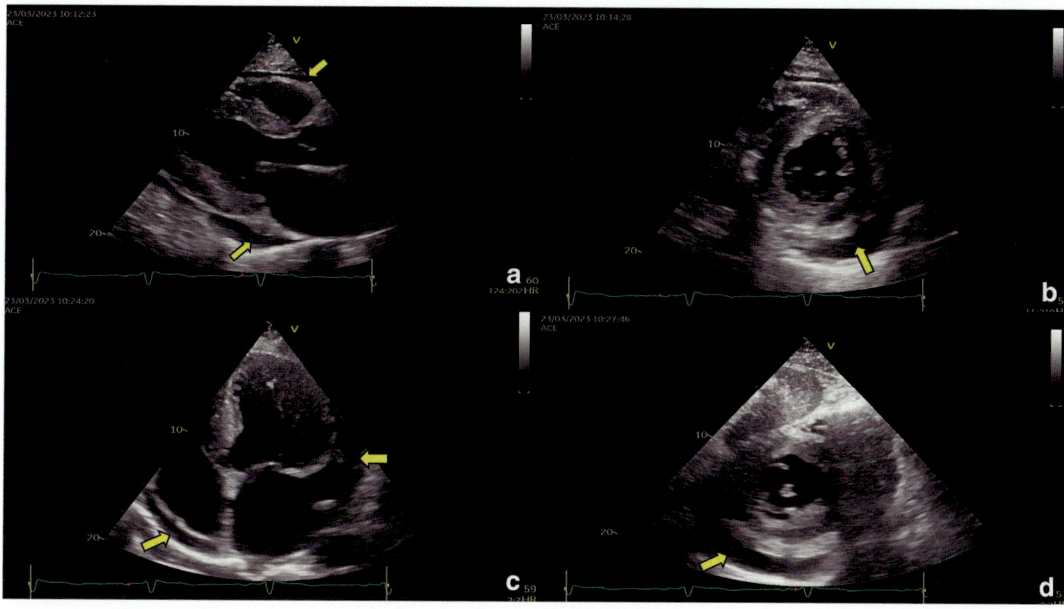

Fig 10.1 Pericardial effusion: **a** parasternal long-axis view; **b** parasternal short-axis view; **c** apical four-chamber view; **d** subxiphoid view

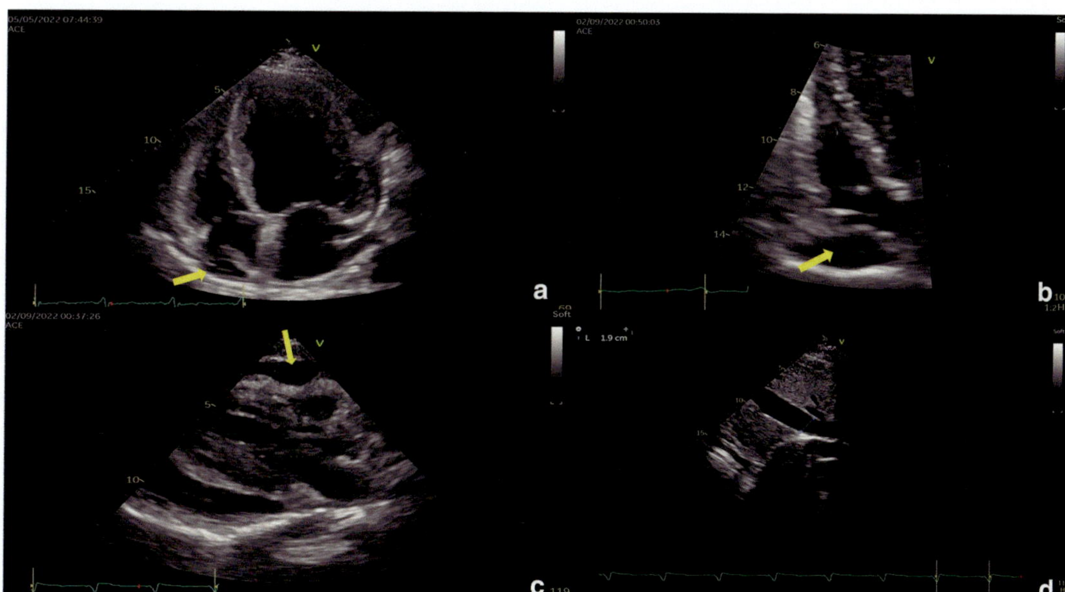

Fig 10.2 Cardiac tamponade signs: **a** right atrial collapse in systole in apical four-chamber view; **b** right atrial collapse in systole in apical four-chamber with zoom; **c** right ventricular collapse in diastole in parasternal long axis view; **d** plethoric inferior vena cava visualized from subcostal view

Conservative management of perforation may associate tamponade over follow-up in patients who initially had no/mild effusion, most of them with antiplatelet drugs and anticoagulants (Acha et al. 2019). Lead repositioning or replacement must be carefully evaluated in patients

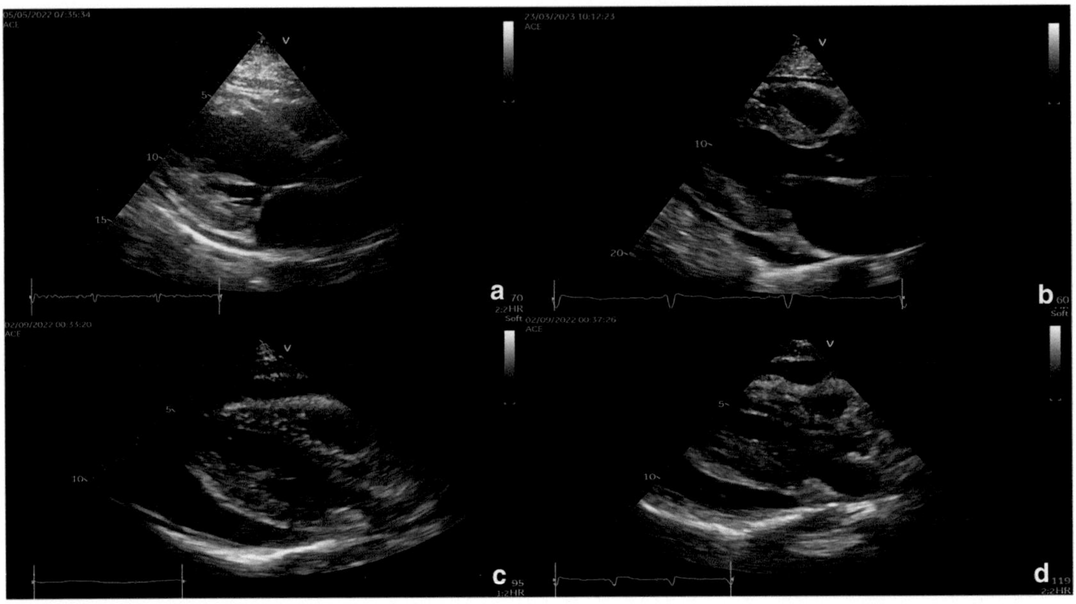

Fig 10.3 Pericardial effusion: **a** small effusion; **b** moderate effusion; **c** large effusion; **d** large effusion with cardiac tamponade signs

with perforation (Acha et al. 2019), and treated in centers with cardiac-thoracic surgery. The risk of infection is high in early reintervention (Tarakji et al. 2019).

Passive atrial leads (Witt et al. 2016; Luria et al. 2007) and VDD pacemaker, if the patient does not need atrial pacing, will be chosen in case of increased risk of perforation (Shurrab et al. 2014).

10.2 Cardiac Device-Related Infective Endocarditis

The evidence of cardiac device-related infective endocarditis (CDRIE) with clinical signs of pocket infection and/or imaging vegetation identification on the pacing lead supports the diagnosis (Delgado et al. 2023; Kerut et al. 2007).

The infection after lead implantation affects 5–20% of patients (Dai et al. 2019; Sohail et al. 2007). CDRIE reported incidence ranges between 0.6 and 3.4% (Blomstrom-Lundqvist et al. 2020) The risk of system infection in patients with a pacemaker (1.19%), ICD (1.7–1.91%)(OlsenT et al. 2019), CRT-P (2.18%), and CRT-D (3.35%) (Greenspon et al. 2018). The risk is higher in patients with reoperations or a previous device-related infection, in men, and younger patients (Greenspon et al. 2018).

Infection associates high morbidity, between 10 to 30% of patients, frequently in patients with systemic infections (Khaloo et al. 2022; Polyzos et al. 2015; Sohail et al. 2011). Mortality depends on the rapidity of diagnosis and adequate management (Duval et al. 2004).

Classification of CDRIE:

- Anatomical: generator pocket or electrodes; infection can occur with or without the involvement of the generator pocket (Delgado et al. 2023). The vegetation can be located on pacemaker leads, pacemaker leads, and cardiac valves, or cardiac valves only (without evidence of pacemaker-lead involvement) (Chua et al. 2000).
- Time of onset following implantation/manipulation: early infection, developing within the first six months, late infection from 1 to

12 months, and delayed infection beyond 12 months of implantation/manipulation (Chamis et al. 2001; Durante-Mangoni et al. 2013).

Risk factors for pacemaker infective endocarditis (IE) are:

Device-related—the risk is higher in patients with two or more leads (Sohail et al. 2011; Lekkerkerker et al. 2009; Herce et al. 2013).

Patient-related—comorbidities increase the risk of infection: immunosuppression, advanced age, cancer therapy, chronic kidney disease, diabetes mellitus, cirrhosis, active infection, chronic obstructive pulmonary disease, heart failure, and reintervention. Males present an increased risk (Sohail et al. 2011; Lekkerkerker et al. 2009; Birnie et al. 2013).

Other clinical conditions associated with risk infection:

- The anticoagulants use increases the risk of pocket hematoma, sometimes requiring percutaneous drainage (Lekkerkerker et al. 2009; Herce et al. 2013; Vaccarino et al. 2009)
- Fever 24 h before intervention, local skin disorders, or history of lead infection (Sohail et al. 2011; Klug et al. 2007)

Procedure-Related

- Postoperative hematoma, reintervention for lead dislodgement, device replacement, lack of perioperative antibiotics prophylaxis, temporary pacing using, operator inexperience, and procedure length (Sohail et al. 2011). Temporary pacing and lack of antibiotic prophylaxis are associated with an increased risk of infection (Uslan et al. 2007; Tarakji and Wilkoff 2014).
- Generator replacement increases the risk of infection by 4% and lead replacement by 15% (Tarakji and Wilkoff 2014). The risk of infection is up to tenfold higher in patients undergoing a lead replacement or a device upgrade (Palmisano et al. 2013).
- Biventricular resynchronization therapy has the highest risk of infection (Bristow et al. 2004).
- Local factors related to the pacing system—erosion of the pacemaker pouch and the number of previously inserted leads (Poole et al. 2010)
- Infection rates are higher with device replacement, upgrade procedures (Rattanawong et al. 2019), CRT, or ICD than with pacemaker implantation (Baddour et al. 2003).

The diagnosis of CDRIE should be considered in a patient with a pacemaker/ICD and unexplained fever (Karchmer and Longworth 2003). Septic pulmonary embolism is a widespread complication and represents a major diagnostic criterion for diagnosing CDRIE (Cook et al. 2005; Victor and Place 1999).

Duke criteria sustain electrode infection diagnosis: positive blood cultures and vegetation on the electrode (Chamis et al. 2001; Karchmer and Longworth 2003), but Duke criteria have low sensitivity in patients with lead implantation (Delgado et al. 2023). Guidelines recommend TTE and TEE in patients with suspected CDRIE (Delgado et al. 2023; Vilacosta et al. 1994; El-Chami et al. 2019).

TTE is the first imaging tool in all patients with suspected device infection (Sandoe et al. 2015) (Fig. 10.4a) (Supplementary material 9). TEE is superior to transthoracic echocardiogram (TTE) for vegetation detection (Fig. 10.4b, c) (Supplementary material 10, 11). In several studies, TEE identified vegetation on the tricuspid valve or device lead in 90–96% of patients with endocarditis; in contrast, TTE identified such findings in only 22–43% (Blomstrom-Lundqvist et al. 2020; Karchmer and Longworth 2003).

Indication for echocardiography in patients with implanted devices and IE suspicion:

1. If IE diagnosis is suspected, echocardiographic evaluation should be carried out as soon as possible (within 24 h) (Joseph et al. 2013)

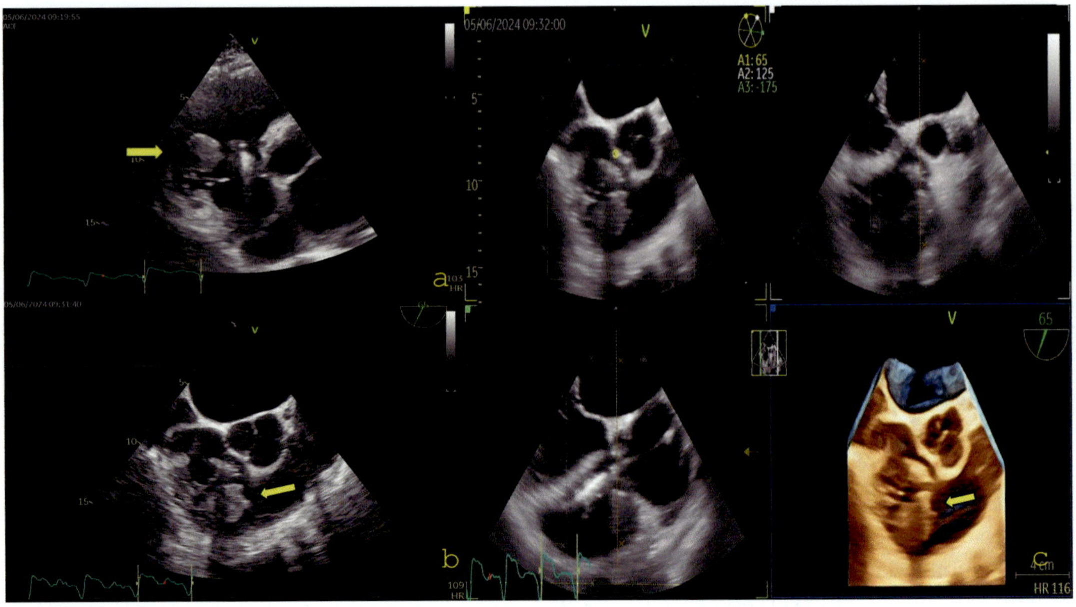

Fig 10.4 Vegetation visualization: **a** Transthoracic echocardiography-apical four-chamber view; **b** Transesophageal echocardiography—bicaval view; **c** four-dimensional echocardiography (arrows)

2. In all patients with generator pocket infection and symptoms or signs of systemic infection/positive blood cultures for diagnosis confirmation (Joseph et al. 2013)
3. In all patients in whom IE infection is suspected clinically (Joseph et al. 2013)
4. Patients with CDRIE and *S. aureus* in one or more blood cultures or other microorganisms in multiple blood cultures (Hochleitner et al. 1990; Athan et al. 2012)
5. After lead removal, repeated echocardiographic imaging is recommended to identify persisting valve or mural vegetations (Joseph et al. 2013)
6. Patients with generator pocket infection and systemic symptoms or signs of infection or positive blood cultures (Joseph et al. 2013)
7. Serial echocardiograms to confirm or exclude IE (Joseph et al. 2013).

TTE and TEE must give detailed information about the tricuspid valve (TV) because concomitant valve infection increases mortality (Ercana et al. 2012) Evaluation should include a TEE examination for patients with permanent pacemakers and fever (Cacoub et al. 1998).

A normal TEE finding does not rule out the involvement of lead IE in the infection process (Chua et al. 2000). TEE is superior to TTE in identifying pacemaker lead and other lead-associated vegetations. TEE's specificity and positive predictive value in vegetation detection is nearly 100% (Vilacosta et al. 1994; Dumont et al. 2003; Rallidis et al. 2003; del Rıo et al. 2003). TTE and TEE are complementary.

TTE usually provides accurate information about left ventricular dimensions and function, right heart size, and pulmonary artery pressure estimation (Delgado et al. 2023).

TEE is the gold standard exam for vegetation detection (Karchmer and Longworth 2003). This imaging technique identifies the masses on the lead, but the blood cultures and inflammation sustain the diagnosis (Lekkerkerker et al. 2009).

Echocardiographic lead vegetation is defined as an oscillating or sessile mass attached to a lead (Fig. 10.5). However, findings should be interpreted in the clinical context because these masses might be non-infected (Joseph et al. 2013). The vegetation may or may not be visible at the level of the TV or leads (Delgado et al. 2023). Usually, the vegetations attach to an

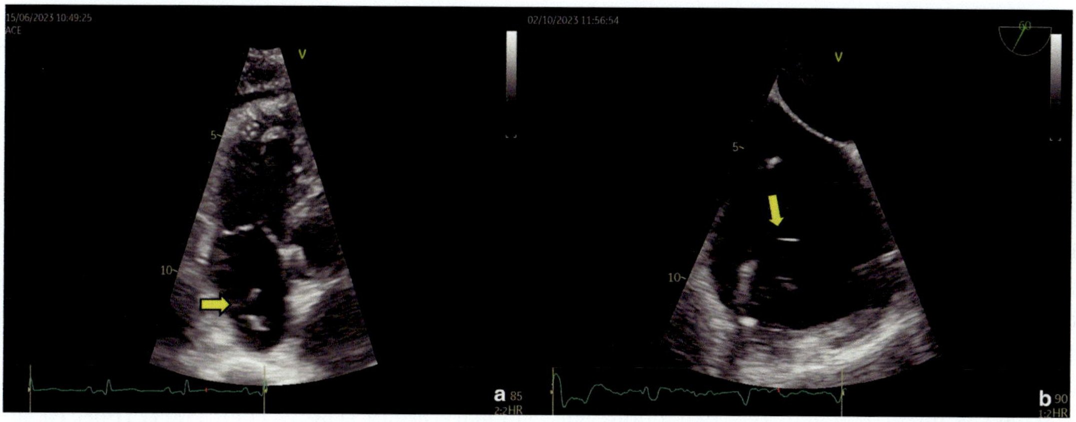

Fig 10.5 Images suggesting thrombus in a patient with pulmonary embolism: **a** transthoracic echocardiography-apical four-chamber view; **b** transesophageal echocardiography—bicaval view

electrode within the right atrium (RA), less frequently in the right ventricle (RV) (Rallidis et al. 2003), but occasionally may arise from the TV leaflet, the atrioventricular plane, or the coronary sinus ostia (Vilacosta et al. 1994).

Sometimes, the vegetations appears on the TV but not the electrode. Also, a pulmonic valve might be involved. Vegetations may be single or multiple, of variable echogenicity and mobility (Vilacosta et al. 1994).

Their size, shape, mobility, and texture should be described in two orthogonal imaging planes (San Filippo et al. 1991; Durack et al. 1994). The vegetation size is an essential parameter because it influences surgical/open device explantation (Joseph et al. 2013).

Echocardiographic diagnostic parameters should also include valve and lead vegetations, new valve regurgitation, and abscess formation (Sawalha et al. 2021). The vegetation is present at the T level and the pulmonary, mitral, and aortic valves. Aortic or mitral valve vegetations are present in 10–15% of patients, increasing in-hospital mortality (Joseph et al. 2013).

Finally, a negative echocardiographic study does not rule out the diagnosis of CDRIE endocarditis (Patel et al. 2023). Recommendation is to repeat TTE and/or TEE within 5–7 days, in case of an initially negative examination, if clinical suspicion of CDRIE remains high (Delgado et al. 2023).

TEE cannot always detect the difference between an infected vegetation and a noninfectedechodense mass (Golzio et al. 2019), such as a thrombus or fibrosis (Joseph et al. 2013). Patients with implanted devices may present fibrinous masses attached to the leads without predicting CDRIE in long-term follow-up (Cleland et al. 2005). Noninfected strands, with 1–2 mm width and 3–5 mm length, are common in patients with implanted devices (Vilacosta et al. 1994; Rallidis et al. 2003), but filaments of 3 mm width and up to 20 mm length are more frequently vegetations (Sawalha et al. 2021).

The blood culture results are positive in 80–100% of pacemaker-related endocarditis.70–90% of lead infections are caused by gram-positive bacteria.

The most frequently detected microorganisms are Staphylococci 78% (coagulase-negative Staphylococci 48%, *S. aureus* 29%) and *Streptococci viridans* 6% (Blomstrom-Lundqvist et al. 2020; Hussein et al. 2016; Mateos Gaitan et al. 2020; Madhavan et al. 2010), Enterococcus spp., β-hemolytic streptococci, oral streptococci group, *Cutibacterium acnes*, and *Corynebacterium* spp. (Madhavan et al. 2010; Arora et al. 2020; Esquer Garrigos et al. 2019; Axell-House et al. 2023). Coagulase-negative staphylococci are more often associated with larger vegetations (> 1 cm) than those in infections with Staphylococcus aureus, which more often causes smaller vegetations (< 1 cm) (Khaloo et al. 2022; Young et al. 2003).

The American Heart Association and Heart Rhythm Society guidelines recommend complete device removal and antibiotic therapy for up to 6 weeks in any patient with a lead infection (Issa and Issa 2021; Karchmer and Longworth 2003). Some cases respond to medical therapy, but the entire pacing system should be removed for infection eradication in some situations (Edelstein et al. 2009). There are two different techniques for lead extraction. The first one is direct percutaneous extraction, and the other option is surgical thoracotomy (Habib et al. 2009).

Percutaneous extraction technique can be used when:

- the vegetation is smaller than 10 mm
- the tricuspid valve is not involved
- the time from implantation is shorter than 1–2 years
- the patient is not pacemaker dependent.

Otherwise, the surgical extraction and placement of an epicardial lead is recommended (Spittell and Hayes 1992; Meier-Ewert et al. 2003).

Due to the risk of pulmonary emboli, large lead vegetations are difficult to extract by percutaneous approach (Karchmer and Longworth 2003).

Septic pulmonary embolism incidence ranges from 31.2 to 55% of patients (Uslan et al. 2007; Said et al. 2016). The most critical risk factor for pulmonary embolic events is the size of the vegetation > 15 mm in diameter (Bailey and Wilkoff 2006; Delewi et al. 2012).

10.3 Lead Thrombosis

The autopsies revealed thrombi on 48% of atrial leads and 33% of ventricular leads (Nowak et al. 2015).

The incidence of thromboembolic events after implantation of intra-cardiac devices is 0.6–3.5% (Delewi et al. 2012). Abnormal left ventricle (LV) apical wall motion induced by RVA pacing can result in thrombosis in the LV cavity and systemic thromboembolism (Shin et al. 2011; Jung et al. 2014; Barakat et al. 2000) (Fig. 10.5). Majority of thrombosis occurs within the first three months after the procedure without clinical sequelae (Feuchter and Katz 2012; Rooden et al. 2004; Domain et al. 2023). RA pacemaker-lead thrombosis (LT) may present as an incidental echocardiographic finding (Wierzbowska et al. 2001) or with symptoms of right-sided heart failure (Brumberg et al. 2012), obstruction, or embolization of the pulmonary artery (Duray et al. 2009) (Fig. 10.5a). The hemodynamic significance of the intracardiac clot depends on its size and location. The RA LT is more dangerous and challenging to manage (Rahbar et al. 2013). Patients with atrial fibrillation (AF) have a higher risk of developing thrombus on endocavitary leads (Fabijani et al. 2005). LT patients may present right-sided heart failure, arrhythmias, or pulmonary artery embolism, but usually, the complication is an echocardiographic finding without any symptoms (Feuchter and Katz 2012; Rooden et al. 2004; Domain et al. 2023; Wierzbowska et al. 2001; Brumberg et al. 2012; Duray et al. 2009; Rahbar et al. 2013; Fabijani et al. 2005; Coleman et al. 2004).

LT may be an incidental echocardiographic finding, or the patients present with symptoms of right-sided heart failure, obstruction, or embolization of the pulmonary artery. Clinical presentation, echocardiographic features, and laboratory findings are essential for differential diagnosis. Thrombotic and embolic rate complications occur in 0.6–3.5% of patients (Feuchter and Katz 2012).

In endocavitary thrombus, TEE is required (Duray et al. 2009; Rahbar et al. 2013) (Fig. 10.5b). LT echocardiographic feature is an immobile solid mass around the lead (Feuchter and Katz 2012; Coleman et al. 2004). The thrombus may range from one to several centimeters in diameter and may cause functional tricuspid stenosis insufficiency or refractory right ventricular failure (Feuchter and Katz 2012; Brumberg et al. 2012; Coleman et al. 2004).

Fibrosis along the electrode is the primary responder for developing thrombi and endocardial vegetation (Chua et al. 2000; Feuchter and Katz 2012). Other risk factors for IE and LT are diabetes, malignancies, immunosuppressive therapy, and local factors such as erosion of the pacemaker pouch and the number of previously inserted leads (Tarakji and Wilkoff 2014; Coleman et al. 2004).

Because no standard guidelines exist for the therapeutic options in LT, the decision should consider the clot size and patients' signs and symptoms (Feuchter and Katz 2012). The therapeutic approach consists in

- surgical extraction in patients with large thrombus
- percutaneous intervention
- medical therapy: anticoagulation or thrombolysis (Xiong et al. 2018; Rahbar et al. 2013; Mazzolai et al. 2018) and depends on clinical practice symptoms and thrombus dimensions.

Oral anticoagulants have low efficacy in preventing embolization from endocavitary thrombi compared to antivitamin K anticoagulants (Konstantinides et al. 2020; Robinson et al. 2020; Mutlak et al. 2009).

10.4 Tricuspid Valve Damage

Another rare lead-related complication is tricuspid damage (Kumar et al. 2022) (Fig. 10.6).

Moderate to severe tricuspid regurgitation is associated with increased mortality in cardiac implantable electronic devices (CIED) patients [167]. The presence of CIED may interfere with TV function (Fig. 10.7) (Suppementary material 12). Many mechanisms can explain CIED-induced tricuspid regurgitation (TR): implantation-related, lead-related, and pacing-related (Addetia et al. 2019; Riesenhuber et al. 2021). Direct interaction of the lead with the TV produces lead-related TR. The probability of significant TR development after implanted devices is due to the lead position at the TV level, usually involving anteroseptal and anteroposterior commissures. Postero-septal commissural or central lead positions seem not to influence the development of TR (Riesenhuber et al. 2021).

The frequency of significant TR following CIED implantation ranges from 7 to 45% (Riesenhuber et al. 2021).

TR worsening after RV lead implant associates a bad outcome (Dreyfus et al. 2015).

TR in patients with implanted devices may be primary (implantation-related, lead-related)

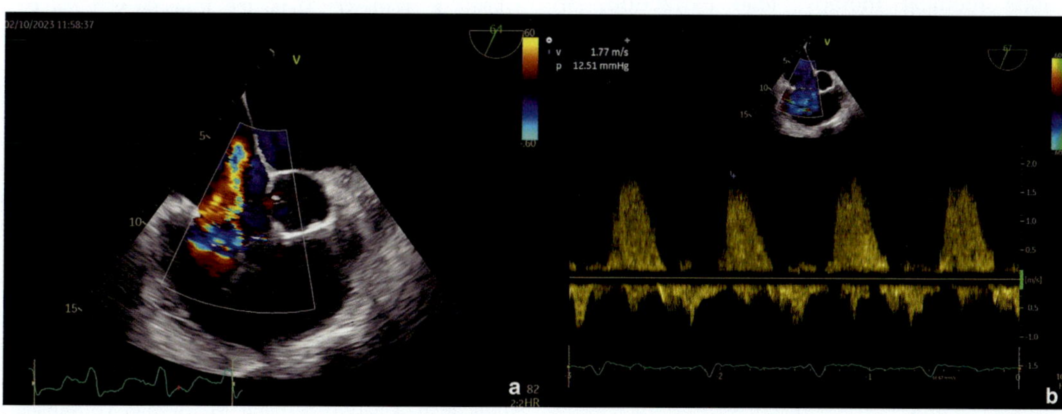

Fig 10.6 Tricuspid regurgitation in a patient with CRT-D; **a** TR color jet visualized from mid esophageal view at 64 degrees; **b** Pulmonary artery systolic pressure calculation from tricuspid regurgitation jet

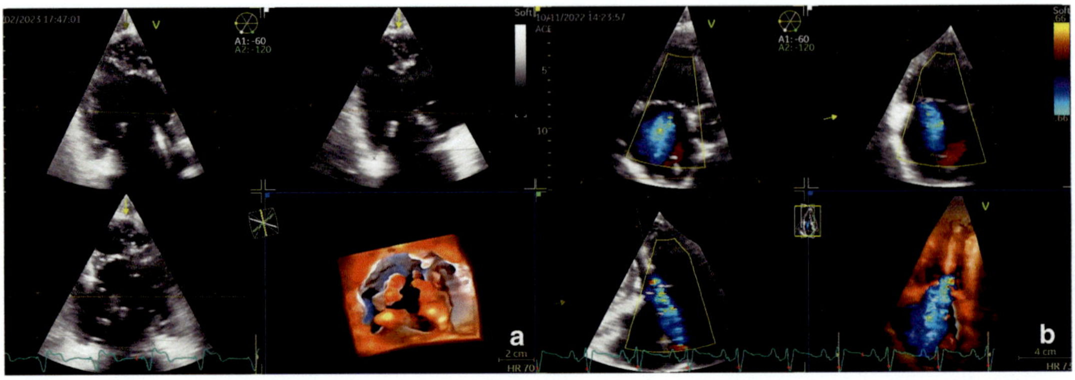

Fig 10.7 Tricuspid damage in a patient with implanted cardio defibrillator: **a** three-dimensional echocardiography of tricuspid valve and lead; **b** tricuspid regurgitation visualized by tridimensional color Doppler echocardiography

and secondary (pacing-related, "functional") (Addetia et al. 2019). Primary CIED-induced TR results from the lead interaction with the TV. Secondary CIED-induced TR results from RV dilatation and dysfunction in patients with a high percentage of RV pacing (Schleifer et al. 2018; Beurskens et al. 2019). It is still debated whether pacing leads positions in the RV apex, RV septum, or LV pacing via the coronary sinus influences TR development (Taramasso et al. 2019).

The guidance for managing TR in patients with CIED leads still needs to be improved. The worsening of HF may result from the effect on tricuspid leaflet mobility or cooptation (Schleifer et al. 2018). The therapeutic options include medical therapy, lead extraction, or alternative pacing strategies (LV pacing via the coronary sinus or epicardial leads). Lead extraction is linked to the risk of damage to the TV and worsening TF [143]. Surgical valve repair or replacement follows the recommendations based on symptoms, the severity of TR, and RV function [144].

10.5 Conclusion

The most frequent complications in patients with implanted devices are pericardial effusion, endocarditis, lead thrombosis, and tricuspid valve damage. Echocardiography is the primary imaging tool for diagnosis. The masses identified on the lads or at the right heart level must be interpreted in the clinical context. TR results from the lead interaction with the tricuspid valve, especially in patients with defibrillators, because of the increased dimension of the lead. All the complications in this group of patients must be diagnosed and treated early because of the bad outcome.

References

Acha MR, Rafael A, Keaney JJ, Elitzur Y, et al. The management of cardiac implantable electronic device lead perforations: a multicentre study. Europace. 2019;21:937–43.

Addetia K, Harb SC, Hahn RT, Kapadia S, Lang RM. Cardiac implantable electronic device lead-induced tricuspid regurgitation. JACC Cardiovasc Imaging. 2019;12:622–36.

Adler Y, Charron P, Imazio M, et al. 2015 ESC guidelines for the diagnosis and management of pericardial diseases The Task Force for the Diagnosis and Management of Pericardial Diseases of the European Society of Cardiology (ESC) Endorsed by: The European Association for Cardio-Thoracic Surgery (EACTS) Authors/Task Force Members. Eur Heart J. 2015;36:2921–2964.

Agarwal N, Mojadidi MK, Ahmed M. Constrictive pericarditis from an endocardial pacemaker lead. BMJ Case Rep. 2017;2017:bcr2016218365.

Allouche E, Chargui S, Fathi M, Bezdah L. Subacute right ventricle perforation: a pacemaker lead complication. BMJ Case Rep. 2021;14(5):e242489.

Arora Y, Perez AA, Carrillo RG. Influence of vegetation shape on outcomes in transvenous lead extractions: does shape matter? Heart Rhythm. 2020;17:646–53.

Athan E, Chu VH, Tattevin P, et al. ICE-PCS ınvestigators. Clinical characteristics and outcome of infective endocarditis involving implantable cardiac devices. JAMA. 2012;307:1727–35.

Axell-House DB, Khalil S, Sohail MR. Clinical approach to evaluation of underlying cardiac device infection in patients hospitalized with bacteremia. Methodist DeBakey Cardiovasc J. 2023;19(4):48–57.

Baddour LM, Bettmann MA, Bolger AF, et al. American Heart Association scientific statement: nonvalvular cardiovascular device-related infections. Circulation. 2003;108:2015–31.

Bailey SM, Wilkoff BL. Complications of pacemakers and defibrillators in the elderly. Am J Geriatr Cardiol. 2006;15:102–7.

Barakat K, Robinson NM, Spurrell RA. Transvenous pacing lead-induced thrombosis: a series of cases with a review of the literature. Cardiology. 2000;93:142–8.

Beurskens NEG, Tjong FVY, de Bruin-Bon RHA, et al. Impact of leadless pacemaker therapy on cardiac and atrioventricular valve function through 12 months of follow-up. Circ Arrhythm Electrophysiol. 2019;12:e007124.

Birnie DH, Healey JS, Wells GA, et al. Pacemaker or defibrillator surgery without interruption of anticoagulation. N Engl J Med. 2013;368(22):2084–93.

Blomstrom-Lundqvist C, Traykov V, Erba PA, et al. European Heart Rhythm Association (EHRA) international consensus document on how to prevent, diagnose, and treat cardiac implantable electronic device infections-endorsed by the Heart Rhythm Society (HRS), the Asia Pacific Heart Rhythm Society (APHRS), the Latin American Heart Rhythm Society (LAHRS), International Society for Cardiovascular Infectious Diseases (ISCVID) and the European Society of Clinical Microbiology and Infectious Diseases (ESCMID) in collaboration with the European Association for Cardio Thoracic Surgery (EACTS). Europace 2020;22:515–549. Prutkin JM, Reynolds MR, Bao H, et al. Rates of and factors associated with infection in 200,909 Medicare implantable cardioverter defibrillator implants: results from the National Cardiovascular Data Registry. Circulation. 2014;130(13):1037–1043.

Boriani G, Biffi M, Martignani C. Uneventful right ventricular perforation with displacement of a pacing lead into the left thorax. J Cardiothorac Vasc Anesth. 2008;22:423–5.

Bristow MR, Saxon LA, Boehmer J, et al. Cardiac resynchronization therapy with or without an implantable defibrillator in advanced chronic heart failure. Nengl J Med. 2004;350:2140–50.

Brumberg GE, Kaseer B, Hemal Shah H, et al. Biventricular defibrillator patients have higher complication rates after revision of recalled leads. Pacing Clin Electrophysiol. 2012;35(6):665–71.

Buszkiewicz K, Greberski K, Luczak M, Angerer D, Poprawka T, Bugajski P. Progressivecardiac tamponade and right ventricular free wall perforation as complications after dual-chamber pacemaker implantation—a case report. Pol Merkur Lek Organ Pol Tow Lek. 2021;49(289):54–6.

Cacoub P, Leprince P, Nataf P, et al. Pacemaker infective endocarditis. Am J Cardiol. 1998;82(4):480–4.

Cano O, Andres A, Alonso P, Osca J, Sancho-Tello MJ, Olague J. Incidence and predictors of clinically relevant cardiac perforation associated with systematic implantation of active-fixation pacing and defibrillation leads: a single-centre experience with over 3800 implanted leads. Europace. 2017;19:96–102.

Carda R, Almería C, Lennie V, et al. What to do with an atrial thrombus? Eur J Echocardiogr. 2008;9:204–5.

Chamis AL, Peterson GE, Cabell CH, et al. Staphylococcus aureus bacteremia in patients with permanent pacemakers or implantable cardioverter-defibrillators. Circulation. 2001;104:1029–33.

Chlabicz M, Jakim P, Zalewska-Adamiec M, Róg-Makal M, Dobrzycki S. A RARE CASE of acute pleuropericarditis as a complication of permanent pacemaker insertion. Am J Case Rep. 2021;22.

Chua JD, Wilkoff BL, Lee I, et al. Diagnosis and management of infections involving implantable electrophysiologic cardiac devices. Ann Intern Med. 2000;133:604–8.

Cleland JGF, Daubert J-C, Erdmann E, et al. for the Cardiac Resynchronization-Heart Failure (CARE-HF) Study Investigators. The effect of cardiac resynchronization on morbidity and mortality in heart failure. N Engl J Med. 2005; 352:1539–1549.

Coleman DB, DeBarr DM, Morales DL, et al. Pacemaker lead thrombosis treated with atrial thrombectomy and biventricular pacemaker and defibrillator insertion. Ann Thorac Surg. 2004;78:e83-84.

Cook RJ, Ashton RW, Aughenbaugh GL, et al. Septic pulmonary embolism: presenting features and clinical course of 14 patients. Chest. 2005;128:162–6.

Cosyns B, Plein S, Nihoyanopoulos P, et al. On behalf of the European Association of Cardiovascular Imaging (EACVI) and European Society of Cardiology Working Group (ESCWG) on Myocardial and Pericardial diseases. European Association of Cardiovascular Imaging (EACVI) position paper: multimodality imaging in pericardial disease. Eur Heart J Cardiovasc Imaging 2014;16:12–31.

Dai M, Cai C, Vaibhav V, et al. Trends of cardiovascular implantable electronic device infection in 3 decades: a population-based study. JACC Clin Electrophysiol. 2019;5(9):1071–80.

Deichl AS, Lacour P, Belyavs E, et al. Case report: assessing the position of pacemaker leads via transthoracic echocardiography: additional value of the subcostal en face view. Front Cardiovasc Med. 2021;8:697052.

del Rıo A, Anguere I, Miro JM, et al. Surgical treatment of pacemaker and defibrillator lead endocarditis: the impact of electrode lead extraction on outcome. Chest. 2003;124:1451–1459.

Delewi R, Zijlstra F, Piek JJ. Left ventricular thrombus formation after acute myocardial infarction. Heart. 2012;98:1743–9.

Delgado V, Marsan AN, de Waha S, et al. 2023 ESC Guidelines for the management of endocarditis developed by the task force on the management of endocarditis of the European Society of Cardiology (ESC) Endorsed by the European Association for Cardio-Thoracic Surgery (EACTS) and the European Association of Nuclear Medicine (EANM). Eur Heart J. 2023;44:3948–4042.

Domain G, Strubé C, Plourde B, et al. Acute transvenous pacemaker lead thrombosis early after implantation: a rare clinical scenario. Pacing Clin Electrophysiol. 2023;46(8):934–8.

Dreyfus GD, Martin RP, Chan KM, Dulguerov F, Alexandrescu C. Functional tricuspid regurgitation: a need to revise our understanding. J Am Coll Cardiol. 2015;65:2331–6.

Dumont E, Camus C, Victor F, et al. Suspected pacemaker or defibrillator transvenous lead infection: prospective assessment of a TEE-guided therapeutic strategy. Eur Heart J. 2003;24:1779–87.

Durack DT, Lukes AS, Bright DK. New criteria for diagnosis of infective endocarditis: utilization of specific echocardiographic findings. Duke endocarditis service. Am J Med. 1994;96:200–9.

Durante-Mangoni E, Mattucci I, Agrusta F, Tripodi MF, Utili R. Current trends in the management of cardiac implantable electronic device (CIED) infections. Intern Emerg Med. 2013;8(6):465–76.

Duray GZ, Schmitt J, Cicek-Hartvig S, et al. Complications leading to surgical revision in implantable cardioverter defibrillator patients: comparison of patients with single-chamber, dual-chamber, and biventricular devices. Europace. 2009;11(3):297–302.

Duval X, Selton-Suty C, Alla F. Endocarditis in patients with a permanent pacemaker: a 1-year epidemiological survey on infective endocarditis due to valvular and/or pacemaker infection. Clin Infect Dis. 2004;39:68–74.

Edelstein S, Yahalom M, et al. Cardiac device-related endocarditis: epidemiology, pathogenesis, diagnosis and treatment—a review. Int J Angiol. 2009;18:167–72.

El-Chami MF, Johansen JB, Zaidi A, et al. Leadless pacemaker implant in patients with pre-existing infections: Results from the Micra postapproval registry. J Cardiovasc Electrophysiol. 2019;30:569–74.

Ercana S, Altunbasb G, Yavuza F, et al. Permanent pacemaker lead endocarditis due to Staphylococcus hominis and review of the literature Cor et vasa. 2012;54:e336–38.

Esquer Garrigos Z, George MP, Vijayvargiya P, et al. Clinical presentation, management, and outcomes of cardiovascular implantable electronic device infections due to Gram-negative versus Gram-positive bacteria. Mayo Clin Proc. 2019;94:1268–77.

Fabijani D, Giunio L, Vuji i M, Vukovi I, Ermacora R, Kneževi N. Right atrial pacemaker lead thrombosis incidentally detected by transesophageal echocardiography. Coll Antropol 2005;29:159–160.

Feuchter AC, Katz KD. Right atrial thrombus secondary to pacemaker wires. J Emerg Med. 2012;43:e185–7.

Gadler F, Valzania C, Linde C. Current use of implantable electrical devices in Sweden: data from the Swedish pacemaker and implantable cardioverter defibrillator registry. Europace. 2015;17:69–77.

Golzio PG, Errigo D, Peyracchia M, et al. Prevalence and prognosis of lead masses in patients with cardiac implantable electronic devices without infection. J Cardiovasc Med (hagerstown). 2019;20:372–8.

Goodman A, Perera P, Mailhot T, Mandavia D. The role of bedside ultrasound in the diagnosis of pericardial effusion and cardiac tamponade. J Emerg Trauma Shock. 2012;5(1):72–5.

Greenspon AJ, Eby EL, Petrilla AA, Sohail MR. Treatment patterns, costs, and mortality among Medicare beneficiaries with CIED infection. Pacing Clin Electrophysiol. 2018;41(5):495–503.

Habib G, Hoen B, Tornos P, et al. ESC Committee for Practice Guidelines. Guidelines on the prevention, diagnosis, and treatment of infective endocarditis (new version 2009): the task force on the prevention diagnosis, and treatment of ınfective endocarditis of the European Society of Cardiology (ESC). Endorsed by the European Society of Clinical Microbiology and Infectious Diseases (ESCMID) and the Interna tional Society of Chemotherapy (ISC) forınfection and cancer. Eur Heart J. 2009;30:2369–413.

Haghjoo M, Alizadeh A, Fazelifar AF, Hajahmadi M, Sadr Ameli MA. Delayed cardiac perforation by one small body diameter defibrillator lead. J Electrophysiol. 2010;43:71–3.

Hanson MG, Chan B. The role o point-of-care ultrasound in the diagnosis of pericardial effusion: a single academic center retrospective study. Ultrasound J. 2021;13:2.

Haq SA, Heitner JF, Lee L, Kassotis JT. Late presentation of a lead perforation as a complication of permanent pacemaker insertion. Angiology. 2008;59:619–21.

Herce B, Nazeyrollas P, Lesaffre F, et al. Risk factors for infection of implantable cardiac devices: data from a registry of 2496 patients. Europace. 2013;15(1):66–70.

Hirschl D, Jain V, Spindola-Franco H, Gross J, Haramati L. Prevalence and characterization of asymptomatic pacemaker and ICD lead perforation on CT. Pacing Clin Electrophysiol. 2007;30(1):28–32.

Hochleitner M, Hörtnagl H, Ng CK, Hörtnagl H, Gschnitzer F, Zechmann W. Usefulness of physiologic dual chamber pacing in drug-resistant idiopathic dilated cardiomyopathy. Am J Cardiol. 1990;66:198–202.

Hosseini SM, Moazzami K, Rozen G, et al. Utilization and in-hospital complications of cardiac resynchronization therapy: trends in the United States from 2003 to 2013. Eur Heart J. 2017;38:2122–8.

Hsu JC, Varosy PD, Bao H, Dewland TA, Curtis JP, Marcus GM. Cardiac perforation from implantable cardioverter-defibrillator lead placement: insights from the national cardiovascular data registry. Circ Cardiovasc Qual Outcomes. 2013;6:582–90.

Hussein AA, Baghdy Y, Wazni OM, et al. Microbiology of cardiac implantable electronic device infections. JACC Clin Electrophysiol. 2016;2:498–505.

Imazio M, Hoit BD. Post-cardiac injury syndromes. An emerging cause of pericardial diseases. Int J Cardiol 2013;168:648–652.

Issa ZF, Issa TZ. Feasibility and safety of percutaneous lead revision for subacute and delayed cardiac device lead perforation. JACC Clin Elec Trophysiol. 2021;7:26–35.

Joseph JP, Meddows TR, Webster DP, et al. Prioritizing echocardiography in Staphylococcus aureus bacteraemia. J Antimicrob Chemother. 2013;68:444–9.

Jung HC, Chung WB, Lee M-Y. Thrombosis in the left ventricle after implantable cardioverter-defibrillator implantation: a rare cause of systemic thromboembolism. Korean J Crit Care Med. 2014;29(1):27–31.

Karchmer AW, Longworth: Infections of intracardiac devices. In Durack DT, Crawford MH (eds) Cardiology clinics—infective endocarditis, Philadelphia, W.B. Saunders Co.; 2003, p. 253–71.

Kerut EK, Hanawalt C, Everson CT. Role of the Echocardiography Laboratory in diagnosis and management of pacemaker and implantable cardiac defibrillator infection, echocardiography. J CV Ultrasound Allied Tech. 2007;24(9):1008–1012.

Khaloo P, Uzomah UA, Shaqdan A, et al. Outcomes of patients hospitalized with cardiovascular implantable electronic device-related infective endocarditis, prosthetic valve endocarditis, and native valve endocarditis: a nationwide study, 2003 to 2017. J Am Heart Assoc. 2022;11(17):e025600.

Khan M, Joseph G, Khaykin Y, Ziada K, Wilkoff BL. Delayed lead perforation: a disturbing trend. Pacing Clin Electrophysiol. 2005;28:251–3.

Kirkfeldt RE, Johansen JB, Nohr EA, et al. Risk factors for lead complications incardiac pacing: a population-based cohort study of28,860 Danish patients. Heart Rhythm. 2011;8:1622–8.

Klein AL, Abbara S, Agler DA, et al. American Society of Echocardiography clinical recommendations for multimodality cardiovascular imaging of patients with pericardial disease: endorsed by the Society for Cardiovascular Magnetic Resonance and Society of Cardiovascular Computed Tomography. J Am Soc Echocardiogr. 2013;26:965-1012.e15.

Klug D, Balde M, Pavin D, et al. People study group. Risk factors related to infections of implanted pacemakers and cardioverter-defibrillators: results of a large prospective study. Circulation 2007;116:1349–1355.

Knopp BW, Gerakopoulos K, Parmar J. Acute pericardial effusion from pacemaker lead 4 perforation of right ventricle identified on bedside emergency department ultrasonography. Curr Res Emerg Med (CREM). 2022;2(5):2832–5699.

Koneru JN, Jones PW, Hammill EF, Wold N, Ellenbogen KA. Risk factors and temporal trends of complications associated with transvenous implantable cardiac defibrillator leads. J Am Heart Assoc. 2018;7:e007691.

Konstantinides SV, Meyer G, Becattini C, et al. 2019 ESC Guidelines for the diagnosis and management of acute pulmonary embolism developed in collaboration with the European Respiratory Society (ERS). Eur Heart J. 2020;41:543–603.

Kumar P, Skrabal J, Frasure SE, Pourmand A, Pacemaker lead related myocardial perforation. Am J Emerg Med. 2022;53:281.e1–e3.

Laborderi J, Barandon L, Ploux S, et al. Management of sub-acute and delayed right ventricular perforation with a pacing or an implantable cardioverter-defibrillator lead. Am J Cardiol. 2008;102:1352–5.

Lekkerkerker JC, van Nieuwkoop C, Trines SA, et al. Risk factors and time delay associated with cardiac device infections: leiden device registry. Heart. 2009;95(9):715–20.

Liang JJ, Killu AM, Osborn MJ, Jaffe AS. Pacemaker lead perforation causing hemopericardium eight years after implantation. Indian Heart J. 2013;65:331–3.

Lin YS, Hung SP, Chen PR, et al. Risk factors influencing complications of cardiac implantable electronic device implantation: infection, pneumothorax and heart perforation a nationwide population-based cohort study. Medicine. 2014;93:e213.

Lopez LR, Brandao L, Carrageta M. Single-step transvenous extraction of a passive fixation lead with delayed perforation of the right ventricle. Europace. 2007;9:672–3.

Luria DM, Feinberg MS, Gurevitz OT, Bar-Lev DS, Granit C, Tanami N, et al. Randomized comparison of J-shaped atrial leads with and without active fixation mechanism. Pacing Clin Electrophysiol. 2007;30:412–7.

Madershahian N, Wipperman J, Wahlers T. The bite of the lead: multiple perforations by an active-fixation permanent pacemaker lead. Interac Cardiovasc Thorac Surg. 2010;11:93–4.

Madhavan M, Sohail MR, Friedman PA, et al. Outcomes in patients with cardiovascular implantable electronic devices and bacteremia caused by Gram-positive cocci other than Staphylococcus aureus. Circ Arrhythm Electrophysiol. 2010;3:639–45.

Mahapatra S, Bybee KA, Bunch TJ, et al. Incidence and predictors of cardiac perforation after permanent pacemaker placement. Heart Rhythm. 2005;2:907–11.

Mateos Gaitan R, Boix-Palop L, Munoz Garcia P, et al. Infective endocarditis in patients with cardiac implantable electronic devices: a nationwide study. Europace. 2020;22:1062–70.

Mazzolai L, Aboyans V, Ageno W, et al. Diagnosis and management of acute deep vein thrombosis: a joint consensus document from the European Society of Cardiology working groups of aorta and peripheral vascular diseases and pulmonary circulation and right ventricular function. Eur Heart J. 2018;39:4208–18.

Meier-Ewert HK, Gray ME, John RM. Endocardial pacemaker or defibrillator leads with infected vegetations: a single-center experience and consequences of transvenous extraction. Am Heart J. 2003;146(2):339–44.

Migliore F, Zorzi A, Bertaglia E, Leoni L, Siciliano M, De Lazzari M, et al. Incidence, management, and prevention of right ventricular perforation by pacemaker and implantable cardioverter defibrillator leads. Pacing Clin Electrophysiol. 2014;37:1602–9.

Mutlak D, Aronson D, Lessick J, Reisner SA, Dabbah S, Agmon Y. Functional tricuspid regurgitation in patients with pulmonary hypertension: is pulmonary artery pressure the only determinant of regurgitation severity? Chest. 2009;135:115–21.

Nowak B, Tasche K, Barnewold L, et al. Association between hospital procedure volume and early complications after pacemaker implantation: results from a large, un selected, contemporary cohort of the German nationwide obligatory external quality assurance programme. Europace. 2015;17:787–93.

Ohlow MA, Lauer B, Brunelli M, Geller JC. Incidence and predictors of pericardial effusion after permanent heart rhythm device implantation: prospective evaluation of 968 consecutive patients. Circ J. 2013;77:975–81.

OlsenT, Jorgensen OD, Nielsen JC, et al. Incidence of device-related infection in 97750 patients: clinical data from the complete Danish device-cohort (1982–2018). Eur Heart J. 2019;40:1862–1869.

Palmisano P, Accogli M, Zaccaria M, et al. Rate, causes, and impact on patient outcome of implantable device complications requiring surgical revision: large population survey from two centers in Italy. Europace. 2013;15(4):531–40.

Parsonnet V, Bernstein AD, Lindsay B. Pacemaker-implantation complication rates: an analysis of some contributing factors. J Am Coll Cardiol. 1989;13:917–21.

Patel NJ, Singleton MJ, Brunetti R, Richardson KM, Bhave PD. Evaluation of lead-based echodensities on transesophageal echocardiogram in patients with cardiac implantable electronic devices. J Cardiovasc Electrophysiol. 2023;34(1):7–13.

Polyzos KA, Konstantelias AA, Falagas ME. Risk factors for cardiac implantable electronic device infection: a systematic review and meta-analysis. Europace. 2015;17(5):767–77.

Poole JE, Gleva MJ, Mela T, et al. REPLACE Registry Investigators. Complication rates associated with pacemaker or implantable cardioverter-defibrillator generator replacements and upgrade procedures: results from the REPLACE registry. Circulation 2010;122:1553–1561.

Rahbar AS, Azadani PN, Thatipelli S, et al. Risk factors and prognosis for clot formation on cardiac device leads. Pacing Clin Electrophysiol. 2013;36:1294–300.

Rajkumar CA, Claridge S, Jackson T, et al. Diagnosis and management of iatrogenic cardiac perforation caused by pacemaker and defibrillator leads. Europace. 2017;19(6):1031–7.

Rallidis LS, Komninos KA, Papasteriadis EG. Pacemaker-related endocarditis: the value of transoesophageal echocardiography in diagnosis and treatment. Acta Cardiol. 2003;58:31–4.

Rattanawong P, Kewcharoen J, Mekraksakit P, et al. Device infections in implantable cardioverter defibrillators versus permanent pacemakers: a systematic review and meta-analysis. J Cardiovasc Electrophysiol. 2019;30:1053–65.

Riesenhuber M, Spannbauer A, Gwechenberger M, Pezawas T, Schukro C, Stix G, et al. Pacemaker lead-associated tricuspid regurgitation in patients with or without pre-existing right ventricular dilatation. Clin Res Cardiol. 2021 Epub ahead of printChang JD, Manning WJ, Ebrille E, Zimetbaum PJ. Tricuspid valve dysfunction following pacemaker or cardioverter-defibrillator implantation. J Am Coll Cardiol. 2017;69:2331–41.

Robinson AA, Trankle CR, Eubanks G, et al. Off-label use of direct oral anticoagulants compared with warfarin for left ventricular thrombi. JAMA Cardiol. 2020;5:685–92.

Sadamatsu K, Enomoto N, Tsuji M, Tashiro H. Progressive atrial lead perforation developed 5 years after pacemaker replacement. J Cardiol. 2009;53:150–3.

Said SAM, Nijhuis R, Derks A, Droste H. Septic pulmonary embolism caused by infected pacemaker leads after replacement of a cardiac resynchronization therapy device. Am J Case Rep. 2016;17:507–11.

Sandoe JAT, Barlow G, Chambers JB, et al. Guidelines for the diagnosis, prevention and management of implantable cardiac electronic device infection. Report of a joint Working Party project on behalf of the British Society for Antimicrobial Chemotherapy (BSAC, host organization), British Heart Rhythm Society (BHRS), British Cardiovascular Society (BCS), British Heart Valve Society (BHVS) and British Society for Echocardiography (BSE). J Antimicrob Chemother. 2015;70:325–59.

SanFilippo AJ, Picard MH, Newell JB, et al. Echocardiographic assessment of patients with infective endo carditis. J Am Coll Cardiol. 1991;18:1191–9.

Sanoussi A, El Nakadi B, Lardinois I, De Bruyne Y, Joris M. Late right ventricular perforation after permanent pace-maker implantation: how far can the lead go? Pacing Clin Electrophysiol. 2005;28:723–5.

Sawalha K, Khan S, Vedala K. Always check the lead!… Unique case of cardiac arrest due to pacemaker infective endocarditis. Arch Clin Med Case Rep. 2021;5(1):216–20.

Schleifer JW, Pislaru SV, Lin G, et al. Effect of ventricular pacing lead position on tricuspid regurgitation: a randomized prospective trial. Heart Rhythm. 2018;15:1009–16.

Shabetai R. Pericardial effusion: haemodynamic spectrum. Heart. 2004;90:255–156.

Shariff REFR, Wen LC, Khir RN, Ibrahim KS, Kasim S. A unique case of non-capture of permanent pacemaker lead: delayed lead perforation and cardiac tamponade. Cardiovasc Imaging Asia. 2021;5(3):110–3.

Shin SN, Yun KH, Ko JS, et al. Left ventricular thrombus associated with takotsubo cardiomyopathy: a cardioembolic cause of cerebral infarction. J Cardiovasc Ultrasound. 2011;19:152–5.

Shingaki M, Kobayashi Y, Suzuki H. Acute pericarditis with cardiac tamponade induced by pacemaker implantation. Asian Cardiovasc Thorac Ann. 2015;23(9):1093–5.

Shingaki M, Kobayashi Y, Suzuki H. Acute pericarditis with cardiac tamponade in duced by pacemaker implantation. Asian Cardiovasc Thorac Ann. 2015;23(9):1093–5.

Shurrab M, Elitzur Y, Healey JS, Gula L, Kaoutskaia A, Israel C, et al. VDD vs DDD pacemakers: a meta-analysis. Can J Cardiol. 2014;30:1385–91.

Singhal S, Cooper JM, Cheung AT, Acker MA. Rib perforation from a right ventricular pacemaker lead. Circulation. 2007;115:e391–2.

Sohail MR, Henrikson CA, Braid-Forbes MJ, Forbes KF, Lerner DJ. Mortality and cost associated with cardiovascular implantable electronic device infections. Arch Intern Med. 2011;171(20):1821–8.

Sohail MR, Uslan DZ, Khan AH, et al. Management and outcome of permanent pacemaker and implantable cardioverter-defibrillator infections. J Am Coll Cardiol. 2007;8;49(18):1851–1859.

Spittell P, Hayes D. Venous complications after insertion of a transvenous pacemaker. Mayo Clin Proc. 1992:67:258–65.

Stefanidis AS, Pnagiotis NM, Kotsakis AA, Papasteriadis EG. Three-dimensional echocardiographic documentation of pacemaker lead perforation presenting as acute pericar ditis. Hellenic J Cardiol. 2009;50:335–7.

Sterlinski M, Przybylski A, Maciag A, et al. Subacute cardiac perforations associated with active fixation leads. Europace. 2008;11:206–12.

Tarakji KG, Wilkoff BL. Cardiac implantable electronic device infections: facts, current practice, and the unanswered questions. Curr Infect Dis Rep. 2014;16(9):425.

Tarakji KG, Mittal S, Kennergren C, Corey R, Poole JE, Schloss E, et al. Antibacterial envelope to prevent cardiac implantable device infection. N Engl J Med. 2019;380:1895–905.

Taramasso M, Benfari G, van der Bijl P, et al. Transcatheter versus medical treatment of patients with symptomatic severe tricuspid regurgitation. J Am Coll Cardiol. 2019;74:29983008.

Tziakas D, Alexoudis A, Konstantinou F, Chalikias G, Stakos D, Bougioukas G. A rare case of late right ventricular perforation by a passive-fixation permanent pacemaker lead. Europace. 2009;11:968–9.

Udo EO, Zuithoff NP, van Hemel NM, et al. Incidence and predictors of short- and long-term complications in pacemaker therapy: the FOLLOW PACE study. Heart Rhythm. 2012;9:728–35.

Uslan DZ, Sohail MR, StSauver JL, et al. Permanent pacemaker and implantable cardioverter defibrillator infection: a population-based study. Arch Intern Med. 2007;167:669–75.

Vaccarino GN, Nacinovich F, Piccini F, et al. Pacemaker endocarditis: approach for lead extraction in endocarditis with large vegetations. Rev Bras Cir Cardiovasc. 2009;24(4):570–3.

van Rooden CJ, Molhoek SG, Rosendaal FR, et al. Incidence and risk factors of early venous thrombosis associated with permanent pacemaker leads. J Cardiovasc Electrophysiol. 2004;15:1258–62.

Victor F, De Place C, et al. Pacemaker lead infection: echocardiographic features, management, and outcome. Heart. 1999;81:82–7.

Vilacosta I, Sarria C, San Roman JA, et al. Usefulness of transesophageal echocardiography for diagnosis of infected transvenous permanent pacemakers. Circulation. 1994;89:2684–7.

Welch AR, Yadav P, Lingle K, et al. Subacute right ventricular pacemaker lead perforation: often talked about in consent forms but very rarely seen. J Innov Card Rhythm Manage. 2011;2:442–5.

Wierzbowska K, Krzemińska-Pakua M, Marszal-Marciniak M, Drozdz J, Zasonka J, Kasprzak JD. Symptomatic atrial pacemaker lead thrombosis: detection by echocardiography and successful surgical treatment. Pacing Clin Electrophysiol. 2001;24:391–3.

Witt CM, Lenz CJ, Shih HH, Ebrille E, Rosenbaum AN, Aung H, et al. Right atrial lead fixation type and lead position are associated with significant variations in complications. J Interv Card Electrophysiol. 2016;47:313–9.

Xiong M, Zhang Z, Hu K, Dong M. Hu W Recurrent, late-onset pleural effusions in elderly patients receiving pacemaker therapy. Medicine. 2018;97(43):e12915.

Young JB, Abraham WT, Smith AL, et al. Combined cardiac resynchronization and implantable cardioversion defibrillation in advanced chronic heart failure: the MIRACLE ICD Trial. JAMA. 2003;289:2685–94.

Zeitler EP, Patel D, Hasselblad V, Sanders GD, Al-Khatib SM. Complications from prophylactic replacement of cardiac implantable electronic device generators in response to United States Food and Drug Administration recall: a systematic review and meta-analysis. Heart Rhythm. 2015;12:1558–64.

MIX
Papier aus verantwortungsvollen Quellen
Paper from responsible sources
FSC® C105338

If you have any concerns about our products,
you can contact us on
ProductSafety@springernature.com

In case Publisher is established outside the EU,
the EU authorized representative is:
Springer Nature Customer Service Center GmbH
Europaplatz 3, 69115 Heidelberg, Germany

Printed by Libri Plureos GmbH
in Hamburg, Germany